The Medical Review Officer's Manual Fourth Edition

Medical Review Officer Certification Council

Robert Swotinsky, MD, MPH
Fallon Clinic, Inc.
Worcester, Massachusetts

Donna Smith, PhD
FirstLab, Inc.
North Wales, Pennsylvania

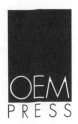

OEM Press
Beverly Farms, Massachusetts

To Donna Bush, PhD, and Jim Swart, MA,
for their dedication and contributions to the federal testing programs

ISBN 978-1-883595-54-8

Library of Congress Cataloging-in-Publication Data

Swotinsky, Robert B.
  The medical review officer's manual / Medical Review Officer Certification
  Council ; Robert Swotinsky, Donna Smith. — 4th ed.
    p. ; cm.
  Includes bibliographical references and index.
  ISBN 978-1-883595-54-8
    1. Employees—Drug testing. 2. Drug testing—Law and legislation—United
  States. I. Smith, Donna, Ph. D. II. Medical Review Officer Certification
  Council. III. Title.
  [DNLM: 1. Substance Abuse Detection—methods—United States—Guideline.
  2. Documentation—standards—United States—Guideline. 3. Laboratory
  Techniques and Procedures—United States—Guideline. 4. Specimen
  Handling—methods—United States—Guideline. 5. Substance Abuse
  Detection—legislation & jurisprudence—United States—Guideline.
  6. Workplace—United States—Guideline. HV 5823.5.U5 S979m 2010]

  HF5549.5.D7S89 2010
  658.3'82—dc22

                                                                2010013734

Printed in the United States of America

OEM Press® is a registered trademark of OEM Health Information, Inc.

Questions or comments regarding this book should be directed to:

OEM Health Information, Inc.
8 West Street
Beverly Farms, MA 01915-2226
978-921-7300
978-921-0304 (fax)
info@oempress.com
5 4 3 2 1

Contents

7 ■ Adulterants, Substitution, and Dilution   95

8 ■ Laboratory Analysis   101

9 ■ Laboratory Results   121

10 ■ MRO Review of Drug Test Results   131

11 ■ Split Specimen Tests and Retests   191

12 ■ Urine and Other Specimens   201

13 ■ Alcohol and Specific Drugs   217

14 ■ Alcohol Testing   269

Preface

The *Medical Review Officer's Manual,* fourth edition is a reference for physicians and other providers of workplace drug and alcohol testing services. This book presents the rules and guidelines and the authors' understanding of best practices. It focuses on the review and interpretation of workplace drug and alcohol test results and related topics important to medical review officers (MROs). The standard operating procedures for MRO practice are well defined by federal regulations and guidelines, primarily those of the U.S. Department of Health and Human Services (HHS) and U.S. Department of Transportation. Many MROs follow the federal procedures when reviewing nonregulated tests because the procedures make sense, and because they are used to them. However, the federal procedures do not cover every scenario nor do they cover drugs beyond the federal five-drug panel and tests performed on nonurine specimens. This book covers the federal procedures *and* other scenarios not covered by the federal procedures.

Four years have passed between this fourth edition and the third edition. This fourth edition has updates for regulatory compliance and technological changes, including changes to the HHS *Mandatory Guidelines* and Federal Drug Testing Custody and Control Form that were scheduled to take effect in 2010 (but were delayed as this book went to press). It also features more information about (1) nonurine tests; (2) prescription opiates and testing for prescription drugs; and (3) specimen validity testing. This fourth edition has updated endnote references. The text includes citations for some of the less well-known parts of the federal rules, so that readers can more easily locate the source material.

We thank the Medical Review Officer Certification Council (MROCC) and Brian Compney, MROCC's executive director, for supporting this project. Excellent comments on drafts of this fourth edition were provided by Sue Clark, MBA; Steven Herbets, MD; Carl Selavka, PhD; and Gilbert Woodall, Jr., MD. We thank Curtis Vouwie at OEM Press, the publisher, for his encouragement and responsiveness.

To those who purchased earlier editions—thanks for coming back!

RS
DS

List of Figures and Tables

Common Acronyms

AAMRO	American Association of Medical Review Officers		COC	chain of custody (*see also* CCF)
ABMS	American Board of Medical Specialties		CPT	current procedural terminology
ACOEM	American College of Occupational and Environmental Medicine		CSA	Controlled Substance Act
			C-SAPA	Certified Substance Abuse Program Administrator
ADA	Americans with Disabilities Act		C/TPA	consortium/third-party administrator
AMA	American Medical Association		DATIA	Drug and Alcohol Testing Industry Association
ASAM	American Society of Addiction Medicine		DEA	Drug Enforcement Administration
ASD	alcohol screening device		DER	designated employer representative
ATF	alcohol testing form			
BAC	blood alcohol concentration		DHS	Department of Homeland Security
BAT	breath alcohol technician			
CAP	College of American Pathologists		DOL	Department of Labor (federal)
CAP–FDT	College of American Pathologists–Forensic Drug Testing		DOT	Department of Transportation (federal)
			DWI	driving while intoxicated (also DUI: Driving Under the Influence)
CBA	collective bargaining agreement			
CCF	custody and control form		EAP	employee assistance program
CDL	commercial driver's license			
CEAP	certified employee assistance professional		EAPA	Employee Assistance Professionals Association
CEU	continuing education unit		EBT	evidential breath testing device
CFR	Code of Federal Regulations			
CME	continuing medical education		EIA	enzyme immunoassay
			E/M	evaluation/management
CLIA	Clinical Laboratories Improvement Amendments (federal)		EMIT	enzyme multiplied immunoassay technique
			EMTALA	Emergency Medical Treatment and Active Labor Act
CMV	commercial motor vehicle			
CPL	Conforming Products List			

EO	Executive Order	NAADATP	Nationally Accredited for Administration of Drug and Alcohol Testing Programs
FAA	Federal Aviation Administration		
FDA	Food and Drug Administration	NHTSA	National Highway Traffic Safety Administration
FFD	fitness for duty		
FMCSA	Federal Motor Carrier Safety Administration	NIDA	National Institute on Drug Abuse
FPIA	fluorescence-polarization immunoassay	NLCP	National Laboratory Certification Program
FRA	Federal Railroad Administration	NRC	Nuclear Regulatory Commission
FTA	Federal Transit Administration	ODAPC	Office of Drug and Alcohol Policy and Compliance (of DOT)
GC/MS	gas chromatography/mass spectrometry	ODOT	Oregon Department of Transportation
GPO	Government Printing Office	ONDCP	Office of National Drug Control Policy
HHS	Department of Health and Human Services (federal)	OSHA	Occupational Safety and Health Administration (federal)
HIPAA	Health Insurance Portability and Accountability Act		
HRP	Human Reliability Program	PHMSA	Pipeline Hazardous Materials Safety Administration
ICRC	International Certification Reciprocity Consortium	PCR	polymerase chain reaction
IITF	Instrumented Initial Test Facility	PIE	public interest exclusion
		POCT	point-of-collection testing
IV	intravenous	QAP	quality assurance plan
KIMS	kinetic interaction of microparticles	RIA	radioimmunoassay
		RVU	relative value unit
LC/MS	liquid chromatography/mass spectrometry	SAMHSA	Substance Abuse and Mental Health Services Administration (of HHS)
LOD	limit of detection		
LORC	letter of regulatory compliance	SAP	substance abuse professional
MIS	management information system	SAPAA	Substance Abuse Program Administrators Association
MRO	medical review officer	SAPACC	Substance Abuse Program Administrators' Certification Commission
MROA	medical review officer assistant		
MROCC	Medical Review Officer Certification Council	STT	screening test technician
		TAC	tetracaine, adrenaline, cocaine
NAADAC	National Association of Alcoholism and Drug Abuse Counselors	TLC	thin-layer chromatography
		TPA	third-party administrator
		USCG	United States Coast Guard

About the Authors

Robert Swotinsky, MD, is chair of Fallon Clinic's Occupational Medicine Department in Massachusetts, where he leads a multisite clinical program. Dr. Swotinsky is board certified in occupational medicine, is certified as a medical review officer (MRO) and substance abuse professional (SAP), and is an aviation medical examiner. This fourth edition of *The Medical Review Officer's Manual* is Dr. Swotinsky's fifth book on workplace drug and alcohol testing. He is also founding editor of the *MRO Update* newsletter, is a coauthor of the Medical Review Officer Certification Council's (MROCC) MRO certification examination, and teaches in national courses for MROs. Dr. Swotinsky's expertise includes workplace drug and alcohol testing, toxicology, and assessment of work (dis)ability. Dr. Swotinsky graduated with chemical engineering and biology degrees from MIT, his MD degree from Vanderbilt University School of Medicine, and a masters in public health from the University of California, Los Angeles.

Donna Smith, PhD, is Regulatory Affairs and Program Development Officer at FirstLab in North Wales, Pennsylvania. Dr. Smith previously served as the Acting Director, Drug Enforcement and Program Compliance, for the U.S. Department of Transportation (DOT) in Washington, D.C. She coordinated the development, implementation, and enforcement of DOT's workplace drug and alcohol testing programs. She was a principal author of the DOT drug and alcohol testing regulations and numerous government publications on drug and alcohol testing procedures. Dr. Smith has provided testimony and statements as an expert witness on behalf of the DOT and HHS procedures for workplace drug testing. Dr. Smith has taught collectors, MROs, and other service agents in training programs throughout the United States and abroad. A graduate of Capital University of Columbus, Ohio, Dr. Smith went on to receive a masters of social work from Hunter College in New York, and a doctorate in counseling psychology from Ball State University in Muncie, Indiana.

The Medical Review Officer (MRO) ∎

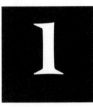

MRO Responsibilities ∎

The MRO is a licensed physician who functions between the laboratory and employer as the gatekeeper of drug test results. The MRO shares responsibility with the laboratory for the review of drug-testing custody and control forms to verify that they are completed correctly. For each non-negative result, the MRO allows the donor (i.e., the applicant or employee who provided a drug test specimen) an opportunity to discuss the result and present explanations, such as use of a prescription medication. If the donor presents a legitimate medical explanation for a positive, adulterated, or substituted result, the MRO reports the result as negative to the employer. If the MRO learns medical information about the donor that suggests a fitness-for-duty or safety issue, the MRO notifies the employer or other appropriate party.

Workplace drug testing is a three-step process:

1. Specimen *collection*, in which a custody and control form (CCF) is used to document the link between the specimen and its donor.
2. *Laboratory* analysis, which consists of a screening test and, if the screening result is positive, a confirmation test.
3. *MRO review* of the test result.

The MRO makes the final and definitive verification decision for each drug test result and reports that decision to the employer. As the final reviewer, the MRO can identify problems in the collection and laboratory steps. The MRO provides feedback to employers, collection sites, laboratories, and federal agency representatives about performance problems when necessary. The MRO is an advocate for the accuracy and integrity of the drug testing process and for workplace safety.

MRO Assistant ■

Most MROs have assistants who perform administrative tasks that do not involve interpreting test results. In federally regulated testing, an MRO assistant may perform the following tasks:

- Receive, review, and report negative results.
- Receive and collate test forms and prepare records of non-negative results for review by the MRO.
- Schedule interviews and verify phone numbers with donors.
- Advise donors of the importance of speaking with the MRO, ask donors to have medical information ready for the MRO, and explain the consequences of not speaking with the MRO.
- *After* a donor has spoken with the MRO and presented a medical explanation for the result, help corroborate that medical explanation.
- Report non-negative results.
- Provide summary reports to employers.

In regulated testing, the MRO assistant must not substitute for or be used to avoid direct discussion between the donor and MRO.

An MRO assistant should be detail oriented, well organized, and reliable. Under the U.S. Department of Transportation (DOT) and Nuclear Regulatory Commission (NRC) drug and alcohol testing rules, the MRO assistant directly reports to the MRO for all drug test-related activities. DOT has stated that the MRO's supervision of the assistant "involves personal oversight of staff members' work; personal involvement in evaluation, hiring, and firing; line authority over the staff for decisions, direction, and control; and regular contact and oversight concerning drug testing program matters. It also means that the MRO's supervision and control of the staff members cannot be superseded by or delegated to anyone else with respect to test results review and other functions staff members perform for the MRO" (65 *FR* 79494).

MRO assistant training is provided by the Drug and Alcohol Testing Industry Association (DATIA), the Substance Abuse Program Administrators Association (SAPAA), and the American College of Occupational and Environmental Medicine (ACOEM). The Medical Review Officer Certification Council (MROCC) offers certification of MRO assistants in collaboration with these organizations. Neither federal nor state laws address the training or certification of MRO assistants.

MRO Coverage While Away ■

Arrangements should be made for an alternate, qualified MRO to review results while the primary MRO is temporarily unavailable (e.g., on vacation, sick). The covering MRO is responsible for each verification determination that he or she handles. While the primary MRO is away, drug test results and forms continue to arrive in his or her office, but the MRO assistant can forward non-negative results to the covering MRO during the primary MRO's absence. Should the covering MRO need to communicate with the laboratory for additional information, the laboratory may require written authorization from the primary MRO. In large practices, MROs sometimes share reviews; for example, one MRO starts a review and, if he or she becomes unavailable, another MRO finishes it.

MRO Qualifications ■

Federal regulations allow only physicians to serve as MROs because federal regulators believe only physicians have the relevant and necessary skills, credibility, and integrity for this role. Federal rules establish the following qualification criteria for serving as an MRO:

1. Either a doctor of medicine (MD) or doctor of osteopathy (DO) degree.
2. A medical license in any U.S., Canadian, or Mexican jurisdiction. A physician licensed in one state or province may perform MRO functions for donors in other states and provinces without holding licenses in those states and provinces. Nevertheless, some contracts for MRO services and some specific state laws and regulations call for MROs to hold medical licenses in specific states.
3. Knowledge about the pharmacology and toxicology of illicit drugs.
4. Knowledge and clinical experience in controlled substance abuse disorders. MROs have this through their medical school and residency training. MROs who see patients have a great deal of relevant knowledge and experience if they perform fitness-for-duty assessments or counsel patients with substance abuse disorders.
5. Knowledge about the federal agency drug testing rules and guidelines under which the MRO operates.
6. Training and knowledge necessary to review workplace drug testing results.
7. Successful completion of a written examination administered by a recognized MRO certification board.

TRAINING

An MRO must complete training before reviewing federally regulated drug test results. MRO training must include instruction about:

1. Specimen collection procedures
2. Chain of custody procedures, reporting, and recordkeeping
3. Interpretation of test results
4. Federal agency rules, guidance, interpretations, and policies affecting the MRO

Initial training must also include assessment tools to help the MRO determine if he or she has learned the material. ACOEM and AAMRO are the two primary organizations that train MROs. Their 1–2 day courses currently cost $350–$600.

DOT requires that MROs complete at least 12 continuing education units (CEUs) relevant to MRO functions every 3 years. (In 2010, DOT proposed dropping MRO CEU requirements from its role.) Continuing education must include instruction about new drug testing technologies, regulatory changes, and other developments in MRO practice as they pertain to DOT-regulated testing. It must also include assessment tools to help the MRO determine if he or she has learned the material. The continuing education can consist of classroom training similar to the initial training course. The Medical Review Officer Certification Council (MROCC) offers texts and self-assessment exams that MROs can complete from a distance for CEUs.

MROs are responsible for maintaining documentation that they meet the training requirements. DOT requires that MROs make this documentation available on request to DOT agency representatives and to employers or service agents using the MRO's services.

CERTIFICATION

The HHS, DOT, and NRC rules require that the MRO passes an examination administered by a nationally recognized MRO certification board or subspecialty board. Two groups—the American Association of Medical Review Officers (AAMRO) and the Medical Review Officer Certification Council (MROCC)—offer these exams and refer to them as certification exams. MROs who pass these exams call themselves *certified MROs*. Use of the term board certified for MROs should be avoided because that term is better used by diplomates of boards recognized by the American Board of Medical Specialties (ABMS). Neither AAMRO nor MROCC are ABMS-approved medical specialty boards.

Two states, Vermont and Florida, have laws that require MRO certification. Vermont requires it for all programs. Florida requires it for programs that participate in the state's workers' compensation premium discount program. Some employer policies also call for use of certified MROs. MRO certification has become increasingly accepted as a necessary credential for MROs participating in workplace drug testing programs.

Certification is intended to recognize qualified MROs, validate their competency, and promote acceptable standards of practice. To be a certified MRO, one must demonstrate the specific competencies necessary to review and properly report the results of drug tests as well as perform related administrative and program management duties.

AAMRO and MROCC began offering certification examinations in 1992. In the mid-1990s, the two groups considered merging but decided to remain separate. MROCC is endorsed by the American Medical Association and several other medical organizations. Chapter 16 provides additional detail about MROCC and its certification program. As of 2009, MROCC had certified more than 9000 MROs and AAMRO had certified about 5500 MROs. AAMRO and MROCC currently charge $400–$600 for MRO certification exams. From 1996 to 2002, the American Society of Addiction Medicine (ASAM) examination added MRO-related questions to its certification exam and offered MRO certification to those who completed MRO training and passed the ASAM exam.

RECERTIFICATION

AAMRO and MROCC encourage MRO recertification to demonstrate current competence in this evolving field. Recertification is a common practice of medical specialty boards; it is not unique to AAMRO and MROCC. The federal drug testing regulations require that MROs participating in their programs obtain initial certification but do not require that they recertify.

AAMRO and MROCC each have tools on their websites to verify an MRO's certification status. AAMRO and MROCC handle this differently:

- When AAMRO certification expires, AAMRO removes the "in good standing" designation from the MRO's listing on its website.

- When MROCC certification expires, MROCC removes the MRO's listing from its website. MROCC keeps the unlisted MROs in an offline database in case anyone contacts MROCC to verify that someone completed certification.

The certifications that ASAM gave to MROs had no expiration date.

MROCC recertifies MROs who have already been AAMRO or MROCC certified, demonstrate current medical licensure, complete at least 12 hours of relevant category 1 CME in the past 3 years, and pass the current version of the MROCC exam. MROCC offers recertification exams onsite after ACOEM and ASAM MRO courses for $395 and offers the test online for MROs to complete at home or at work for $495 (fees as of 2009).

AAMRO recertifies MROs who take its on-line test. AAMRO offers CME for taking this exam; it does not separately ask the MRO to demonstrate completion of CME. AAMRO recertification costs $450.

STATE REQUIREMENTS

Laws in several states (Hawaii, Iowa, Louisiana, Montana, Oklahoma, and Vermont) and Puerto Rico mandate medical review of positive workplace drug test results. Laws in several other states (Connecticut, Maryland, New York, and Oregon) require that physicians order or review drug tests—or, more broadly, laboratory results—but do not specifically mention MROs. Many states offer employers incentives to use MROs. The most common incentives include discounts on workers' compensation insurance and revocation of workers' compensation benefits for any worker who has a positive post-accident drug test.

Several state laws set forth qualification requirements of MROs. Most of these parallel the federal requirements. States with special MRO requirements include the following:

- Florida [*Florida Drug-Free Workplace Act. Chapter 59A-24.008(1)(c)*]. Florida's Drug-Free Workplace Program standards, which apply to employers who participate in the workers' compensation discount program, require that MROs be certified by AAMRO, ACOEM, or ASAM. However, there was misunderstanding on the part of the authors of this law: ACOEM and ASAM do not certify MROs; rather they helped develop MROCC, which is independent. So, the Florida law's intent is to recognize certification by either AAMRO or MROCC.
- *Hawaii* [*Hawaii Administrative Rules. Title 11, Chapter 113*]. A Hawaiian MRO license is required to review positive drug test specimens collected in Hawaii. The license application can be obtained from:

State of Hawaii Department of Health
State Laboratories Division
Attn: Substance Abuse Testing
2725 Waimano Home Road
Pearl City, HI 96782-1496
(808) 453-6658

The applicant submits a four-page form with a picture, documentation of training and experience, a photocopy of his or her MD diploma, and verification of medical licensure in Hawaii or another state. The MRO license must be renewed every 24 months. The Hawaii Department of Health can revoke the license if the MRO is addicted to drugs or alcohol, reviews results while impaired by drugs or alcohol, is grossly negligent in functioning as an MRO, or is convicted of a crime directly related to functioning as an MRO.

- *Iowa [§730.5(1)(f)].* The MRO can be "a licensed physician, osteopathic physician, chiropractor, nurse practitioner, or physician assistant."
- *Oklahoma [Workplace Drug and Alcohol Testing Act, Chapter 638, Section 310, Oklahoma Administrative Code, 1995].* The MRO must have a medical license or hold a doctoral degree in clinical chemistry, forensic toxicology, or a similar biomedical science. The MRO must also have completed at least 12 hours of MRO training.

Other Roles of Physicians Who Serve as MROs ■

A few physicians are full-time MROs and work for large consortium/third-party administrators (C/TPAs). Most MROs are physicians who primarily do other things, often in occupational health clinics. These clinics usually offer a variety of services related to drug and alcohol testing. MROs are sometimes asked to provide expert testimony for tests that are being legally challenged. Employers sometimes ask MROs to help develop or revise their policies. The following two sections address litigation support and policy development.

LITIGATION SUPPORT

MROs involved in legal challenges can find themselves in any of the following situations:

1. Defendant. Avoid this.
2. Fact witness. The employer or another party asks the MRO to testify about the facts in an administrative or legal proceeding about a drug test result policy or related issue. The MRO may be asked to identify the specific actions he or she took in reviewing and interpreting a drug test result and the decision-making process. The MRO would attest to the content of the review, reason for the decision, and report to the employer. The MRO as fact witness presents only the facts as he or she knows them and offers no opinion or other interpretative information. For example, the MRO might acknowledge that the laboratory result states "positive for marijuana," but would not be expected to speculate as to what caused this result.
3. Expert witness. If the MRO is retained as an expert witness, the MRO can present the facts *and* offer opinions. For example, the MRO might acknowledge that the laboratory result states "positive for marijuana" and such results are almost always due to smoking marijuana, although prescription dronabinol is a distant second possibility.

POLICY AND PROCEDURES DEVELOPMENT

Employers may ask their MROs for help in developing their policy and procedures, establishing employee assistance programs (EAPs), coordinating employee and supervisory training, reviewing reasonable suspicion determinations, and monitoring compliance with federal or state laws and regulations. These consultative roles require a broad knowledge base beyond the core elements of reviewing, interpreting, and reporting drug test results. MROs can provide valuable insights because of their technical knowledge and experience with the issues that arise. Employers sometimes ask MROs for help with policies and other drug testing issues beyond interpretation of drug test results. The MRO may want to caution the employer to also consult with an attorney for help with legal issues.

Independence Between Laboratories and MROs ■

The MRO must feel free to report significant laboratory problems to the appropriate parties. To this end, in regulated testing the MRO must be financially independent from the laboratory, as follows:

- The MRO cannot be employed by, be a contractor for, or have a direct financial interest in the laboratory that analyzes tests that the MRO reviews.
- The laboratory cannot recommend or direct its clients to use particular MROs, nor can the laboratory derive a financial benefit by having an employer use a specific MRO. (A laboratory can, however, refer employers to large, categorical lists of MROs, such as all MROs who have been certified by AAMRO or MROCC.)

An MRO can manage the laboratory contract on the employer's behalf and bill the employer for those laboratory services. A laboratory can bill an employer for MRO services if the laboratory itemizes the MRO's services separately and distinctly on each invoice.

It is common for MROs to work within clinics that perform on-site screening tests for drugs. The federal conflict-of-interest restrictions between MROs and laboratories refer to the off-site, certified laboratories that are required to be used by federally mandated testing programs.

Risk Management ■

Drug-testing litigation has focused more on collectors, laboratories, and employers than on MROs. Courts have allowed donors to proceed with lawsuits against collection sites for alleged procedural errors, reasoning that the face-to-face relationship and clinical setting help create an expectation of responsibility to the donor. By contrast, courts have usually held that drug testing laboratories owe no duty to donors and on this basis have dismissed donor's lawsuits against laboratories. Donors have challenged employers over alleged wrongful discharge, civil rights and disability discrimination, and other traditional tort causes of action. Drug testing service agents can be dragged into legal actions against employers.

Federal rules impose requirements on federally mandated testing. Federal guidelines supplement and explain these rules. These rules and guidelines help establish standards of practice. Some state laws reference the HHS *Guidelines* or DOT Part 40 rule as the standard for workplace drug testing conducted in those states. MRO training courses and literature also help establish standards of practice. The MRO Code of Ethical Conduct presented in Appendix B provides guidelines for appropriate conduct. Adherence to published rules and guidelines can serve as a defense in litigation. Employers and MROs may have good reason(s) for deviating from those procedures—e.g., for not conducting split specimen tests—but should be prepared to explain those reasons if challenged.

The MRO and the MRO's staff should maintain and follow written standard operating procedures. These establish their usual practices and provide the staff with guidance in emergency or unfamiliar situations. The MRO and MRO's staff should treat the records as confidential information that can be released only to designated recipients.

Workplace drug testing is a paper-intensive process. The MRO should meticulously document the process and the reasoning employed in reaching each decision. Each record is a potential courtroom exhibit. Furthermore, complete records may persuade a litigious donor or a plaintiff's attorney that no case exists.

Any MRO who serves in DOT-regulated programs should have ready access to the DOT Part 40 procedures, applicable agency regulations, and DOT's guidelines. MROs must keep abreast of new information. Technology and federal regulations continue to evolve, and an increasing body of case law and state legislation has developed. DOT rules require MRO continuing education, as previously described in this chapter. A number of newsletters and journals feature information about workplace drug and alcohol testing. The DOT Office of Drug and Alcohol Policy and Compliance (ODAPC) posts current information about its workplace drug testing rules on its website, and sends e-mail updates to those who subscribe through the website. The Division of Workplace Programs at HHS also posts information on its website. Appendix A lists these and other sources of information.

INSURANCE COVERAGE

Most MROs have malpractice insurance for their work as physicians. Most of these policies cover most MRO-related claims. If a medical malpractice insurer balks in accepting an MRO-related claim, the MRO might in a worst-case scenario have to sue the carrier for coverage. The court would probably find that medical malpractice insurance covers MRO services. After all, MRO work is a core part of occupational medicine practice and is defined by federal regulation as a service that can be performed only by a licensed physician. As a precaution, an MRO may want to send his or her medical malpractice insurer a description of MRO services and invite the carrier to respond if there are questions or concerns.

Some claims against MROs are atypical for medical malpractice. These include violations of Constitutional rights and unwarranted interference with employment. Medical malpractice insurers are more likely to question these types of claims as nonmedical. Many MROs are employees of organizations that have errors and omissions insurance, which should cover claims that are deemed nonmedical. Errors and omissions insurance is cheaper than medical malpractice insurance.

In the mid-1990s, in response to uncertainties about medical malpractice coverage of the new field of MRO work, a few carriers offered insurance coverage specifically for MROs. Few MROs purchased these policies. Few, if any, insurers offer MRO insurance anymore.

CONTRACTS

MROs often provide services without written contracts in place. If there is a contract between the MRO and an employer or third-party administrator, it should include a statement of work that sets forth the duties of each party. The contract offers an opportunity to clarify the client's responsibility for payment for necessary laboratory tests, including split specimens and amphetamine isomers. A short contract (e.g., letter of agreement) may suffice for a low-volume client, while a more detailed contract may be needed for a high-volume client. Figure 1-1 presents a sample contract. The DOT rule states that any contract or

---

Figure 1-1. Sample Agreement Between MRO and Employer ■

Section 1. Scope of Services provided by the medical review officer (MRO):

A. Qualifications. The MRO:

1. Is knowledgeable of the requirements for the MRO in compliance with the regulations of the U.S. Department of Transportation (DOT).

2. Is a licensed doctor of medicine or osteopathy with knowledge of drug abuse disorders.

3. Has the requisite level of experience to interpret positive, adulterated, substituted, and invalid drug test results.

4. Will comply with applicable regulations governing the conduct of the MRO.

B. Receipt, review, and reporting of drug test results conducted through the COMPANY's program.

1. The MRO will receive results from the laboratory that analyzes drug test specimens on behalf of the COMPANY. The MRO will report as "canceled" to the COMPANY those tests that have significant procedural or technical errors.

2. The MRO will review and interpret each positive, adulterated, substituted, and invalid result. The MRO will determine if there is a legitimate medical explanation for the result. In carrying out this responsibility, the MRO will make a reasonable effort to contact the specimen donor and conduct an interview and review of his/her medical history and other relevant factors. The MRO will review all medical records and reasonable explanation made available by the donor for a positive, adulterated, or substituted result. The MRO may also arrange for a medical evaluation to determine if the individual has clinical signs of drug abuse that correlate with opiate abuse, except when 6-acetylmorphine is detected or when the morphine or codeine concentration exceeds 15,000 ng/mL. Only those laboratory-positive results that have no legitimate medical explanation will be reported to the employer as positive. The MRO will be available to the COMPANY for consultation regarding the use of prescribed medications.

3. The MRO will furnish to the COMPANY a report of the results of each test.

C. Recordkeeping. The MRO will maintain certain drug test records on behalf of the COMPANY. These records will include the laboratory reports, custody and control forms, and documentation of the MRO's evaluation for positive, adulterated, substituted, and invalid results. The MRO will maintain these records for at least 5 years for verified positive, adulterated, and substituted results and at least one year for other test results. If requested in writing, the MRO will maintain these records for longer periods.

D. Consultation and expert testimony. The MRO will be available for telephone consultation concerning drug test procedures and will provide expert testimony in drug test-related cases on an as-requested basis.

Figure 1-1. Continued ■

Section 2. Employer Responsibilities: The COMPANY will:

A. Provide the MRO with a copy of the COMPANY's current drug abuse/drug testing policy and procedures; the name and phone and fax numbers and address of a representative to assist with contacting individuals and to whom results should be reported.

B. Before performance begins, inform the MRO of applicable drug testing regulations and the MRO's responsibilities, if any, with regard to the COMPANY's employee assistance program.

C. Assure that the means of receiving results from the MRO (e.g., fax transmissions) are secure and confidential and that individual drug test results will be maintained confidentially and will be disclosed only to individuals with a business need for the information or otherwise in accordance with law.

D. Assume responsibility for the performance of the collection site(s) and/or laboratory, if the COMPANY has contracted directly with these providers for services.

E. Be responsible for costs of split specimen analyses and other required additional tests performed on specimens.

F. Have sole responsibility for decisions about the employment, termination, retention, or disciplining of any employee, former employee, or applicant for employment.

---

agreement between an MRO or other service agent and a DOT-regulated employer presumes that the service agent will follow the DOT procedures [49 *CFR* §40.11(c)].

MRO WORK AND THE DOCTOR-PATIENT RELATIONSHIP

The existence of a "doctor-patient relationship" can be unclear as it relates to services provided on behalf of third parties. In general, a doctor-patient relationship develops when a person seeks the assistance of the physician for the purpose of obtaining a diagnosis or treatment. When a physician reviews a workplace drug test result, he or she is providing neither a diagnosis nor treatment. According to DOT, MRO review of a donor's drug test result does not establish a doctor-patient relationship [49 *CFR* 40.123(d)]. The Americans with Disabilities Act (ADA) has a similar statement: "A test to determine the illegal use of drugs shall not be considered a medical examination" [42 *CFR* §126.12114(d)(1)]. The Clinical Laboratory Improvements Amendments of 1988 also exclude from coverage forensic drug and alcohol tests. ("Forensic tests" includes workplace tests.) These federal rules reflect a consensus that workplace drug tests are not medical exams. MRO work does not establish the position of patient advocacy that is typical of a traditional doctor-patient relationship. Furthermore, the federal drug testing rules impose requirements for MROs to report test results to appropriate designees without regard to donor consent. This also supports the notion that workplace drug tests differ from medical services where patient information is kept confidential.

If a physician reviews a drug test result on a donor who is that physician's patient, the physician may perceive a conflict of interest between those two roles. If a physician feels his or her MRO role compromises his or her professional responsibility to a patient, the physician may want another MRO to review that person's test result. If the physician works alongside another qualified MRO, the physician could refer the case to that MRO. Some companies with in-house physicians contract out for MRO services because of concern that MRO services may place in-house physicians in an adversarial role against employees. If any MRO wishes to refer a case to another MRO whom the employer has not already agreed to use, the MRO should first ask the employer for permission.

Laws, Guidelines, and Policies ■

2

Military Testing Programs ■

Workplace drug testing has its roots in military testing programs of the 1960s and early 1970s, when soldiers were tested upon return from Southeast Asia to identify heroin and hashish users and refer them to treatment. In the early 1970s, military testing was broadened to include all personnel reporting for active duty. The military services established forensic urine drug testing laboratories capable of analyzing large numbers of specimens. These tests used chain-of-custody procedures. The laboratories were subject to external proficiency monitoring and on-site inspections to ensure accuracy and reliability of test results.

Federal Drug and Alcohol Testing Laws ■

In 1986, the federal government increased efforts to stop illegal drug trade as part of the Reagan Administration's "War on Drugs." The government tried to reduce supply and reduce demand. As part of the latter, the government developed federal workplace programs to deter drug abuse. In 1986, President Ronald Reagan signed Executive Order (E.O.) 12564, declaring all federal agencies drug-free workplaces and prohibiting federal employees from use of illegal drugs. E.O. 12564 defined illegal drugs as Schedule I and II drugs whose possession was unlawful. E.O. 12564 required each executive-branch federal agency to establish a comprehensive drug-free workplace program that included the following elements:

- Formal written policy;
- Employee assistance program;
- Supervisory training;
- Provisions for self-referral to treatment; and,
- Provisions for detecting illicit drug users, including drug testing of federal employees in safety-sensitive and security-critical positions.

These programs were patterned after the military testing programs. Testing of civilian workers was rationalized by data that showed that about three-quarters of illicit drug users in the civilian population held jobs. These programs were intended to deter use of illicit drugs and identify drug abusers and refer them to treatment. They were not expected to identify every abuser or eradicate drug abuse. These programs struck a balance between concerns about drug misuse and the need to maintain reasonable privacy protections and safeguard against false accusations of drug abuse.

DEPARTMENT OF HEALTH AND HUMAN SERVICES
MANDATORY GUIDELINES

E.O. 12564 directed the Department of Health and Human Services (HHS) to develop guidelines and procedures for the federal drug testing programs. The Supplemental Appropriations Act of 1987 reinforced E.O. 12564 by requiring a more formal laboratory certification program and the publication of the guidelines in the Federal Register. HHS published its *Mandatory Guidelines for Federal Workplace Drug Testing Programs* in final form in April 1988 (53 *FR* 11970). These regulations were referred to as the *National Institute on Drug Abuse (NIDA) Guidelines*. They established a standard drug panel—then called the *NIDA 5*—for testing of amphetamines (amphetamine, methamphetamine), cocaine, marijuana, opiates (emphasizing detection of heroin), and phencyclidine. They established initial and confirmation cutoff values for these analytes. They also established detailed procedures for specimen collection and handling, introduced the concept of the physician medical review officer (MRO) who interprets drug test results, and established a comprehensive certification program for drug testing laboratories. HHS chose tests of urine rather than other specimens because, thanks to the military programs, there were already laboratories capable of testing urine reliably and at high volume and because urine testing was well understood at the time. HHS included confirmation testing by gas chromatography/mass spectrometry (GC/MS), which was the gold standard for accuracy.

In 2004, HHS issued a proposed set of procedures for testing of hair, sweat, and oral fluid specimens, and for conducting point of collection tests (71 *FR* 19673). This proposal met with much controversy and was dropped. Speculation remains that HHS will eventually expand its testing procedures to include one or two, but not all, of the aforementioned non-urine specimens. In 2008, HHS issued changes to the *Guidelines* that were scheduled to take effect in 2010, and that included addition of several designer amphetamines to the test panel and allowing use of screen-only laboratories that would send positive specimens elsewhere for confirmation testing (73 *FR* 71858).

The HHS *Guidelines* apply to federal agency employee drug testing programs. About 2.1 million federal employees and job applicants are covered under this program. Not everyone in the federal government is tested. There are about 400,000 testing-designated positions, with about 210,000 urine drug tests conducted per year [1]. Other federal testing rules, such as those of the U.S. Department of Transportation (DOT), evolved from the HHS *Guidelines*, and require use of laboratories that follow the procedures of, and are certified under, the HHS *Guidelines*. The *Guidelines* have also been incorporated into many state laws and are referenced in many employer policies.

U.S. DEPARTMENT OF TRANSPORTATION *PROCEDURES*

In 1989, DOT finalized its drug testing rule, 49 *CFR* Part 40, *Procedures for Transportation Workplace Drug Testing Programs* (54 *FR* 49854). The rule is often called *Part*

40 or *The DOT Procedures.* Part 40 was originally based on the HHS *Guidelines* and remains similar but not identical. Part 40 requires use of laboratories that follow the procedures of, and are certified by, HHS. Part 40 states *how* to conduct testing and *how* to return employees to safety-sensitive duties after they violate a DOT drug and alcohol regulation. Each DOT agency regulation states *who* is subject to testing, and *when* and in *what* situations for that particular transportation industry. DOT drug and alcohol testing is conducted in six sectors of the transportation industry:

1. Commercial motor carriers (Federal Motor Carrier Safety Administration, FMCSA)
2. Aviation (Federal Aviation Administration, FAA)
3. Railroad (Federal Railroad Administration, FRA)
4. Public transportation (Federal Transit Administration, FTA)
5. Pipeline (Pipeline and Hazardous Materials Safety Administration, PHMSA)
6. Maritime (United States Coast Guard, USCG) (The USCG was a DOT agency but is now in the Department of Homeland Security. The USCG uses Part 40 procedures for *drug* testing, but not for *alcohol* testing.)

Appendix G summarizes each DOT agency rule. More than 12 million private-sector employees are subject to DOT agency drug and alcohol testing rules. Almost 90% of these are subject to the FMCSA rule [2]. Under the North American Free Trade Agreement, which was implemented in 1994, Canadian and Mexican trucking firms must comply with DOT/FMCSA drug and alcohol testing rules and other U.S. regulations to be allowed access to U.S. roadways. Canadian and U.S. trucks now travel freely in either country. Because of disagreements between Mexico and the United States, Mexican trucks are limited to about 20 miles within the U.S. border.

After a series of fatal accidents associated with illegal drug use or alcohol misuse, Congress expanded the scope of DOT testing programs with passage of the Omnibus Transportation Employee Testing Act of 1991. The Omnibus Act added alcohol tests, split specimen collection procedures for urine, and created the role of the substance abuse professional (SAP) as part of return to duty process. The Omnibus Act covered aviation, commercial motor carriers, railroads, and public transportation but not pipelines or maritime. Thus, the alcohol testing regulations in pipeline and maritime industries differ from those of other transportation agencies. For example, the pipeline and maritime industries do not conduct random alcohol tests. The Omnibus Act also expanded the scope of testing to include intrastate commercial vehicle operators (i.e., drivers holding a commercial drivers license). The Omnibus Act recognized the close relationship between the HHS *Guidelines* and Part 40 and required DOT to "incorporate" the HHS *Guidelines* and amendments into DOT testing procedures, while leaving DOT authority to make other changes. In 1994, DOT issued additional drug and alcohol testing rules that implemented the requirements of the Omnibus Act.

In 2000, DOT issued a complete rewrite of Part 40 with many new features (65 *FR* 79462). These included a process for employers to be allowed to stand down employees pending completion of the test verification process; a process for banning noncompliant service agents from providing DOT-mandated testing services; MRO review of adulterated and substituted specimens; and a requirement that employers check with previous employers for drug and alcohol testing results of applicants with safety-sensitive jobs.

In 2003, DOT changed the substituted criteria by lowering the creatinine cutoff to 2 mg/dL (68 *FR* 31624). This was in response to challenges brought by several airline employees who claimed they normally produced urine with creatinine values in the 4's—i.e., below the previous creatinine cutoff of 5 mg/dL—and had thereby been unjustly accused of substituting their specimens. HHS made the same change in its *Guidelines* shortly thereafter (69 *FR* 19644). In 2008, DOT issued rule changes that focused on preventing specimen tampering during collections (73 *FR* 35961). These changes included a more explicit procedure for directly observed collections, mandatory validity testing using HHS standards, and clarified MRO procedures for: (1) invalid specimens, (2) two specimens at test event, and (3) one specimen with multiple results.

DEPARTMENT OF DEFENSE

The Department of Defense (DOD) testing programs for civilian DOD employees and certain contractors are essentially consistent with the HHS *Guidelines*. DOD testing programs for uniformed personnel have several differences from HHS and DOT, including:

- Batch chain of custody documentation.
- Active duty testing at least once a year; Reserve and Guard at least biennially.
- All specimens are tested for marijuana, cocaine, and amphetamines (including MDMA).
- Pulse testing for opiates, PCP, barbiturates, and LSD.
- Steroid testing by commander request.
- Cutoff levels are, for certain drugs, lower than those of DOT and HHS.

DEPARTMENT OF ENERGY

The Department of Energy (DOE) drug testing procedures (10 *CFR* Part 707) apply to DOE contractors and subcontractors working at nuclear reactors. The procedures call for pre-employment, random, post-accident, and reasonable suspicion testing. Testing generally follows the HHS *Guidelines*.

The DOE Human Reliability Program (HRP) (10 *CFR* Part 712) governs DOE contractors and subcontractors with access to nuclear explosives and in certain other positions responsible for national security. The HRP requires random alcohol testing, at least once every 12 months, in addition to post-accident and reasonable-suspicion testing. Under the HRP, failure to appear for random testing within 2 hours of notice is a refusal to submit to a test. The HRP requires abstinence from drinking alcohol 8 hours prior to working. Any HRP-covered employee who tests at or above an alcohol concentration of 0.02% cannot perform covered duties for 24 hours.

NUCLEAR REGULATORY COMMISSION

The Nuclear Regulatory Commission (NRC) Fitness for Duty (FFD) Programs rule (10 *CFR* Part 26) requires all nuclear power plant licensees (approximately 65 in the United States) to implement drug and alcohol testing of personnel (including contractors) having access to nuclear operations. NRC's rule took effect in 1989 (73 *FR* 24468). NRC produced a new rule in 2008 with more detailed procedures aligned with the HHS and DOT rules, particularly for MRO review, specimen validity testing, Substance Abuse Professional evaluation, and breath alcohol testing procedures (73 *FR* 16966). NRC's rule differs from those of other federal agencies in several ways. First, NRC drug and alcohol testing is part of a comprehensive program to address a broad range of other worker fitness issues as well as drug abuse. NRC's emphasis on fitness for duty is illustrated by its allowance for screening tests on site. Access to the nuclear facility is denied if an employee screens positive for THC or cocaine, pending the laboratory's confirmation. The NRC program includes several provisions aimed at improving detection of drug use:

- Allowing testing to the limit of detection on dilute urine specimens.
- Employer options to use more stringent cutoff levels than specified by HHS and to test for Schedule III, IV, and V controlled substances.
- Broad-scope "for-cause" testing programs after workplace accidents, incidents, and safety violations.
- The MRO and other FFD program staff must be part of the drug and alcohol testing program and meet all the requirements including background checks and testing.

Split specimens are optional under the NRC rule; but, if a single specimen is collected, the donor has the right to reanalysis of that single specimen.

COORDINATION BETWEEN FEDERAL AGENCIES

The federal agencies develop their rules in a coordinated manner, particularly whereas they all rely on HHS to certify and monitor laboratory performance. The federal agencies periodically update their rules and guidelines as significant developments occur in the technology and practice of drug testing. They get help from federal advisory groups, such as the Drug Testing Advisory Board, which meets periodically in Rockville, Maryland. Many of the published guidelines are eventually incorporated into the rules through formal rulemaking processes, including publication of the proposed changes and review of public comments before issuing final changes that get codified in the *Code of Federal Regulations*. The rules are more authoritative than the guidelines. For example, the government can successfully prevail in enforcement action or court action only for violations of published, final rules, and not for violations of guidelines.

Nonregulated Testing ■

Nonregulated, or non-DOT, tests comprise 80–85% of all workplace drug tests. A small portion of non-DOT tests are performed to comply with state laws. Most non-DOT tests are performed by choice. Employers choose to conduct drug tests for various reasons, including safety, avoidance of liability, image, productivity, and avoidance of hiring workers who cannot get jobs at other companies that conduct testing. An employer may have both DOT and non-DOT testing programs. An employer may either include or exclude DOT-covered employees from its non-DOT testing program.

The term "nonregulated" implies no rules, but even nonregulated programs are subject to certain state and city laws. The Americans with Disabilities Act and certain other federal laws, while not focused on drug testing, indirectly affect workplace testing programs. These are discussed later in this chapter.

The federal procedures provide an industry standard for workplace drug testing. The content of MRO training courses, MRO textbooks (like this one), and MRO certification exams are based on the federal procedures. Many service agents and employers who conduct nonregulated testing choose to follow many or most aspects of the federal procedures because of their sound reputation. Most nonregulated drug testing programs differ from regulated testing in various aspects, including:

- Tests for additional drugs beyond the five-drug panel used in regulated programs.
- Tests at different (usually lower) cutoffs than the regulated programs.
- Single-specimen tests rather than split specimen tests.
- On-site tests.
- Use of test specimens other than urine.
- Immediate removal of workers from duty pending review by the MRO if they have laboratory-positive results.
- Collection of prescription medication information at the time of specimen collection.

Those who challenge nonregulated test results often cite the *DOT Procedures* as an industry standard. While the *DOT Procedures* are an excellent standard, few employers adopt them *in toto* for non-DOT programs. There are well-designed non-DOT programs that do not follow the *DOT Procedures*.

State Drug and Alcohol Testing Laws ■

Some states and cities have laws about workplace drug and/or alcohol testing. Some state laws affect all employers. Others establish voluntary standards and offer incentives for employers who comply (e.g., discounts on workers' compensation insurance premiums). Common provisions in state drug testing laws include the following.

TEST TYPES

Some state laws restrict when employers can test, for example:

- Limited or no random testing. (This is relatively common.)
- Required random testing for certain groups, e.g., school bus drivers.
- Post-accident testing only if the employer has established "reasonable suspicion" or "probable cause."
- No return-to-duty or follow-up testing if the employee has self-referred for substance abuse treatment.
- Pre-employment testing only if a job offer has already been made. (The offer would be contingent on passing the test.)

PROCEDURES AND POLICIES

Some state laws address the testing procedures, for example:

- Employers must pay for testing.

- Directly observed collections are prohibited.
- Only certain types of specimens can be tested, e.g., urine, hair, or oral fluid.
- Tests must be analyzed by certified laboratories. (Those states that require use of HHS certified laboratories implicitly limit testing to urine, because HHS laboratory certification applies only to urine drug testing processes.)
- Positive results must be reviewed by MROs.
- Employees can obtain copies of test records.
- Employers must offer rehabilitation and cannot fire employees after the first positive test.

DENIAL OF WORKERS' COMPENSATION BENEFITS

Under the laws of most states, an employee forfeits workers' compensation benefits for an injury caused by intoxication or being "under the influence." In some states, a positive post-accident drug or alcohol test result creates a rebuttable presumption that use of that substance caused or contributed to the workplace injury.

DENIAL OF UNEMPLOYMENT BENEFITS

If an employee is fired (or not hired) for a positive test, unemployment benefits may be denied because he or she was fired for misconduct, or because state law specifically calls for denial of benefits if the employee is fired for a positive test. Some states deny benefits only if the employer can prove "impairment on duty" or if the employer's policy defines a positive test as gross misconduct.

CRIMINALIZE TEST SUBVERSION

A few states have criminalized the manufacture, sale, distribution, or use of adulterant or substitution products to defraud or manipulate a workplace drug test.

OVERLAP OF STATE AND FEDERAL LAWS

Each state's laws apply to tests conducted in that state, without regard to where the employer is headquartered. Where they conflict, federal drug testing laws or regulations preempt state and city laws. However, employers may have to conduct nonregulated tests differently in different states to comply with state laws. For example, an employer may be able to conduct non-DOT random tests in one state but not in another. Case law (i.e., past decisions made by courts) is also relevant because it establishes precedent that courts may apply to similar cases.

Canadian Human Rights Act ■

Workplace drug and alcohol testing is less common in Canada than in the United States. Under the Canadian Human Rights Act, drug and alcohol dependence are considered disabilities, much like the Americans with Disabilities Act (ADA). The Canadian Human Rights Act protects even workers who test positive for illicit drugs. The Canadian Human Rights Commission Policy on Alcohol and Drug Testing states that if a worker tests positive, the employer must make reasonable accommodations for that worker's needs, including, if needed, reassignment to a nonsafety-sensitive job [3]. The policy allows testing of drivers covered by U.S.

DOT requirements. Otherwise, the policy limits testing as follows:

Prohibited:

- Preemployment drug and alcohol testing
- Random drug testing
- Random alcohol testing of employees in nonsafety-sensitive positions is prohibited

Allowed:

- Random alcohol testing or employees in safety-sensitive positions
- Reasonable cause testing
- Post-accident testing if it appears that the accident occurred due to impairment from drugs or alcohol
- Follow-up testing if it is part of a broader program of monitoring and support

Employer Policies, Collective Bargaining Agreements ■

Policies and collective bargaining agreements help establish the rules for the workforces to which they apply. They may be the only written rules for nonregulated testing programs. They may supplement applicable federal or state rules. In a unionized workplace, the collective bargaining agreement (CBA) between the employer and employees typically sets the rules for any drug and alcohol testing. Where there is any conflict between an employer policy or CBA and DOT regulation, the regulation prevails. See also the "Employer Policy" section in Chapter 4.

Americans with Disabilities Act ■
WHO IS PROTECTED BY THE ACT AND WHO IS NOT?

The Americans with Disabilities Act (ADA) protects qualified individuals with disabilities from employment discrimination (29 *CFR* §1630). An individual with a disability is someone who "has a physical or mental impairment that substantially limits one or more major life activities" (e.g., caring for oneself, walking, seeing, hearing, speaking, working), "has a record of such impairment, or is regarded as having such an impairment."

An individual currently using illegal drugs *is not* a "qualified individual with a disability" under the ADA. *Current* illegal drug use means recent enough to believe that the drug use is an ongoing problem. *Current* is not limited to use within a certain period of time. Current use of a controlled substance without medical authorization is not a protected behavior under ADA. Current alcohol use, or at least alcoholism, *is* protected under the ADA except to the extent it is incompatible with one's job.

EMPLOYER INQUIRES ABOUT SUBSTANCE ABUSE

An employer may ask an applicant if he or she currently drinks alcohol or uses illegal drugs, because such use is not protected under the ADA. Prior to extending a job offer, the employer may not ask about an applicant's history of drug or alcohol abuse. After a job has been offered, the employer may conduct an examination or make other inquiries into the applicant's history of drug or alcohol abuse and other medical issues. If the employer is going to conduct this type of post-offer assessment, the employer should offer the job contingent on passing the post-offer assessment.

HIRING, FIRING, AND SUBSTANCE ABUSE

An employer can fire or refuse to hire a person with a history of drug or alcohol abuse, even if the person stopped using drugs or alcohol, if the employer can show that its policy is job related and consistent with business necessity. The employer must be able to demonstrate in this case that the person cannot perform the essential duties of the job or the person poses a "direct threat" to health or safety. A direct threat would be based on the high probability that he or she would abuse drugs or alcohol and thereby pose a likely risk to him- or herself or someone else that cannot be reduced or eliminated with a reasonable accommodation. An employer cannot prove a direct threat simply by referring to statistics indicating that addicts or alcoholics, in general, are likely to suffer a relapse. The risk must instead be based on an individualized assessment of that person and the nature of the job. For some jobs, a history of substance abuse may make the person unable to properly perform his or her job. For example, a law enforcement agency may exclude a person with a history of illegal drug use from a police officer position because such illegal conduct could undermine his or her credibility, such as when serving as a witness for the prosecution in a criminal case. The employer may be obliged to offer a reasonable accommodation. Examples of accommodations may include a last-chance agreement that includes random testing, increased supervision at work, or a modified work schedule that would permit the person to attend treatment.

The ADA permits an employer to discipline or discharge an employee for current illegal use of drugs. The ADA permits an employer to discipline or discharge an employee for current use of alcohol if the employee uses or is under the influence of alcohol while at the workplace or if the use of alcohol adversely affects job performance. An employee's or job applicant's immediate enrollment in a treatment program does not preclude the employer from imposing disciplinary action after a positive test result.

DRUG AND ALCOHOL TESTING

Tests for illegal use of drugs are not considered medical examinations under the ADA and thus are not subject to the ADA's restrictions on medical examinations [42 CFR §12114(d)]. An employer who discriminates against someone based on a test that has identified a legally prescribed drug may be in violation of the ADA. Use of an MRO to review drug test results can sort out which results are caused by legally prescribed drug use and which are not, and thereby help prevent charges of discrimination.

The ADA permits removal of employees who test positive for illegal drugs. Some employers fire these employees and will not rehire them ever or for a period of time, for example, 12 months. In 2003, the U.S. Supreme Court ruled on this issue, finding that an employer could refuse to rehire someone who had previously tested positive for drugs because the employer based its refusal on that person's history of workplace misconduct [4].

Tests for alcohol *are* considered medical exams under the ADA. Alcohol tests are thus subject to the restrictions the ADA places on medical exams, such as prohibiting them in a pre-offer setting. Employers *can* require alcohol tests in a post-offer setting if the tests are job related and consistent with business necessity.

The ADA does not preempt an employer's responsibility to comply with the U.S. Department of Transportation Part 40 rule or other applicable federal drug and alcohol testing rules.

Clinical Laboratory Improvement Amendments ■

The Clinical Laboratory Improvement Amendments of 1988 (CLIA) establish rules to ensure the accuracy, reliability, and timeliness of patients' laboratory test results. The CLIA rules apply to diagnostic testing performed by clinical laboratories. They do *not* apply to the laboratories certified by the Substance Abuse and Mental Health Services Administration (SAMHSA) for the tests they perform under the HHS *Guidelines* [42 *CFR* §493.3(b)(3)]. Workplace drug and alcohol tests are considered forensic tests, and this category of testing is exempt from CLIA rules [42 *CFR* §493.3(b)(1)].

Point-of-collection (i.e., instant) drug tests and saliva alcohol tests are "waived" from CLIA requirements because of their simplicity. HHS has taken the position that breath alcohol testing is not a diagnostic test and therefore is not covered by CLIA. A facility that performs no testing covered under CLIA can obtain a general certificate of waiver. The facility would then be exempt from routine inspections but may be inspected as part of a compliance investigation or on a random basis to determine whether or not only waived tests are being performed.

Emergency Medical Treatment and Active Labor Act ■

The Emergency Medical Treatment and Active Labor Act (EMTALA) was passed by Congress in 1986 to assure that hospitals provide care to anyone needing emergency health care treatment regardless of citizenship, legal status, or ability to pay [42 *U.S.C.* §1395dd]. EMTALA requires that the hospital perform appropriate screening to determine whether the patient has a medical condition constituting an emergency. The initial screening may include drug and/or alcohol tests.

Food and Drug Administration ■

The Food and Drug Administration (FDA) regulates point-of-collection drug test (POCT) kits as diagnostic medical devices. FDA requires manufacturers to obtain marketing approval or clearance from FDA for their POCTs. FDA review of POCTs includes an evaluation of both performance data and labeling. FDA reviews performance data to ensure that the assay meets current standards for accuracy and reliability when used as intended. FDA reviews labeling to help ensure that intended users can understand the instructions for use and that the labeling conveys other important information, such as the importance of confirmatory testing when a screening result is positive.

FDA has issued draft guidance to manufacturers to help them prepare their

POCTs for premarket submission and review by the FDA [5]. In these recommendations, FDA suggests that on-site testing operators receive training from an MRO or other physician. FDA does not specifically recommend MRO review of positive on-site test results, but does suggest that people who receive results consult with a doctor or another qualified professional to help understand these results.

Health Insurance Portability and Accountability Act ■

The Health Insurance Portability and Accountability Act of 1996 (HIPAA) establishes standards by which health plans, health care clearinghouses, and certain health care providers must maintain the privacy of individually identifiable health information (45 *CFR* Part 164). The HIPAA is intended to prevent improper access to "protected health information," which essentially means medical records. It allows an exemption under which protected health information can be released without written authorization if the release is required or permitted by other regulation or law. The HHS *Guidelines* and DOT *Procedures* are two examples of regulations that mandate certain releases of information. Several state laws direct MROs to report DOT test results to state transportation agencies (see Chapter 10, Table 10-7).

It is unclear if HIPAA covers nonregulated drug test information. Some of this ambiguity is because drug tests can be performed as part of patient evaluation and treatment, and not just for employment purposes. An interpretation issued by HHS recommends that a HIPAA-compliant release be obtained prior to releasing protected health information concerning drug and alcohol test tests in workplace programs that are not mandated by federal or state law [6]. Most clinics that perform drug test collections use HIPAA-compliant release forms for every patient visit, and treat drug and alcohol test subjects no differently, i.e., have them complete the forms. The form offers an opportunity to document that the donor has been informed that the result will be released to the employer. However, failure to complete such a form should not preclude reporting the result to the employer.

HIPAA-compliant releases often come up when MROs are trying to obtain corroborating medication information from health care providers. Some health care providers (with justification) demand HIPAA-compliant releases prior to disclosing personal health information to MROs.

Student Drug Testing ■

Approximately one-quarter of public school districts containing middle or high schools have adopted a student drug testing policy, according to data published by the Centers for Disease Control and Prevention in 2007 [7]. Grant programs from the Office of National Drug Control Policy (ONDCP) have encouraged student drug testing programs. Court decisions have upheld the legality of student drug testing programs, at least when targeted at students participating in athletics and extracurricular activities or students given driving and parking privileges on school property.

Almost all student testing programs include random and reasonable suspicion testing. Many programs also include initial (e.g., at the beginning of a sports season) and periodic testing. Periodic testing programs are for the remainder of the term or the sport season and are generally at least biweekly or monthly. Random programs are typically conducted weekly, biweekly, or monthly, and they test 25–50% of eligible students each term or sports season. Random selections are usually generated by a school nurse or program administrator. A parent or guardian and the student should both be asked to sign a consent and authorization form at the start of the program. If they refuse to sign or if they test positive, the student is ineligible for the privilege (e.g., parking) or the extracurricular activity.

Most school programs use urine specimens and test for the HHS 5 panel and alcohol. Some programs test for designer amphetamines, i.e., MDA, MDMA, and MDEA. Few programs routinely test for steroids, in part because it is expensive. Most programs collect specimens at school facilities using school nurses or drug program coordinators as collectors. MROs review and interpret test results and then contact a parent or guardian and the student if the result is non-negative. In contrast to workplace testing where MROs just speak with donors, in school testing MROs often wind up speaking with parents or guardians of students. The MRO reports final results to the designated school representative.

The ONDCP and other proponents of student drug testing have recommended that positive tests be used to identify students who need education, counseling, or treatment. They have discouraged punishing students who test positive for the first time, and have encouraged limiting reporting of results to those who "need to know." Actual practices among schools vary widely [8].

Impaired Professional Follow-Up Testing ∎

States that license professionals who provide services to the public have an interest in assuring those professionals practice unimpaired. Health care professionals are of particular concern because they have access to drugs, knowledge of drug testing procedures, and, in some cases, relationships with laboratory personnel. All 50 states have impaired physicians programs. They are often sponsored by the medical society in conjunction with the licensing board. All 50 states also have impaired attorney programs, most sponsored by state supreme courts or bar associations. Impaired professional programs refer people to treatment and monitor their compliance with treatment. They also monitor sobriety, typically for 5 years with random testing coordinated by a third-party administrator. Most tests are conducted with urine. Many use a 20+ "health professional drug panel" that includes various prescription opiates. About two-thirds test for ethyl glucuronide, an indirect indicator of alcohol use.

Nicotine Testing ∎

No federal or state laws specifically address workplace testing for nicotine. Nicotine testing is infrequent in workplace testing and is more typical of exams for life insurance. Nicotine tests do not specifically identify smokers because they also detect nicotine from use of snuff and nicotine gum.

There are some state laws that prohibit smoking at work. There are also some state laws that prohibit employment discrimination against those who smoke outside of work.

Pain Clinic Testing ∎

Some health care providers test patients who are on long-term pain medications to help monitor compliance. The prescribing health care providers conduct these tests to help verify that their patients are taking medications as prescribed and not taking unauthorized drugs. A negative test result for a prescribed drug may indicate non-use. A positive result for a drug that has not been prescribed may indicate abuse. Some pain clinic testing programs use POCT devices, which provide results that are inexpensive and rapid, albeit with sacrificed accuracy. Some laboratories offer specialized programs for monitoring patients receiving pain medications. The health care provider indicates on the requisition form the prescribed drug(s) and, with some programs, frequency and dose. The laboratory then reports whether test results are consistent with the information recorded on the forms.

Effectiveness of Workplace Drug Testing ■

A landmark study on the effectiveness of workplace drug testing was conducted in the late 1980s at Boston's U.S. Postal Service. In that study, new employees had preemployment drug tests and the results were not viewed or acted upon until the end of the study, when they were compared to the employees' first-year work records. In comparison to those with negative preemployment test results, those with positive pre-employment test results had higher rates of accidents, injuries, job turnover, and other adverse employment outcomes [9]. A cost-benefit analysis showed a cost saving of $162 per applicant hired over 1 year [10]. This type of study has not been replicated because it is a rare employer that would agree to drug testing without viewing or acting on the results.

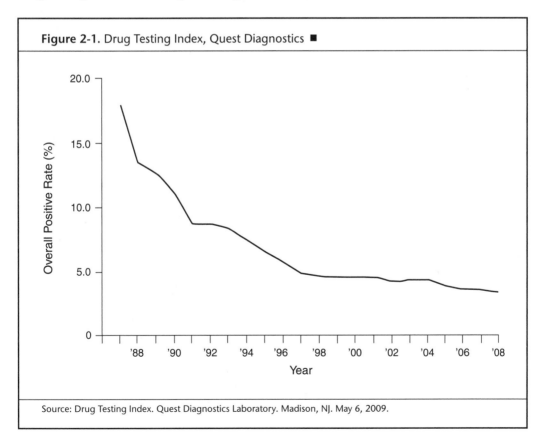

Figure 2-1. Drug Testing Index, Quest Diagnostics ■

Source: Drug Testing Index. Quest Diagnostics Laboratory. Madison, NJ. May 6, 2009.

As Figure 2-1 illustrates, the positive rates in workplace drug testing have declined since 1987. During this same period, workplace drug testing became prevalent. The decline in positive rates may be because drug testing has deterred drug abuse by employees. Other factors may also contribute to the decline, including societal changes in rates of abuse for those drugs commonly included in test panels, and increased sophistication of drug-abusing donors at evading detection. The data in Figure 2-1 are from the *Drug Testing Index* published biannually by Quest Diagnostics, the largest laboratory provider of workplace drug testing services.

References ■

1. Bush D. Presentation at the Drug Testing Advisory Board Meeting. Rockville, MD. June 2, 2009.
2. Swart J. DOT Program Update. Presentation at the Drug and Alcohol Testing Industry Association. 8th Annual Conference. Seattle, WA. April 16, 2004.
3. Canadian Human Rights Commission. Policy on Alcohol and Drug Testing. Ottawa, Canada, June 2002.
4. *Raytheon Company v. Hernandez.* U.S. Supreme Court, No. 02-749. December 2, 2003.
5. U.S. Food and Drug Administration. *Draft guidance for industry and FDA staff: Premarket submission and labelling recommendations for drugs of abuse screening tests.* Rockville, MD, December 2, 2003.
6. Office for Civil Rights, U.S. Department of Health and Human Services. Q&A: Does the HIPAA Privacy Rule's public health provision permit covered health care providers to disclose protected health information concerning the findings of pre-employment physicals, drug tests, or fitness-for-duty examinations to an individuals employer? March 13, 2006. http://www.hhs.gov/ocr/privacy/hipaa/faq/.
7. Jones S, Fisher C, Greene B, et al. Health and safe school environment, part I. Results from the School Health Policies and Program Study 2006. *J Sch Health* 2007;77:522–43.
8. Ringwalt C, Vincus A, Ennett S, et al. Responses to positive results from suspicionless random drug tests in US public school districts. *J Sch Health* 2009;79:177–83.
9. Zwerling C, Ryan J, Orav E. The efficacy of pre-employment drug screening for marijuana and cocaine in predicting employment outcome. *JAMA* 1990;264:2639–43.
10. Zwerling C, Ryan J, Orav E. Costs and benefits of pre-employment drug screening. *JAMA* 1992; 267:91–3.

Test Types ■

Workplace drug and alcohol tests can be categorized by when they are performed, as follows.

Pre-employment ■

A pre-employment drug test is performed before hiring or before placing a current employee in a position that is subject to drug testing. This is the most common type of workplace drug test. It is relatively easy for employers to schedule and manage. It carries low liability exposure for employers because applicants do not have the same rights as employees and are less likely to sue over adverse actions. Pre-employment testing serves to screen out potentially problematic employees.

Each DOT agency requires pre-employment drug testing and, except for the United States Coast Guard (USCG), allows pre-employment alcohol testing. Each DOT agency specifies which positions are subject to pre-employment testing. DOT requires a negative pre-employment drug test result prior to performing safety-sensitive duties. Thus, if an employee is changing from a nonsafety-sensitive position to one in which he or she may perform DOT-covered, safety-sensitive duties, that employee first needs a negative pre-employment test result. In DOT-regulated testing, the employer must wait to receive the negative test report from the MRO—that is, may not assume "no news is good news"—prior to allowing someone to perform safety-sensitive work.

PRE-EMPLOYMENT TESTING WHEN CHANGING EMPLOYERS

The Federal Motor Carrier Safety Administration (FMCSA) rule allows employers to forgo pre-employment drug testing if the driver has participated in a DOT testing program within the previous 30 days and, while participating in that program, was either tested within the past 6 months *or* was in a DOT random testing pool for the previous 12 months. The employer would have to obtain documentation of the driver's participation in that previous DOT testing program, including the dates of any tests conducted.

PRE-EMPLOYMENT TESTING AFTER EXTENDED LEAVE

A pre-employment test may be required if an employee returns to covered activity following an extended leave during which he or she has not been subject to testing. The FMCSA rule requires a pre-employment test if an employee returns from temporary leave and has not been subject to DOT random drug testing for

30 days or more. The Federal Transit Administration (FTA) rule requires a pre-employment test if an employee returns from temporary leave and has not been subject to DOT testing for at least 90 consecutive days.

Reasonable Suspicion/Cause ■

In DOT-regulated programs, "reasonable suspicion" arises when one or more trained supervisors has observed an employee engaging in workplace behaviors often associated with drug or alcohol misuse or abuse. Most non-DOT employers use similar criteria. The observation must be specific, contemporaneous, and articulable and must be documented. DOT requires supervisor training on determining reasonable suspicion, as described in the "Supervisor Training" section of Chapter 4. DOT states that reasonable suspicion determinations must be made by supervisors and cannot be delegated to service agents. An employee selected for reasonable suspicion testing should be escorted to the collection site and—particularly if the alcohol result is positive—helped with transportation home, rather than allowing him or her to drive while impaired. Reasonable suspicion tests generate a high frequency of challenges, often about the basis for reasonable suspicion and claiming that the test was really ordered for discriminatory reasons. Reasonable suspicion testing generates the highest positive rates. Still, most reasonable suspicion test results are negative, but a negative reasonable suspicion test result does not mean that the test was improperly ordered or that the employee was not under the influence of drugs or alcohol.

Post-accident ■

Post-accident testing may be required of a surviving employee after occurrence of an accident or other adverse event in which the employee's performance may have caused or contributed to the event. It is also referred to as *post-incident* or *unsafe practice* testing. Some employers mistakenly call post-accident tests "reasonable suspicion," but this is incorrect and fails to acknowledge that post-accident tests are triggered by accidents and not by suspicion of drug or alcohol abuse. Each DOT mode sets forth criteria for which accidents warrant post-accident testing (see Appendix G). Some state laws also set thresholds for when accidents should prompt post-accident testing. Post-accident testing is addressed in many workers' compensation laws and regulations and is generally required to qualify for workers' compensation insurance premium discounts.

Post-accident tests should be performed as soon as practical. DOT wants DOT alcohol tests performed within 2 hours of the accident. If more than 8 hours elapses, the employer documents the reason for the delay and keeps trying, up to 8 hours. After 8 hours, the employer stops trying and no alcohol test is performed. DOT wants post-accident urine drug testing performed within 32 hours of the accident. If more than 32 hours elapses, the employer documents the reason for the delay and stops trying, i.e., no urine drug test is performed. FMCSA and FTA allow post-accident breath or blood alcohol tests performed by federal state, and local law enforcement officials (e.g., police officers) to substitute for DOT tests if the employer can obtain the results of those non-DOT tests. The Federal Railroad Administration (FRA) operates a post-accident drug and alcohol program that predates DOT's Part 40 rule, and which authorizes blood testing for drugs and alcohol and testing of deceased employees.

An unconscious donor cannot voluntarily submit specimen(s) for workplace testing, and thus should not be tested. DOT explicitly prohibits testing of unconscious people.

Random ■

Random tests are performed on employees selected by chance and with minimal advance notice. Random drug testing is believed to have a strong deterrent effect.

The DOT requires random testing of workers who perform certain safety-sensitive duties. These workers can be selected for random drug tests to take place even at times when they are not actually performing or about to perform safety-sensitive duties. Illicit drug use by these workers is never acceptable. By contrast, random alcohol tests may only be conducted shortly before, during, or shortly after the performance of safety-sensitive duties. Alcohol use is legal and is prohibited only with respect to its potential affect on safety-sensitive duties.

A number of state laws prohibit or restrict random testing. The most common restriction is to limit random testing to "safety-sensitive" employees. DOT requirements for random testing supersede any state prohibitions or restrictions. Under DOT, an employee who is not performing covered activities but may be called upon to perform such activities is included in the random testing pool. Some employees object to random testing, complaining that it is intrusive and is performed without cause or reasonable suspicion. However, random testing is not intended to confirm suspected substance abuse. It instead serves as a deterrent to those who might otherwise abuse drugs or alcohol. This might not characterize most workers in any group, but may characterize at least some.

RATES

In federally regulated programs, random testing is conducted to achieve minimum annual rates. A rate is the number of tests per year divided by the average size of the testing pool over the year, multiplied by 100 to make a percentage. For example, if the employer conducts 50 tests per year from a pool of 100 covered employees, the annual test rate is 50%. Immediately after each employee is tested, he or she remains in the selection pool and has an equal chance of being selected again. Some employees may be selected more than once and others may not be selected at all during a given year. Thus, if 50 tests are conducted, probably fewer than 50 different employees will be tested.

DOT agencies adjust minimum test rates as often as every year based on industry-wide positive rates during the preceding 2 years. Random rates under DOT's random rates for calendar year 2010 are listed in Table 3-1. Note that USCG and the Pipeline Hazardous Materials Safety Administration (PHMSA) do not authorize random alcohol testing. Under the Nuclear Regulatory Commission drug testing rule, the random rate is 50% and tests are conducted at least weekly and at various times during the day.

SELECTIONS

Random selections must be conducted using a scientifically valid method, for example, a random-number table or a computer-based random number generator

Table 3-1. DOT Random Rates, 2010 ■

Agency	Random Drug	Random Alcohol
FAA	25%	10%
FMCSA	50%	10%
FRA	25%	10%
FTA	25%	10%
PHMSA	25%	N/A
USCG*	50%	N/A

*USCG is part of the Department of Homeland Security, not DOT.

Source: Office of Drug and Alcohol Policy and Compliance. U.S. Department of Transportation. Washington, DC. 2009.

that is traceable to a specific employee (or with FRA, to a train number, and thereby all covered employees on that train). Unacceptable random selection practices include selecting numbers from a hat, rolling dice, throwing darts, picking cards, or selecting ping pong balls. Use of a random pool consisting of social security numbers or other numeric identifiers, rather than names, can help ensure unbiased selections. The employer should document the selections, including numbers or names drawn, test dates, and date and time that each selected employee was notified and submitted to testing.

DOT asks employers to randomly select individuals (except for FRA, which allows employers to randomly select employees individually or in groups). Some nonregulated programs randomly select groups of employees. An employer may overselect to help assure that the minimum random rate is achieved. For example, an employer using a 50% test rate, a pool of 100 covered employees, and quarterly random testing events may select 15 people four times a year, thereby selecting 60 people to help assure that at least 50 tests are performed. The frequency of selection events is left to the employer; however DOT rules require at least four selection events spread throughout the year. More frequent selections improve deterrence and allow more opportunity to adjust the number of selections to help ensure hitting the target, which is especially important if the pool of covered employees varies or if tests get cancelled. (Cancelled tests do not count toward the required annual test rates.) For maximum deterrence value, and to reduce the ability of drug users to take measures for defeating their tests, random testing dates should be unpredictable and spread out. Employers should consider special needs of employees who have scheduled medical or childcare commitments directly after work, for example, by trying to avoid scheduling of testing during the last 3 hours of their work shifts.

Random pools must be kept up to date. When a pool is missing employees who are subject to random testing or includes ex-employees or employees who are on leave, the covered employees remaining in the pool will have to be selected more frequently to achieve the target annual rate. This is among the reasons why some employees are disproportionately selected for random testing.

The FMCSA requires owner-operators to be in a random testing pool of two or more persons (62 *FR* 16382). This essentially requires owner-operators covered by FMCSA to be in a consortium for purposes of random testing.

TEST PROMPTLY AFTER NOTIFICATION

Random alcohol and drug tests must be unannounced. Because of this, the person selecting employees for random testing cannot be among those in the pool from which selections are made. Each employee who is notified by the program administrator or his/her delegate that he or she has been selected for random testing must proceed immediately to the test site unless he or she is absent due to illness, vacation, or disability. If an employee is selected for testing on a particular day but is not notified (e.g., because it is his or her day off), the employer should notify and test the employee as soon as possible within that selection cycle. Efforts to test a selected employee stop once the next selection cycle begins. However, if an employee is told to report for testing and the test does not take place, the employer does not reschedule the test and instead merely documents why the test did not take place (e.g., employee refused testing, or collection site closed).

Return-to-Duty ■

A return-to-duty test is conducted after a drug or alcohol rule violation and prior to reinstating the employee to safety-sensitive duties. Under DOT rules, the employer orders a return-to-duty test only after receiving a letter indicating the employee has complied with the substance abuse professional (SAP) recommendations. The DOT rule requires collection of return-to-duty tests under direct observation. The return-to-duty test may include drugs, alcohol, or both, and includes whatever the employee previously tested positive for. In DOT testing, the return-to-duty test is typically a DOT five-drug panel and/or an alcohol test.

An employee who returns to work after extended leave may be subject to a pre-employment test, as described earlier in this chapter. The employer may mistakenly call this a *return-to-duty* test, but DOT calls this a *pre-employment* test and does not require collection under direct observation.

Chapter 15 has more information about return-to-duty testing.

Follow-up ■

Follow-up testing is conducted for a period of time after an employee is reinstated (e.g., to work, or to safety-sensitive duties) after a drug or alcohol test violation. It serves to deter substance abuse and provide the employer with some assurance that the employee has not relapsed. The odds are not good—more than half of substance abusers relapse within a year after the first time they undergo treatment [1]. Rates of positive results in follow-up testing are high, second only to those in reasonable suspicion testing.

Employers order follow-up tests. In DOT-mandated testing, employers do so according to the SAP's recommendations, e.g., six tests in the first 12 months after return to duty. Follow-up tests supplement any random testing the employee may also be subject to. The DOT rule requires collection of return-to-duty tests under direct observation.

A few states restrict the frequency or duration of non-federal follow-up testing. Several states prohibit follow-up testing of employees who have "self-referred" for substance abuse treatment.

Chapter 15 has more information about follow-up testing.

Periodic ■

Periodic tests are performed on a regular basis, for example, annually. Periodic tests were part of the original DOT rules that took effect in 1989, but were largely phased out after the implementation of random testing. The USCG still requires periodic drug tests for the original issuance, renewal, or upgrade of a USCG-issued credential. The credential-holder, rather than an employer, is responsible for assuring that he or she undergoes a periodic test and submits the test result, signed by a DOT-qualified MRO, with each renewal application to USCG. The periodic test is often performed with the donor designated as the "employer." Regional USCG centers may require use of a CG 719P "DOT/USCG Periodic Drug Testing Form" with the MRO's signature.

The federal custody and control form (CCF) does not list "periodic" as a reason for testing. The collector checks the "other" box in "reason for test" on the CCF and prints "periodic" on the adjacent line.

Reference ■

1. Maddux JF, Desmond DP. Relapse and recovery in substance abuse careers. In: FM Tims and CG Leukefeld (eds). *Relapse and Recovery in Drug Abuse.* NIDA Research Monograph 72. Rockville, MD: National Institute on Drug Abuse, 1986, pp. 49–71.

Employer Responsibilities ■

Employer Policy ■

In U.S. Department of Transportation (DOT) mandated testing, employers must have written policies and make them available to employees subject to DOT-mandated testing. Written policies are also required or recommended under certain state laws and are generally a good practice. MROs and other service agents should encourage employers to have written policies. They should not, however, refuse to provide services just because an employer has no written policy.

An employer's policy supplements but does not supersede applicable DOT rules. DOT-regulated employers can incorporate Part 40 by reference and do not need to restate it within their policies.

Employers and consortium/third-party administrators (C/TPAs) performing testing under U.S. Coast Guard (USCG) rules can send their drug testing policies to USCG for review. If the policy is consistent with its rules, USCG will issue a letter of regulatory compliance (LORC), which acknowledges that the policy has been reviewed and is not deficient in its requirements and procedures. Marine employers and C/TPAs are not obligated or required to obtain a LORC for their testing programs. Several federal agencies (HHS, Department of Labor, and most DOT-covered agencies) have published model policies for public use. Drug testing policies can also be found by web search. Employers who are creating policies from scratch will often want to use these kinds of policies as starting points. The types of issues that employers may want to address in their policies may include the following:

- Handling of negative dilute results.
- Cutoff levels for drugs and for alcohol (in nonregulated programs).
- Payment for split specimens, *d*– and *l*–isomers separation.
- Use of borrowed prescription medications.
- Use of drugs legitimately obtained or purchased from foreign countries.
- Acceptability of medical marijuana where allowed by state law (in nonregulated programs).
- Availability and use of a substance abuse professional (SAP).
- Treatment policies and available services.
- Submission of blind performance testing specimens.

- Employment consequences of a positive, adulterated, or substituted result or of a refusal to test.

An employer may have its policy reviewed by an attorney or other expert familiar with labor and case law related to drug testing. The employer may also want to have its policy reviewed by the MRO, who offers expertise in technical and procedural issues.

Employee Training ■

DOT requires employers to provide employee drug and alcohol abuse education and training. This education should include the following information:

- The name and phone number of persons assigned to answer questions about the program.
- The duties of the employees who are subject to the program.
- Employee conduct that the regulations prohibit.
- The requirement for drug and alcohol testing of employees.
- When and under what circumstances employees will be tested.
- The testing procedures that will be used.
- An explanation of what constitutes a refusal to test.
- An explanation of the consequences of refusing a test.
- The consequences of violating DOT rules.
- Information on the affects of drugs and alcohol on a person's health, work, and personal life.
- The signs and symptoms of drug use and alcohol misuse.
- The name, address, and phone number of a person or organization that can provide counseling and access to treatment programs.

Appendix G describes employee training requirements specific to each DOT agency.

Supervisor Training ■

DOT requires employers to train supervisors who may make reasonable suspicion determinations. The training covers the specific, contemporaneous physical, behavioral, and performance indicators of probable drug and alcohol use. Two hours of supervisor training—1 hour on alcohol, the other on drugs—is standard, although the USCG agency rule calls for just 1 hour of supervisor training. The Federal Aviation Administration (FAA) requires recurrent (e.g., annual) supervisor training. Appendix G describes supervisor training requirements specific to each DOT agency.

Designated Employer Representative ■

A designated employer representative (DER) is a key company employee for many drug and alcohol program functions. This is a task that cannot be contracted out to a service agent. The only exception is when a consortium/third-party administrator (C/TPA) functions as a DER for an owner-operator truck driver.

The DER gets test results from the medical review officer (MRO) and breath alcohol technician (BAT). The DER ensures that any employee who refuses or fails a drug or alcohol test is promptly removed from safety-sensitive duties and referred to a substance abuse professional (SAP). The DER has additional roles as reflected in the following list. An employer must give its service agents the DER name and phone number in case they need to promptly and directly speak with the DER. The DER's name and phone and fax numbers are also printed on the custody and control form and alcohol testing form, to help facilitate communication with the DER if necessary during a specimen collection or alcohol test.

DERs should be familiar with the testing procedures and the employer's policies with regard to drug and alcohol testing. DERs should know what to do in each of these situations:

- A collection-site representative or BAT calls to inform the employer of a donor with insufficient volume, suspicion of tampering or adulteration, test refusal, observed collections, or the donor's late arrival at the collection site.
- A collection-site representative or BAT calls because the donor fails to provide proper identification.
- The MRO asks the DER to inform a donor that the MRO needs to speak to him/her immediately.
- The MRO reports a positive test result or a refusal to test.
- Request by the MRO to retest the donor.
- The DER is asked to help decide if post-accident or reasonable-suspicion testing should take place.
- The DER receives a written report and follow-up testing plan from the SAP for an employee that has completed treatment after a test violation.

Employer Actions After Receiving Test Results ■

DOT agency rules set forth certain employer responsibilities for each test outcome (see Table 4-1). Actions that occur "immediately" should take place upon the employer's receipt of the test result by phone, fax, or hardcopy, whichever happens first. An employer should designate one or more backup DERs so that required actions can be accomplished immediately if the primary DER is unreachable.

REMOVAL FROM SAFETY-SENSITIVE DUTIES

Upon notification of a violation of a DOT agency drug and alcohol testing rule, a covered employer must immediately remove the employee from safety-sensitive duties (or not place an applicant in such duties) and give that person the name(s) of one or more substance abuse professionals (SAPs). Certain other federal and state rules impose additional requirements on covered programs. For example, the FAA rule provides for a lifetime ban from the employee's current aviation occupation (e.g., pilot, flight attendant, etc.) after that person's second rule violation.

DOT agencies define rule violations as any of the following:

- Positive or positive-dilute drug result.
- Refusal to test (including adulterated or substituted specimen).
- Breath alcohol result of 0.04 or more.

Table 4-1. Employer Actions After Receiving Results in DOT-Regulated Testing ■

Result	Employer Action
1. Negative	No action.
2. Negative dilute	No action *or* collect a new specimen, but not under direct observation.
3. Negative dilute, creatinine 2–5 mg/dL	No adverse employment action; immediately collect a new specimen under direct observation.
4. Breath alcohol result of 0.02–0.039	Immediately remove the individual from safety-sensitive duties for a defined period of time or until retested below 0.02, as defined by DOT agency rule.
5. Positive or positive-dilute; or refusal to test (including adulteration or substitution); or breath alcohol result of 0.04 or more	Immediately remove the donor from safety-sensitive duties and provide the donor with a list of substance abuse professionals (SAPs). Do not reinstate the donor to safety-sensitive duties until he or she has met return to duty requirements.
6. Split specimen reconfirmed	No further action.
7. Test cancelled (because of collector or laboratory error or because the laboratory result was invalid and the MRO found an explanation for this)	No adverse employment action. Immediately collect a new specimen, not under direct observation, if a negative result is required, i.e., in a pre-employment, return-to-duty, or follow-up setting.
8. Test cancelled (because the laboratory result was invalid and the MRO found no medical explanation for this, or because a split specimen test was requested and the split specimen was unavailable)	No adverse employment action. Immediately collect a new specimen under direct observation.
9. Failed to reconfirm: drug(s)/metabolite(s) not detected	Cancellation of both the primary and split results and immediately collect a new specimen if a negative result is required, for example, in a pre-employment, return-to-duty, or follow-up setting.

- Using alcohol on duty.
- Being on duty within 4 hours (for a flight crew, 8 hours) after using alcohol.
- Using alcohol within 8 hours following an accident and before testing if the employee knows of the accident and an alcohol test is required.

HIRING AND FIRING

The federal drug and alcohol testing rules do not address hiring, firing, or other employment actions. Employers make those decisions and may be governed by company policy, state laws, and any collective bargaining agreements. Some employers fire employees the first time they test positive. Some employers fire after the second time. Some employers take an individualized approach, deciding each case as it occurs. If the employer takes a case-by-case approach to decision making, the employer should try to use objective criteria that do not infringe on protected characteristics, such as race, sex, age, or national origin.

Some employers respond to a positive test by sending the donor back for another test. That second test is typically negative, but not because the first result was wrong. This practice is explicitly prohibited in regulated testing and undermines the value of any testing program. The employer would be better advised to refer the donor to a SAP or EAP and restrict the donor from safety-sensitive duties until treatment is complete and the donor agrees to follow-up testing.

REFERRAL TO A SAP

DOT-covered employers must provide any donor who has a DOT drug or alcohol rule violation with the names, telephone numbers, and addresses of SAPs who are accessible to the employee and acceptable to the employer. The employer provides the list of SAPs even if the employer has decided to fire the employee. A service agent (e.g., MRO or C/TPA) may provide the list on the employer's behalf. DOT requires that the list be given to the donor at no charge. DOT does *not* require the employer to schedule or pay for the SAP assessment or for treatment recommended by the SAP.

Background Checks ■

A prospective employer must check each applicant's past record for drug and alcohol test violations prior to allowing him or her to perform safety-sensitive duties. Background checks help prevent assignment of people to safety-sensitive duties if they have past drug and alcohol test violations and have not completed the return-to-duty process. Part 40 requires checking 2 years of past records. The FMCSA rule extends this to 3 years (49 *CFR* §391.23) for motor carriers. The background check requirement applies both to applicants who have never worked for the prospective employer and to those who are being re-employed after having previously left. An employer can perform the background history check itself or can delegate this task to a service agent.

BACKGROUND HISTORY CHECK FORM

The prospective employer asks the applicant to sign a release to obtain past drug and alcohol testing information from each DOT-regulated employer for whom the person has worked within the past 2 years (3 years if covered under FMCSA). If the applicant does not sign the release(s), the employer cannot assign him or her to safety-sensitive duties. The release form asks the past employer to provide information about DOT rule violations and, if applicable, documentation of successful completion of the return-to-duty process. An applicant cannot perform safety-sensitive duties if the employer receives verification of a testing violation without documentation of completion of the return-to-duty process. Figure 4-1 is an example of a background history verification form. The prospective employer would ask the applicant to complete this form (or its equivalent) for each past DOT-regulated employer. The prospective employer would then mail or fax the forms to those past employers.

The prospective employer also asks the applicant if he or she has tested positive, or refused to test, on any pre-employment DOT drug or alcohol test for a job that he or she did not take. If "yes," the employer will need documentation of successful completion of the return-to-duty process before assigning the applicant to safety-sensitive duties. The prospective employer may need to obtain the SAP's follow-up report directly from the SAP and would need the applicant's permission to contact the SAP for this.

An applicant cannot perform safety-sensitive duties for more than 30 days unless the employer has obtained, or made a demonstrable good-faith effort to obtain, drug and alcohol testing information from the applicant's prior employers. The employer who requests the previous information must maintain for 3 years records of the information obtained or the good-faith effort made to obtain them.

PREVIOUS EMPLOYERS' RESPONSE TO BACKGROUND CHECKS

The previous employer who receives a request for past information must confirm that the release signed by the former employee is adequate. If it is, the previous employer provides the prospective employer with all information in its possession concerning that prior employee's DOT drug and alcohol violations that occurred in the 2 (or 3) years preceding the inquiry. This includes information that may have been received from former employers if it is within the time frame. The previous employer keeps records of the information it releases to the prospective employer. The previous employer may not withhold information from the prospective employer pending payment of a fee for responding. If the previous motor carrier does not respond to a request for information, the prospective employer may contact the state office of FMCSA and ask for help resolving this.

STATE DATABASES

Applicants who have drug or alcohol test violations for prior employers may not mention this when they apply for jobs. The FAA keeps track of unresolved test violations through a national database of those who hold flight certificates. There is no other national database that can be queried for test violations. Because of concern that truck drivers with test violations might start driving for other employers without going through the return-to-duty requirements, a growing number of states have developed their own tracking systems for drivers with drug and alcohol violations. (See "Reporting MRO Results" in Chapter 10.) FMCSA has considered creating a national database of truck driver test information, but as of 2010 this remains on the horizon.

Standing Down ■

Standing an employee down refers to an employer temporarily removing an employee from the performance of safety-sensitive duties *after* the laboratory reports a positive, adulterated, or substituted test and *before* the MRO has reported the result. Standing down an employee before receipt of the MRO report undercuts the rationale for the MRO review, can compromise confidentiality, and may unfairly stigmatize the employee. Recognizing, however, that some employers advocate standing down to enhance safety and reducing liability, DOT allows employers to stand employees down if the employers meet certain conditions. Any employer wanting a stand-down waiver must apply in writing to the DOT agency under which they are regulated. The employer's waiver application must include the following:

- Data supporting the safety need for a stand-down policy.
- Drug testing statistics.

- Information about the workplace situation:
  - Size and organization of work units.
  - Process to inform employees of stand-down.
  - Whether there is an in-house MRO.
  - Whether there is a medical disqualification or stand-down policy for matters other than drug testing.
- A written company stand-down policy, distributed to each employee, that ensures:
  - Equal treatment for all employees in a particular job category.
  - Confidentiality of the pending result.
  - Continued pay and benefits for the employee during the stand-down period.
  - A 5-day time limit on the stand-down period (unless the MRO needs more time).
  - Removal of any record of the positive, adulterated, or substituted laboratory result if the MRO verifies the result as negative or cancelled.

These criteria represent a balance between employee rights and public safety. These criteria do not establish a litmus test for granting a waiver. Instead, the appropriate DOT agency decides the merits of each application on a case-by-case basis. To date, only a few employers have received stand-down waivers.

The DOT agency provides a written response to the employer's waiver request. If an employer is granted a stand-down waiver, the MRO or MRO's staff must notify the DER upon receipt of a confirmed positive, adulterated, or substituted result from the laboratory. The MRO does not reveal to the DER any specifics about the test result. Once notified, the DER can remove the employee from safety-sensitive duties pending receipt of the MRO's report.

Some employers who do not fall under DOT rules stand employees down under their own policies. They do so both to limit their liability from having a drug-positive employer at work, and to motivate the employee to contact the MRO.

Some employers remove employees from safety-sensitive duties after an accident or a reasonable suspicion incident and before receipt of the test result. This type of removal is not stand-down and is neither authorized nor prohibited by DOT.

Management Information System Reports ■

DOT-covered agencies collect drug and alcohol program data each year as part of DOT's Management Information System. Some agencies (e.g., FAA) collect data from all covered employers and others (e.g., FMCSA) collect data from a random sampling of employers. Employers submit past calendar year data by March 15th on a one-page form (see Figure 4-2). C/TPAs may submit these forms on behalf of their clients. An employer who is covered by multiple DOT agency rules must be able to submit multiple forms, each with data corresponding to that agency.

Blind Samples ■

A blind performance test sample is a predetermined negative, positive, adulterated, or substituted sample intended for submission to a laboratory as if it was a real donor's specimen. An open performance test sample is similar except it is identified as such when sent to the laboratory. The sample result from the laboratory is

Figure 4-2. Management Information System Report Form ∎

U.S. DEPARTMENT OF TRANSPORTATION DRUG AND ALCOHOL TESTING MIS DATA COLLECTION FORM

Calendar Year Covered by this Report: _____   OMB No. 2105-0529

I. Employer:

Company Name:_____

Doing Business As (DBA) Name (if applicable):_____

Address:_____ E-mail: _____

Name of Certifying Official: _____ Signature: _____

Telephone: (____) _____ Date Certified: _____

Prepared by (if different): _____ Telephone: (____) _____

C/TPA Name and Telephone (if applicable): _____ (____) _____

Check the DOT agency for which you are reporting MIS data; and complete the information on that same line as appropriate:

___ FMCSA – Motor Carrier: DOT #: _____ Owner-operator: (circle one) YES or NO   Exempt (Circle One) YES or NO

___ FAA – Aviation: Certificate # (if applicable): _____ Plan / Registration # (if applicable):_____

___ RSPA – Pipeline: (Check) Gas Gathering__ Gas Transmission__ Gas Distribution__ Transport Hazardous Liquids__ Transport Carbon Dioxide__

___ FRA – Railroad: Total Number of observed/documented Part 219 "Rule G" Observations for covered employees: _____

___ USCG – Maritime: Vessel ID # (USCG- or State-Issued): _____ (If more than one vessel, list separately.)

___ FTA – Transit

II. Covered Employees: (A) Enter Total Number Safety-Sensitive Employees In All Employee Categories: [ ]

(B) Enter Total Number of Employee Categories: [ ]

(C)

Employee Category	Total Number of Employees in this Category	If you have multiple employee categories, complete Sections I and II (A) & (B). Take that filled-in form and make one copy for each employee category and complete Sections II (C), III, and IV for each separate employee category.

III. Drug Testing Data:

Type of Test	1 Total Number Of Test Results [Should equal the sum of Columns 2, 3, 9, 10, 11, and 12]	2 Verified Negative Results	3 Verified Positive Results – For One Or More Drugs	4 Positive For Marijuana	5 Positive For Cocaine	6 Positive For PCP	7 Positive For Opiates	8 Positive For Amphetamines	Refusal Results 9 Adulterated	10 Substituted	11 "Shy Bladder" ~ With No Medical Explanation	12 Other Refusals To Submit To Testing	13 Cancelled Results
Pre-Employment													
Random													
Post-Accident													
Reasonable Susp./Cause													
Return-to-Duty													
Follow-Up													
TOTAL													

IV. Alcohol Testing Data:

Type of Test	1 Total Number Of Screening Test Results [Should equal the sum of Columns 2, 3, 7, and 8]	2 Screening Tests With Results Below 0.02	3 Screening Tests With Results 0.02 Or Greater	4 Number Of Confirmation Tests Results	5 Confirmation Tests With Results 0.02 Through 0.039	6 Confirmation Tests With Results 0.04 Or Greater	Refusal Results 7 "Shy Lung" ~ With No Medical Explanation	8 Other Refusals To Submit To Testing	9 Cancelled Results
Pre-Employment									
Random									
Post-Accident									
Reasonable Susp./Cause									
Return-to-Duty									
Follow-Up									
TOTAL									

compared to the expected result to help monitor the laboratory's performance. A positive performance test sample contains one or more drugs or metabolites at concentrations 1.5–2 times the initial drug test cutoff concentration. A blind negative sample contains no drugs. An adulterated or substituted performance test sample meets the laboratory's adulterated or substituted criteria but with allowance for some margin of analytic variability, e.g., the nitrite concentration should exceed the cutoff and then some. Performance test samples must be certified by immunoassay and gas chromatography/mass spectrometry (GC/MS). Stability data must verify their performance over time. The Substance Abuse and Mental Health Administration (SAMHSA), Division of Workplace Programs, maintains a list of vendors that sell performance test samples or that purchase them and arrange for their submission on behalf or client companies. This list is posted on SAMHSA's website (see Appendix A).

Regulatory authorities submit both open and blind samples to monitor performance of certified laboratories. The laboratories themselves insert performance test samples into each batch of specimens as an internal quality control measure. The HHS *Guidelines* require each federal agency to submit at least 3% blind samples based on the projected total number of donor specimens processed per year. The DOT *Procedures* require each covered employer or C/TPA with an aggregate of 2000 or more DOT-covered employees to submit blind samples to each laboratory to which it sends at least 100 specimens in a year, at a 1% rate up to 50 blind samples per calendar quarter. The blind samples can be submitted and monitored by the MRO, C/TPA, or employer, but the employer is responsible for making sure they are submitted.

Blind samples are purchased in batches with blank and spiked samples distributed as requested by the purchaser. The employer should purchase negative, positive, adulterated, and substituted blind samples. The federal regulations direct the employer to submit blind samples as approximately 75% negative, 15% positive for one or more drugs, and 10% either adulterated or substituted.

Blind samples are submitted like real specimens. Whoever submits them completes a CCF, splits the sample if applicable, and labels the bottle(s). That person generates a fictitious social security number or employee identification number and writes fictitious initials on each specimen-bottle label or seal. Blind samples should be distributed throughout the year, and, if applicable, over multiple collection sites. To help the MRO recognize the result as coming from a blind sample, "blind QC sample" or some other statement should be printed where the donor would normally sign (Step 5 on Copy 2 of the federal CCF). Copy 5 of the CCF (the donor copy) may be discarded or kept with Copy 3 of the CCF (the collector copy).

Under the federal rules, it is sufficient to make sure that the result of each blind sample falls in the appropriate category, i.e., negative blinds produce negative results, positive blinds for drug x produce positive results for drug x, and adulterated or substituted blinds produce adulterated or substituted results. Some programs also obtain and compare the reported laboratory concentrations against the expected concentrations of the blind samples. Results should be within 20% of the expected concentrations.

FALSE-NEGATIVE BLIND SAMPLE RESULTS

A false-negative result is one in which the laboratory reports a negative result when a positive result was expected. This can represent an error in sample preparation, laboratory analysis, or specimen handling. In response to a false-negative result, the laboratory should be asked for the immunoassay value, even if it is below the cutoff. The specimen cannot be retested because the laboratory will have already discarded it. However, other specimens that were prepared from the same batch of material may be available from the manufacturer, and these can be tested. If the laboratory states that no drug/metabolite/adulterant was identified at or above the limit of detection, both the vendor who prepared the blind sample and the laboratory who performed the analysis should be notified and asked to investigate the error. False-negative results are a serious concern if they occur frequently.

FALSE-POSITIVE BLIND SAMPLE RESULTS

A false-positive result is that in which the laboratory reports a positive result when a negative result is expected. A false-positive result is a serious discrepancy. In DOT-regulated testing, the employer or service agent that submitted the blind specimen phones or e-mails the discrepancy to the Office of Drug and Alcohol Policy and Compliance (ODAPC). ODAPC in turn notifies HHS, which investigates the discrepancy. The employer or service agent also notifies the laboratory, including the expected results per the supplier of the blind sample. The laboratory will probably retest the specimen or its split specimen as part of the investigation. If the laboratory is HHS certified, it will share its findings with HHS. If a specific cause is identified, the laboratory must take corrective action to prevent it from happening again.

Employer Recordkeeping ■

Under the DOT rule, employers must maintain the following documents:

- Test results.
- Testing process administration.
- Return-to-duty process administration.
- Employee training.
- Supervisor training.

An employer may also need to submit summary annual reports to its corresponding DOT agency, as described in the Management Information Systems section of this chapter.

Employers should store drug and alcohol test records in a secure location with controlled access, e.g., in locked file cabinets. Access to any electronic records should be password protected. An employer may arrange to have a consortium or third-party administrator keep some or all of these records and reports. The employer does not have to maintain a duplicate set of records, but the employer is ultimately responsible for ensuring that accurate and current records are saved according to DOT regulations. If the employer has both DOT and non-DOT testing programs, it must separately store DOT and non-DOT test records.

DOT agencies each have specific requirements for how long employers must keep records, as summarized in Table 4-2.

Table 4-2. Employer Recordkeeping Under DOT Agency Rules ■

Years	FMCSA	FTA	FAA	PHMSA	FRA	USCG
1	— Negative drug test results — Alcohol test results less than 0.02	— Negative drug test results — Alcohol test results less than 0.02	— Negative drug test results (except for pilot records) — Alcohol test results less than 0.02 (except for pilot records)	— Negative drug test results — Alcohol test results less than 0.02		— Negative drug test results — Alcohol test results less than 0.02
2	— Records related to the alcohol and drug collection process	— Education and training records — Records related to the alcohol and drug collection process	— Education and training records — Records related to the alcohol and drug collection process	— Training records, alcohol only — Records related to the alcohol and drug collection process	— Negative drug test results — Alcohol test results less than 0.02 — Education and training records — Record related to the alcohol and drug collection process — Employee dispute records	— Records related to the alcohol and drug collection process
3	— Previous employer records	— Previous employer records	— Previous employer records	— Previous employer records — Training records, drug only	— Previous employer records	— Previous employer records

4

— Annual MIS reports
— Employee evaluation and referrals to SAPs
— Follow-up tests and follow-up schedules
— Refusals to test
— Alcohol test results 0.02 or greater
— Verified positive drug test results
— EBT calibration documentation

Indefinite period: — Education and training records, plus 2 years after ceasing to perform functions

— Annual MIS reports
— Employee evaluation and referrals to SAPs
— Follow-up tests and follow-up schedules
— Refusals to test
— Alcohol test results 0.02 or greater
— Verified positive drug test results

— Annual MIS reports
— Employee evaluation and referral to SAPs
— Follow-up tests and follow-up schedules
— Refusals to test
— Alcohol test results 0.02 or greater
— Verified positive drug test results
— Employee dispute records
— Negative drug test results for pilots
— Alcohol test results less than 0.02 for pilots

— Annual MIS reports
— Employee evaluation and referral to SAPs
— Follow-up tests, and follow-up schedules
— Refusals to test
— Alcohol test results 0.02 or greater
— Verified positive drug test results
— EBT calibration documentation

— Annual MIS reports
— Employee evaluation and referrals to SAPs
— Follow-up tests and follow-up schedules
— Refusals to test
— Alcohol test results 0.02 or greater
— Verified positive drug test results

— Employee evaluation and referrals to SAPs
— Follow-up tests and follow-up schedules
— Refusals to test
— Alcohol test results 0.02 or greater
— Verified positive drug test results

DOT requires employers to keep paper records, but employers may also keep these records in electronic format. DOT authorities find paper records are better (more legible) for resolving questions that may arise about the federal custody and control form. Also, DOT inspectors have found some companies reluctant to allow them access to their computer systems that hold electronic records.

Service Agents ∎

5

A service agent is anyone, other than an employee of the employer, who provides services for employers and/or employees in connection with drug and alcohol testing. This includes but is not limited to consortia/third-party administrators (C/TPAs), specimen collectors, breath alcohol technicians (BATs), screening test technicians (STTs), laboratories, medical review officers (MROs), and substance abuse professionals (SAPs).

Consortium/Third-Party Administrator ∎

A third-party administrator (TPA) is a service agent that provides or coordinates the provision of a variety of drug and alcohol testing services for employers. This may include policy review, educational materials, training programs, random sampling of employees, and/or drug and alcohol tests. TPAs may be referred to as *consortia* if they provide services for more than one program. The federal rules use a single, blended term, *consortium/third-party administrator* (C/TPA). This term includes but is not limited to groups of employers who join together to administer, as one entity, their drug and alcohol testing program.

C/TPAs offer packages of services such as urine collection and breath alcohol testing, complete drug tests (collection, laboratory, and MRO), after-hours testing, and SAP services. Local employers often use their local occupational health clinics for drug and alcohol testing services. These clinics can be considered C/TPAs because they coordinate testing services for multiple employers. C/TPAs with regional or national coverage are well suited for employers who need services across a wide area. C/TPAs are also well suited for small employers that conduct random testing, because the C/TPA can combine employees from multiple companies into a common pool for the purpose of random selections. The FMCSA requires each owner-operator to belong to a consortium for random testing purposes [1].

The largest TPAs employ one or more in-house MROs. C/TPAs that do not have an in-house MRO use "contract" MROs who are named on the CCFs, supervise C/TPA employees in terms of their MRO staff duties, review non-negative results, and serve as resources to the C/TPA and its clients.

C/TPAS AND DRUG TEST RESULTS

In regulated testing, laboratories must report results directly to MROs. C/TPAs may get results from MROs and re-report them to employers. If the C/TPA is serving as an intermediary between the MRO and employer, requirements for prompt, confidential reports to the employer apply to the C/TPA just as they apply to the MRO. Federal drug testing regulators require that laboratory results flow directly to MROs because federal regulators want MROs firmly in the driver's seat of the review process. Direct reporting to the MRO assures the MRO's rapid receipt of results and helps preserve confidentiality by minimizing transfers of and access to the results.

In some nonregulated programs, laboratories report results directly to the C/TPA or to the employer. The C/TPA or employer then sends results that need review to the MRO. Any MRO who serves in this capacity should consider the following:

- Limit such involvement to nonregulated programs because this practice is prohibited in federally regulated programs.
- Seek assurance that the TPA's staff who receive laboratory results and MRO copies of the CCF will be supervised by and take direction from the MRO with regard to reviews of all results, and confidentiality and maintenance of the records.
- For DOT results, the MRO needs to personally review 5% of the negatives and provide timely feedback. This requires periodic (e.g., quarterly) visits. The MRO should get to know the TPA's staff and understand how they handle results.
- The MRO can charge a fixed fee for review of each positive, adulterated, substituted, or invalid result. The MRO cannot readily bill for the quality assurance of negative results because the MRO will not know how many negative results the TPA handles.

In regulated testing, C/TPAs may not serve as intermediary in routing of results from laboratory to MRO (as just described), medical information from MROs to employers, alcohol test results of 0.02 or higher from BATs to employers, or SAP reports from SAPs to employers.

C/TPA PROFESSIONAL ORGANIZATIONS

The Drug and Alcohol Testing Industry Association (DATIA) and Substance Abuse Program Administrators Association (SAPAA) each represent member C/TPAs who provide and manage drug and alcohol testing services. Each offers training courses and periodic national conferences. DATIA offers the Nationally Accredited for Administration of Drug and Alcohol Testing Programs (NAADATP) program for TPAs. The program recognizes organizations that complete the DATIA Drug and Alcohol Testing Program Management Seminar and pass an examination on key information presented during the seminar. The Substance Abuse Program Administrators' Certification Commission (SAPACC) awards certified substance abuse program administrator (C-SAPA) status and credentials to SAPAA members who have required credentials and pass SAPACC's certification exam. Appendix A lists the addresses of DATIA and SAPAA.

Public Interest Exclusion ■

A public interest exclusion (PIE) is DOT's procedure for excluding from participation service agents who fail to comply with its regulations or to cooperate with

DOT oversight and enforcement efforts. DOT reserves PIE proceedings for cases of serious noncompliance with the drug and alcohol testing rules or failure to co-operate with a DOT agency representative. Examples of serious misconduct would include:

- An MRO's verifying tests as positive without interviewing the donors.
- An MRO's practicing without meeting the qualifications of an MRO, as stipulated by DOT.
- A laboratory's refusal to provide information to DOT.
- A SAP's providing SAP services when not meeting the qualifications.
- A SAP's not providing face-to-face assessments.
- Any service agent's disclosure of an employee's test result information to any party not authorized by DOT agency regulations or without written consent from the employee.

PIE proceedings may be started by the DOT agency or DOT's Office of Drug and Alcohol Policy and Compliance (ODAPC). The DOT initiating official contacts the service agent to get its side of the story. The official then sends a correction notice to the service agent. If, within 60 days of receiving the notice, the service agent documents the changes set forth in the correction notice to the satisfaction of the DOT official, the matter is concluded. If not, the initiating official issues a notice of proposed exclusion (NOPE), which recommends that the ODAPC director issue a PIE. The ODAPC director decides whether to issue a PIE and, if so, its duration and scope. The *duration* is 1–5 years and depends on the seriousness of the noncompliance and the need to protect other participants. The *scope* is DOT's decision about the divisions, types of services, affiliates, or people to which a PIE applies.

A service agent may, within 30 days of receiving a NOPE, contest the issuance of a PIE by presenting evidence, documentation, and arguments in writing or in person to the ODAPC director, and the agent can ask for voiding or a reduction in the penalty of the PIE. The director can shorten or stop a PIE if noncompliance has been eliminated. The burden of proof for issuing a PIE rests with DOT, which must demonstrate, by preponderance of the evidence, that the service agent was in serious noncompliance with DOT's drug and alcohol testing regulations.

DOT maintains a list of "Excluded Drug and Alcohol Service Agents" on its website and publishes a notice in the *Federal Register* when a service agent is added to or removed from the PIE list. Service agents must notify their DOT-regulated clients within 3 business days of receiving notice of a PIE and include information about the issuance, scope, duration, and effect of the PIE. The service agent must transfer any and all testing documents to the employer or the employer's new service agent(s) when requested to do so. Within 90 days of the PIE issuance, employers must stop using the services of a service agent for whom a PIE has been issued. Issuance of a PIE does not result in cancellation of tests conducted by the service agent and does not apply to drug and alcohol testing that DOT does not regulate.

DOT's PIE provisions took effect in 2001. As of 2009, just one PIE had been issued—against a non-physician who acted as an MRO (74 *FR* 59,340). DOT does not have the authority to levy fines against noncompliant service agents, but can levy fines against employers for use of noncompliant service agents.

Fees ■

Workplace drug and alcohol testing is a mature market. Many buyers consider tests a commodity; that is, a product undistinguished by quality and purchased based on price and convenience. Table 5-1 lists ranges of typical fees for drug and alcohol testing services. Many service agents charge the same fees for regulated and nonregulated tests, and for five-drug panel and extended panel tests.

SPECIMEN COLLECTION FEES, ALCOHOL TEST FEES

A drug test specimen collection or breath alcohol test takes about 20–30 minutes. Client setup, scheduling, billing, and responses to client questions take additional time and effort. Specimen collections and alcohol tests can be most profitable if performed efficiently, at high volume, and by entry-level staff. Some collection sites charge an additional fee if the specimen collection must be directly observed.

AFTER-HOURS TEST FEES

After-hours tests justify fees as high as $200–500 per test. In much of the country, reliable sources of after-hours testing are hard to find. Few service providers have been able to make money from after-hours tests because they take place sporadically and the service providers must always be on call. Most after-hours service agents charge on a per-test basis, and spend a lot of on-call time without providing any billable service. Other after-hours service agents charge clients an

Table 5-1. Fees for Drug and Alcohol Testing Services ■

Test	Fee Range ($)
Urine drug test:	
■ Collection only	10–25
■ Collection, lab analysis, and MRO, blended fee	35–50
■ Laboratory analysis, blended fee, low volume	13–20
■ Laboratory analysis, blended fee, high volume	9–12
■ Laboratory analysis, confirmation test, only	90–110
■ Laboratory analysis, split specimen	90–120
■ Laboratory analysis, d– and l–isomers	30–100
■ MRO, non-negative result	35–70
■ MRO, blended fee (i.e., all results)	8–18
■ Point-of-collection test, blended fee, all inclusive	30–60
Hair drug test:	55–90
■ Collection only	10–25
■ Laboratory analysis	40–60
Breath alcohol test:	
■ Breath alcohol test (bill for screen and, if positive, bill again for confirmation)	20–30
After-hours test	200–500
Substance abuse professional, all inclusive	300–500
Expert testimony by MRO, hourly rate	250–500

annual retainer to help cover costs of coordinating and paying staff to be on call. Many employers will not agree to retainers. In general, few employers will pay for tests that have not, and may not, take place.

One should expect the after-hours service agent to provide Custody and Control Forms (CCFs) preprinted with that service agent's account, rather than the employer's preprinted CCFs. The after-hours technician cannot reasonably be expected to carry around supplies for every client. Also, while employers may direct drivers and other employees who work outside the office to carry the company's preprinted CCFs with them in case they have an accident, employees sometimes lose these forms or forget to bring them to the collection site. Also, one CCF does not suffice if a second collection is required, e.g., because of a cold specimen. It is the responsibility of the DER or the employer's TPA, if it is coordinating the after-hours testing, to ensure that the specimen collector and breath alcohol technician have the correct employer/DER information and MRO information so that test results and the CCF or ATF can be appropriately routed.

LABORATORY FEES

Many drug testing laboratories only perform tests for clients that have set up accounts. Employers and service agents who conduct both DOT and non-DOT testing need separate laboratory accounts for each. Employer-specific accounts can help with tracking costs and data. For example, the laboratory may set up multiple accounts for a C/TPA so that the C/TPA can assign each employer its own laboratory account.

Laboratories have standard fees, but usually negotiate fees with clients that perform tests in volume. Most laboratories offer blended fees, charging the same fee for both negative and non-negative results. Blended fees are easier to budget and track. A blended fee normally assumes there will be a 96–97% rate of negative results and a 3–4% rate of non-negative results. A blended fee can be calculated by adding 96–97% of the fee of a negative result and 3–4% of the fee of a non-negative result. For example:

1. $100.00 fee per non-negative
2. $10.00 fee per negative
3. Estimated rates of 3.5% non-negative and 96.5% negative
4. Blended fee = ($100.00)(.035) + ($10.00)(.965)
    = $3.50 + $9.65
    = $13.15 per test

Costs of CCFs, collection kits, and shipment of specimens to the laboratory are usually included in the laboratory's per-test fees. Laboratories offer lower fees to high-volume clients because of the volume and because high-volume clients can usually send multiple specimens per courier shipment, thus reducing courier costs. Each agent that provides drug testing services usually contracts with one laboratory that it uses for clients that do not have their own laboratory accounts. Through volume discounts and experience in negotiating laboratory fees, service agents can usually obtain lower laboratory prices than employers. Service agents then mark up laboratory fees to cover indirect costs and profit.

When ordered separately, confirmation testing costs approximately $100 per test. Fees for split specimen tests are higher—approximately $150—because of additional handling by both the sending and recipient laboratories and because of shipping costs (and, perhaps, the problems inherent in collecting these fees).

Point-of-collection testing increases the laboratory's per-test costs because a greater proportion of specimens received by the laboratory require the more expensive validity and confirmation tests. Laboratories usually charge their bundled fees based on anticipated low rates of non-negative results. If the laboratory starts receiving only those specimens that have screened non-negative by POCT, the laboratory's per-test expenses will rise. If the laboratory knows the POCT specimen screened non-negative, it may charge more. However, laboratories often do not know. Few POCT technicians indicate on the chain of custody forms that the specimens were screened and were screen-positive.

MEDICAL REVIEW OFFICER FEES

The cost of MRO services depends in part on the volume of tests and the number of reporting designates. Efficiency is highest for a high-volume client with a single reporting contact. Efficiency is lowest for a low-volume client with many reporting contacts. In the latter situation, the MRO can spend a lot of effort trying to identify the correct reporting contacts.

MROs, like laboratories, often charge the same fee for negative and non-negative results. MROs rarely try to charge based on the complexity and amount of time required per review. Charging by the hour is more complex and invites unwanted questioning about the amount of time the MRO spends on the reviews. To preserve confidentiality, MROs should not list names of tested subjects on invoices but should instead list social security numbers or specimen IDs. Service agreements or contracts between the MRO and the employer should also identify the MRO's fees for litigation support and expert testimony. A blended MRO fee can be calculated by determining the fee per positive, adulterated, substituted, or invalid result (i.e., result requiring MRO interview and review) and the fee per negative, multiplying each fee by the estimated percentages of results requiring MRO review and results that do not, and adding the two products.

MROs who provide expert testimony usually bill by the hour for their time, although some bill in half- or full-day rates for meetings and depositions, particularly where travel is involved. Some MROs bill at reduced rates for travel time. Some MROs ask for an up-front retainer—a good-faith deposit—against which future charges will be deducted. Charges are typically billed monthly. MROs should be wary about working directly for donors who are challenging their tests. The relationship is always better if the MRO instead offers his or her expert opinion on behalf of the attorney representing the donor.

POINT-OF-COLLECTION TEST FEES

POCTs can cost service agents more than laboratory-based drug tests. Service agents incur costs of training, device costs, time spent conducting and recording and reporting POCTs, courier and laboratory costs for presumptive positive specimens, and, if applicable, costs of performance testing. The service agent should therefore charge as much, if not more, for POCT tests than laboratory-based tests. The service agent should charge a single, blended fee for both negative and non-negative results. Otherwise, it can be difficult to reliably track and bill laboratory-based charges for specific tests. Employers may object to the laboratory fees without further explanation, and employers will be able to recognize which tests screened positive because those tests will have laboratory fees, even when the MRO may have reported them as negative. The single, blended fee incorporates the cost of any needed laboratory analyses and MRO review, averaged out across all tests. This is similar to how laboratories and most MROs charge for drug tests. For example, the service agent might decide it wants to charge $X for the POCT, and $Y for each specimen that goes to the laboratory and then the MRO. If about 5% of POCT specimens goes to the laboratory, the service agent's blended fee is then $X + (0.05)($Y).

THIRD-PARTY ADMINISTRATOR

Fees charged for workplace drug testing are approximately $35–$50 per test for the entire process (collection, analysis, review, reporting, and recordkeeping). These are bundled prices; that is, they include any necessary confirmation testing and MRO review of non-negative results. In some nonregulated testing programs, the C/TPAs get all the results and send only the positive, adulterated, substituted, and invalid files to an MRO for review. Fees for random selections, summary reporting, and other expanded services vary widely.

SUBSTANCE ABUSE PROFESSIONAL FEES

Most SAPs charge $200–$500 for an initial and follow-up evaluation. This fee covers the two (or more) office visits and the communication, document review, and report preparation in between the office visits. Some SAPs ask for advance payment for both the initial and follow-up evaluation; this prevents payment issues from resurfacing later. Also, people who pay up front are likely to complete the process and unlikely to view the initial SAP visit as merely an opportunity to challenge the test result or try to get cleared for immediate reinstatement. In most cases, the worker and not the company pays for SAP services.

CPT CODES

Many medical practices use CPT (current procedural terminology) codes and descriptors for billing. The American Medical Association (AMA) developed and maintains CPT codes. The AMA has not developed CPT codes for workplace drug and alcohol testing. Medical groups that use CPT codes for billing may need to establish CPT-like codes for any drug and alcohol testing services they provide. Table 5-2 lists CPT codes that could be used for workplace drug and alcohol testing.

The services and CPT terminology listed here are inexact matches for codes 99080 and 99001. If this CPT terminology were to appear on bills to clients, this may be confusing to clients. Ideally, the billing system would associate a better descriptor with those CPT codes, or fake "CPT codes" with better descriptors could be incorporated into the bill system, e.g., 99080.1 and 99001.1. Unlike medical treatment, workplace drug and alcohol testing services are not reimbursed under state or federal fee schedules, and thus use of CPT codes does not limit the provider to fees from those schedules.

Table 5-2. CPT Codes for Drug and Alcohol Testing Services ■

Service	CPT Code	CPT Terminology
Collection	99000	Handling and/or conveyance of specimen for transfer from the physician's office to a laboratory
Laboratory analysis	80100	Drug, screen multiple drug classes, each procedure
MRO	99080	Special reports such as insurance forms, more than the information conveyed in the usual medical communication or standard reporting form
Collection, laboratory analysis, and MRO	99001	Handling and/or conveyance of specimen for transfer from the patient in other than a physician's office to a laboratory
Breath alcohol test	82075	Alcohol (ethanol); breath

RVUS

The Centers for Medicare & Medicaid Services (CMS) maintains and updates the relative value unit (RVU) schedule. RVUs are used as a measure of provider productivity in terms of volume and intensity of services provided. CMS has not assigned RVU values to MRO work or, for that matter, to many other occupational medicine services; for example, independent medical exams, DOT physicals, etc. This is among the reasons that many groups do *not* compensate occupational physicians based on RVUs; the RVU system does not adequately address occupational medicine services. If the group insists on compensating physicians based on RVUs and has physicians that do MRO work, the group can set aside a separate stipend for MRO work if this work has no assigned RVUs, or the group can create an RVU value for MRO work. This assumes that the group can accurately count the number of tests for which the MRO was responsible. For some MROs, this is a mix of accounts, some in which the MRO is responsible for both negative and positive results, and others in which a third-party administrator handles the results (e.g., non-DOT) and sends just non-negative results to the MRO for review.

MRO RVU values can be calculated by working backwards from fee to RVU. Table 5-1 lists a typical fee for MRO review of around $55 for a non-negative result and a blended fee of around $13 for negative and non-negative results. In 2009, an RVU was worth $36. CMS refers to this value as a "conversion factor." The $55 and $13 fees are thus equivalent to 1.5 and 0.36 RVUs, respectively, using the 2009 conversion factor of $36. If needed, these total RVU values can be further broken down into work RVUs (i.e., RVUs representing the physician's compensation), practice expense RVUs, and malpractice RVUs. The proportion allocated to work RVUs, i.e., the portion directly attributable to the physician's work, varies by type of service under the RVU system. For evaluation and management (E/M) services (typical officer visits), the physician work component RVU is about 55% of the total. Using that percentage in this example, the physician's compensation would be about $30 per test for review of non-negative results and $7 per test for both negatives and non-negatives. If the practice overhead for MRO work is very different than that for E/M work, these values would need adjustment accordingly.

Payment for Tests ■

The employer normally pays for the drug test, although not necessarily for any split test, reanalysis of a single specimen, or other tests performed in follow up of a test violation. Guidance from DOT points out that employers are responsible for regulatory compliance, and this includes assuring that required tests are paid for. Several state laws require employers to pay for required drug and alcohol tests. Some state laws prohibit employers from making applicants and employees pay for work-required medical exams, which presumably includes drug and alcohol tests. Also, time spent having a required drug test is generally considered hours worked (and thus compensable time) under the Fair Labor Standards Act.

If someone pays the MRO for his or her own drug test, the MRO should report the result(s) to that person. That person may complete a release directing that a copy of the result also be sent to a third party.

Service Agents and Noncompliant Employers ■

Many employers, particularly small employers, expect their service agents to understand the regulations and help the employers meet their obligations. Employers are ultimately responsible for their programs' compliance. When the noncompliance involves a service agent, regulatory authorities may hold responsible the employer, the service agent, or both. When an employer is noncompliant, the service agent can notify regulatory authorities. However, the service agent is under no obligation to do so, and most service agents instead try to educate and coax their clients into compliance. A hard copy letter from the service agent to the employer will often get the employer back on track, lest regulators later identify the employer's noncompliance despite helpful, written instructions.

Finding Work as a Medical Review Officer ■

Most physicians get their MRO work from local employers for whom they provide other services and from regional TPAs that contract out for MRO services. Large, national employers often seek out large, national TPAs that provide national coverage and, in most cases, already have MROs on staff or under contract. New MROs looking for business may want to contact smaller, newer TPAs. New TPAs can be identified by checking membership announcements of TPA organizations, and by asking drug-testing–laboratory sales representatives for leads. The few physicians who serve as full-time MROs work for, or own, national firms that offer drug testing services.

MROs competing for business can sometimes distinguish themselves from others by their:

- Certification (although this has almost become "a given").
- Experience with testing in the arena that the particular employer operates under, e.g., aviation, gaming, construction.
- Proximity to the business, particularly if it is a small business.

- 800 telephone number capability.
- Accessibility, including off-hours and vacation coverage.
- Computerized tracking and reporting capabilities.

Reference ■

1. Federal Motor Carrier Safety Administration. *Interpretation for Part 382: Controlled Substances and Alcohol Use and Testing.* Washington, DC: U.S. Department of Transportation.

Specimen Collection ■

6

Collection procedures are designed to strike a balance between evidential standards and individual privacy rights. There are three main objectives:

1. Ensure the proper identification of the specimen with the donor.
2. Ensure the security of the specimen and maintain an intact chain of custody throughout the process.
3. Protect the integrity of the process by deterring adulteration or substitution of the specimen.

Some parts of the procedures are designed to protect the donor's rights. For example, a donor provides a urine specimen in privacy unless there is reason to believe the donor has attempted or may attempt to tamper with a urine specimen and thus directly observed collection is justified. Some parts of the procedures are designed to prevent tampering the specimen by adulteration or substitution. For example, bluing agent is added to the toilet bowl to dissuade donors from placing toilet water into their urine specimen container.

Most of this chapter describes procedures for collecting urine drug test specimens. These procedures are generally applicable to collection of non-urine specimens, too. Separate sections near the end of this chapter present procedures specific to hair, oral fluid, and blood specimen collection. The last part of this chapter discusses point of collection tests, which are also known as *on-site* or *rapid* tests, and which are performed at collection sites.

Collector ■

The collector instructs and assists the donor at a collection site, receives and inspects the specimen, and completes the Custody and Control Form (CCF) for the specimen. Collectors always have face-to-face interaction with the donor. Competent and trained collectors can help assure donors that their specimens will be handled properly throughout the collection process.

THE COLLECTOR AND DONOR SHOULD NOT BE FRIENDS OR COWORKERS

To maintain neutrality, the collector (or observer or monitor) and donor should not be closely related to each other, close friends with each other, or coworkers.

Use of the employee's direct supervisor to collect the specimen is a last resort, i.e., if no one else is available when testing after hours or in remote areas.

Laboratory testing facility staff should not collect specimens if they also perform accessioning, analyses, or can otherwise link the specimen or result with the donor. By contrast, the donor is face-to-face with the technician who performs the test. If the donor tests positive, this can create an awkward situation.

THE COLLECTOR AND MRO MAY WORK TOGETHER

It is common and permitted for MROs to review tests collected by their coworkers or employees. When the MRO and collector work together, one might question the MRO's ability to objectively review the collector's work. However, the CCF is first reviewed by the testing laboratory, which contacts the collector if there is a problem. The MRO's review of the CCF takes place after the laboratory's review of the CCF. There are several potential advantages to having collectors and MROs work together. The MRO can more readily get copies of the CCF and, if needed, corrective memoranda from collectors. The MRO can more easily provide prompt, direct feedback to the collector about problems.

COLLECTOR TRAINING

DOT and HHS require that each individual who serves as a collector be knowledgeable about the collection procedures in the applicable regulation(s) and guidelines(s). DOT and HHS also require that the individual first complete a qualification training program followed by five hands-on, simulated mock collections. Some trainers give certificates to those who take their courses, but there is no regulatory requirement for collector or collection site "certification." A collector's qualifications are not site specific; that is, if the collector changes jobs, the qualifications follow him or her to the next site. Employers and third-party administrators often ask for a collector's certification, but what they really need is documentation of the collector's training, documentation that should include some form of proficiency checksheet. DOT and HHS require that training include the following subjects:

- All steps necessary to complete a collection properly and the proper completion and transmission of the federal CCF.
- Problem collections.
- Fatal flaws, correctable flaws, and how to correct problems in collections.
- The collector's responsibility for maintaining the integrity of the collection process, ensuring the privacy of individuals being tested, ensuring the security of the specimen, and avoiding conduct or statements that could be viewed as offensive or inappropriate.

The training may be conducted in person, by video, by computer programs, via the Internet, by video conference, or by other means. Many collectors are trained with a computer-based course or by viewing videos or reading manuals. The training program's length is at the trainer's discretion. The course should include a post-course test or other tool to reinforce the material and ascertain the required content has been learned. Collectors who do federally regulated drug test specimen collections should also have ready access to current copies of relevant federal regulations and collection guidelines. It is important that collectors be updated with relevant rules and guideline changes.

HHS states that an individual is qualified to train collectors if he or she has personally trained as a collector and regularly conducted drug test collections for at least a year or has successfully completed a "train the trainer" program.

DOT and HHS require collectors to complete refresher training and mock collections every 5 years. These are like the initial training and mock collections and should reflect current rules and practices.

MOCK COLLECTIONS

After successfully completing the qualification training program, the student must complete five consecutive error-free mock collections. The five mock collections must include the following scenarios in any order:

1. Two uneventful/routine.
2. One insufficient volume of urine.
3. One temperature out of range.
4. One refusal to sign the CCF paperwork and refusal to initial the bottle seal.

The trainer or trainer's designee monitors the mock collections. The trainer should provide real-life drug collections and may act as the donor. The trainer may conduct role-play scenarios for each mock collection either in person or remotely but in real time by a video link that allows direct interaction between the monitor and student. It is recommended that the collector use a "checklist" during the mock collections and in real-life tests to ensure that collections are performed completely and correctly. If the mock collections are error-free, the monitor attests to this in writing.

ERROR CORRECTION TRAINING

Any collector who makes an error causing a DOT test to be canceled must undergo error correction training within 30 days of notification of the error. The employer or service agent designated by the employer is responsible for notifying the collection site manager of the error and the retraining requirement and for ensuring that error correction training takes place. The collector may perform DOT collections during this 30-day period but is no longer qualified to perform DOT collections once the 30 days have elapsed unless he or she has successfully completed error correction training.

Error correction training includes a review of the collection procedure related to the error and must include three consecutive error-free mock collections, two related to the area in which the error was made and one uneventful collection. The mock collection monitor attests in writing that these mock collections were error-free.

TRAINING RECORDS

Collectors must maintain records of their training (or refresher training) and their mock collections. In addition, many collection sites maintain training records regarding their collectors. DOT requires that the collector be able to provide his or her training records within a short, reasonable time of a request by a DOT representative, service agent, or employer.

Collection Site ∎

A collection site is a place where donors go to provide specimens for drug testing or undergo alcohol testing. The donor must go to the site designated by the employer or employer's service agent, not a site selected by the donor. If allowed to select the collection site, a donor who uses drugs or alcohol might select a site with lax procedures. The donor might go to his or her own physician's office, which has the primary responsibility of serving the patient's interests rather than the integrity of the testing program.

A collection site is typically located at the employer's facility or at an off-site clinic. Vans or other mobile units can be brought to the worksite and used for collections. A collection site should include a clean surface for the collector to use as a work area. Collection of urine specimens requires a restroom. Collection of non-urine specimens requires an area that affords visual and auditory privacy for the donor.

SITE REQUIREMENTS

The basic requirements for a urine collection site are as follows:

- No unauthorized access into the collection areas. No possible undetected access, e.g., through a door not in view.
- Potential adulterants, places for hiding contraband (e.g., ledges, ceiling tiles), and all sources of water besides the toilet must be disabled or secured unless it is a monitored collection, i.e., one in which a monitor enters the restroom but remains outside the toilet stall while the donor urinates.
- Water in the toilet and tank (if applicable) must have a bluing (coloring) agent in it. If the tank has a movable top, it must be taped or otherwise secured shut.
- The site must be inspected to ensure it has no foreign or unauthorized substances.

The single toilet restroom is the preferred collection area. This facility is the simplest to secure. Privacy is ensured by means of a full-length privacy door and allowing only the donor in the room unless a direct observation collection is required. It is preferable that the source of water for washing hands be outside the closed room where urination occurs. Entry and exit to this room should be restricted to one door.

A multi-stall collection facility can be used if there is no single toilet restroom. Monitored collections are performed in most multi-stall collection facilities because it is usually impractical to disable or secure all potential adulterants and sources of water. A monitored collection is when a medical professional or the same-gender collector, or their designee, stands in the restroom just outside of the closed stall door. The monitor need only blue the water and tank of the one stall being used for the collection. If the monitor hears sounds or makes other observations indicating an attempt by the donor to tamper with a specimen, a second collection is conducted under direct observation. Usually, the same person serves both as collector and monitor. If not, then the monitor's name should be entered on the "Remarks" line of the CCF, and the monitor is not supposed to handle the urine specimen.

SECURING THE FACILITY

The collector secures a urine collection facility to prevent adulteration or tampering of the specimen.

Secure Water Sources

The collector secures all water sources by turning off water supplies or taping the handles of faucets and toilets with tamper-evident tape. The preferred method for securing the water source is at the water shutoff valves, especially if those valves are outside the bathroom. One alternative is to secure the shutoff valves under the sink or the faucet handles with tamper-evident tape. This latter approach often becomes impractical over time as multiple layers of tape are applied over broken and old tape, creating a mess. Another alternative is to remove the handles from the faucet so that it cannot be turned on. If the toilet has an auto-flush valve, its power should be turned off or a solid piece of tape should be placed over the detection lens.

Bluing Agent

The collector must add a bluing agent to the toilet bowl. If using a tank toilet, the collector must put a bluing agent in the tank too and secure the tank lid to prevent access. Enough bluing agent must be added to get a deep blue color that allows the collector to easily identify any attempt to add toilet water to the specimen.

Soap Dispensers

The collector should remove or secure all soaps and dispensers located in the collection room. For example, the collector could remove the liquid soap dispenser bag from the dispenser. Alternatively, the collector could secure the distribution handle from dispensing the liquid.

Check/Secure Hiding Areas

The collector removes any cleaning supplies located in the urine collection area. The collector secures or removes any items that could be used by the donor to hide adulterants, e.g., trash bins, paper towel and toilet paper dispensers, and air conditioning vents. It is important to secure the paper towel and toilet paper dispensers because adulterants could be hidden inside. The collector removes cleaning agents located in the urine collection area so that they cannot be used for adulteration. If air conditioning vents or floor drains are removable, they could be used to hide contraband and therefore should be secured to prevent unauthorized access.

Single Entry Point

The collector ensures there is a single point of entry to the room. If the urine collection area has a window or has multiple doorways, the collector must secure the window and all doorways not in use during the collection process. Do Not Enter signs are recommended. The collector must ensure no one enters the collection facility either before or during the time the donor provides his or her specimen.

Inspect the Collection Room

The collector inspects the urine collection area before and after each collection. The collector inspects that every item is secure and no tampering has occurred. The collector inspects the faucets, towel, paper and soap dispensers, toilet, and any areas in the ceiling that have been secured.

Collection Supplies ■

Typical collection supplies include the following:

1. Custody and Control Forms. These usually include peal-off, self-adhesive, tamper-evident labels/seals for the specimens, preprinted with the same specimen ID number that appears on the form.
2. Extra tamper-evident seals for use in case the seals provided with the chain of custody form tear or otherwise need to be replaced.
3. Plastic bags to hold the sealed specimen(s) and paperwork during transit. For shipment of liquid(s) (urine, oral fluid, or blood), these bags should have two sealable compartments or pouches—one for the specimen(s) and the other for the paperwork—and should contain absorbent material in case the specimen(s) leak in transit.
4. Outer shipping containers/mailers for transporting the specimens to the testing facility and protecting them in transit.
5. Storage box, area, or place where specimens can be stored before shipment to the testing facility.
6. Single-use disposable gloves. The collector should wear a new pair of disposable gloves for each collection both for hygienic reasons and so the collector cannot contaminate the specimen with materials under his or her fingernails or on the skin.
7. The collector's identification badge. This can be the employee identification badge. It does not have to be a picture ID or driver's license.
8. The name and phone number of the designated employer representative (DER) and, where applicable, the consortium/third-party administrator (C/TPA) to contact if significant problems arise during the collection.

Collection supplies corresponding to particular types of specimens include the following:

URINE

1. Single-use collection container/cup that is capable of holding at least 55 mL. This is typically wrapped or sealed in a plastic bag or shrink-wrap.

2. Specimen bottle(s). Kits for split tests contain two bottles that can be sealed for transport; one of which can hold at least 35 mL and the other at least 20 mL. These are typically wrapped or have shrink-wrap seals.
3. Temperature strip(s) capable of temperature readings between 90°–100°F (32°–38°C). The strip is either affixed to the outside of the collection container as supplied or placed by the collector of the collection container. The collection site may want to keep extra strips on reserve, in case a strip from a kit fails.
4. Bluing or other coloring agent to add to the toilet bowl or tank to prevent substitution or dilution of the specimen.

HAIR

1. Collection envelope with foil.
2. Scissors.
3. Alcohol wipes (or other means of cleaning scissors between use).

ORAL FLUID

1. Collection kit.
    a. An absorbent-cotton-fiber pad on a stick, or
    b. A container into which the donor can spit.

BLOOD

1. Non-alcohol skin cleanser.
2. Syringe.
3. Vacutainers.
4. Tube labels and seals.

Custody and Control Form ■

A CCF, also known as a *chain of custody (COC) form,* is used to document the specimen collection procedure and link the specimen to the donor. Every COC form has a sequence of signature lines for recording the transfers of the specimen from person to person. The donor signs the form attesting that he or she provided the specimen and gave it to the collector. The collector signs the form attesting that he or she received the specimen from the donor and is transferring it to the delivery service. The accessioner signs or initials the form attesting that he or she received the specimen from the delivery service. This sequence of signed transfers is referred to as "chain of custody."

Federally regulated programs use the five-page carbonless Federal Drug Testing Custody and Control Form (CCF) (see Appendix E). This is also called the *DOT form* because it is most widely used in DOT-mandated testing. The front of copies 2 through 5 look the same. The back of copy 5, the donor's copy, has instructions for completing the form. The purpose of these instructions is to provide the donor with an overview of the specimen collection process. Copy 1 looks different than copies 2 through 5. Copy 1 goes to the test facility. The donor's name is not entered on copy 1—the test facility is not supposed to know whose specimen they are analyzing. Copy 1 also has a section in which the test facility enters the result, e.g., negative or positive for <drug>.

Nonregulated programs use forms that do not reference the federal requirements. These are sometimes called *non-DOT forms*. Some non-DOT forms look like DOT forms and others do not. A test that is not conducted under authority of DOT or another federally regulated program may not use DOT forms, because doing so would imply that the tests are conducted under federal authority. Because urine is the predominant and thus default type of specimen used in workplace drug testing, when a test is conducted on a non-urine specimen, the type of specimen should be identified on the CCF.

DOT allows the use of non-English versions of the CCF only if the Office of Drug and Alcohol Policy and Compliance (ODAPC) has approved the non-English version and if both the donor and collector understand and can use the form in that language. An alternative approach is to use an interpreter to explain the English CCF and collection procedures to the donor. If the donor is blind, someone other than the collector can read the certification statement to the donor and ask the donor to sign it. The reader would then enter his or her name in the Remarks section with an explanatory comment.

Laboratories preprint CCFs with account-specific information for their clients. Most collection sites store their client's preprinted CCFs. When the donor arrives for a test, the collector pulls the CCF for that client. Alternatively, the donor may bring the CCF to the collection site. If the collection site does not have a CCF preprinted with information for the client, the collector can use a different CCF, line through the incorrect information, and legibly insert the correct information. The corrections may include employer, MRO, collection site, testing facility, and account number information. Most collection sites maintain a supply of CCFs under their own "house" accounts and use these for self-pay donors and for employer clients who do not have preprinted CCFs.

The following sections discuss the demographic information printed in Step 1 of the CCF.

EMPLOYER

The employer's name, telephone number, and fax number are printed in Step 1 of the federal CCF. For tests where a particular employer has not been identified—for example, most periodic tests performed on USCG licensed or documented mariners—the collector can print the donor's name instead of the employer's name. If a C/TPA has been designated to receive the results from the MRO, the C/TPA's address may be printed instead of the employer's address. However, the employer's name, telephone number, and fax number must always be printed on the form.

A C/TPA can use CCFs preprinted under one account for multiple employers if that C/TPA can sort test results and generate employer-specific summaries of laboratory results. Some accounts have subaccounts for each employer, site, or other business unit. An alternative approach is to use one account and include on the CCF a blank line (e.g., "Employer: _____") for entry of the employer name, business unit code, or site code. The laboratory would then be asked to capture information from this line and print it on the individual drug test reports. If the C/TPA has multiple employer accounts under one laboratory account, the

C/TPA would then be responsible for producing the employer-specific summaries that laboratories would otherwise produce as account-specific summaries.

MRO

The MRO's name, address, and phone and fax numbers are printed in Step 1 of the federal CCF. The printed address must include a street address. A post office box is insufficient because the CCF may be delivered to the MRO by courier and couriers require street addresses. The address must be the MRO's principal place of business. If the MRO and C/TPA are located at the same place, the C/TPA's name can be listed with the MRO's address, for example, "Dr. John Smith, c/o (C/TPA's name and address)." A company name can appear as part of the address, but the MRO's name must also appear. When several MROs work together and cover the same clients, one of their names can be printed to represent the group. If a different MRO in the group does the review, his or her name need not appear on the form. The MRO who reviews the result and signs off on the verification decision is wholly responsible for that decision.

COLLECTION SITE

The collection site address and phone and fax numbers are printed in Step 1 of the federal CCF. The collection site address is the location where the collection takes place. For example, if the collection site is part of a multi-site clinic, the address printed in Step 1F is the collection site's address and not the corporate or "main office" address. If the collection takes place at the employer's site, that address should be printed. If the collection takes place in a "mobile unit" or takes place at an accident site, the collector should enter the approximate location, e.g., "Intersection of Broad and Main St." The phone and fax numbers should be the numbers at which the collector can be most readily contacted. If, upon inspecting an incoming specimen and paperwork, the test facility needs a corrective statement, it will fax the request to the collector at the fax number listed on the form.

Release and Consent Forms ■

Release and consent forms are used to document the donor's agreement to undergo testing and have the results sent to the designated recipient. Figure 6-1 is an example of a release and consent form. Use of such forms became especially prevalent with implementation of the Health Insurance Portability and Accountability Act (HIPAA) and its requirements for written consent to release information. Even though HIPAA probably does not cover workplace drug testing (as discussed in Chapter 1), most collection sites use these forms. Part 40 allows use of release and consent forms with DOT tests under certain conditions, but:

1. Donors cannot be compelled to sign them.
2. DOT-authorized disclosures of drug or alcohol test information must take place without regard to these forms. The donor's consent for testing and release of test results is implicit by his or her signature on the CCF and submission of a specimen. The specimen, once submitted, is part of the employer's

NAME

APPT TIME, IF APPLICABLE

EMPLOYER

HOME ADDRESS

SOCIAL SECURITY NUMBER

In accordance with and subject to the terms and safeguards of the above-referenced employer's substance abuse prevention policy, I hereby consent to give specimen(s) to the employer's service agents, including any medical facility or laboratory, for testing for the presence of alcohol and/or prohibited drugs. I further consent and agree that the testing facility or laboratory will provide the results of any tests performed on such specimens to the employer's designated medical review officer, to the designated employer representative, and, where required by regulations or public safety concerns, to the appropriate federal and state agencies. I also authorize the release of this information to any health care provider needing it to determine my physical qualification in accordance with applicable federal regulations. This authorization will remain valid for 12 months from the signature date.

I understand that the employer's agents will hold the test results confidential and not release them except in accordance with this release form and the employer's substance abuse prevention policy.

DONOR'S SIGNATURE

testing program. A donor who has already submitted a specimen for an employer's testing program cannot stop the result from being reported to the employer.

3. The forms *cannot* be used to ask donors for indemnification, e.g., agree not to sue the collector, employer. (The DOT procedures generally prohibit employers from asking employees for indemnification. This includes asking employees to indemnify service agents who act on the employer's behalf.)

4. The forms *cannot* be used to obtain a blanket release of information. A blanket release is a release an employee signs, giving permission to release a category of information (e.g., all test results) or to release information to a category of people. Releases must be specific, indicating exactly what information is to be released (i.e., which drug test), specifically to whom this information is to be released, and for how long the release remains valid.

5. The forms *cannot* be used to obtain a list of medications each donor took. The collector may not require a donor to disclose medical information as part of the specimen collection. This is intended to protect the privacy of those who do not use illicit drugs, i.e., most donors. Furthermore, asking about medications is a medical inquiry and, as such, is prohibited in a pre-offer setting under the ADA. The donor can list his or her medications on the back of the

Donor Copy (#5) of the CCF but should not list them on other copies of the CCF. This list (on the donor's copy) can serve as a convenience to refresh the donor's memory if he or she is later contacted by the MRO. It is not to be transmitted to anyone else. In general, the listing of medications serves little value because the self-reported medication use is uncorroborated and, if untrue, potentially misleading should the result come under medical review.

Testing of Minors ■

In many states, "mature minors" or "emancipated minors" can consent to medical procedures that are low risk. The definition of mature minor varies by state, and typically starts between 12 and 15 years of age. The right to consent is often accompanied by the right to confidentiality. Workplace drug and alcohol tests are not medical procedures and are not high risk. If a minor is undergoing a federally mandated test (DOT, HHS, NRC), parental consent is not required and the minor cannot be compelled to provide it. The law does not specifically address whether parental consent is necessary for workplace drug testing of minors in nonregulated settings. Some collection sites believe parental consent is prudent and require it before collecting specimens from minors. Alerting the parent to the drug test can help if the minor has a positive result and does not know the medicines he or she took or is too intimidated to cooperate. Alerting the parent can create a problem for the MRO if the parent demands that the MRO breach confidentiality and reveal the child's test result.

There are several approaches to getting parental consent. Although inconvenient, one can require that parents accompany their children to the collection site or one can get the parents' consent by phone if they are available at the time of collection. The minor can be asked to bring a consent form with the parent's signature to the collection site, but the minor might forget or might bring one with a forged signature.

School-imposed drug testing of students typically *does* require parental consent. Typically, the school obtains the parent's consent to participate in the testing program, rather than getting individual consents for each specimen collection.

On-Time Arrival for Testing ■

A person who is selected for testing may delay arriving at the collection site to take steps to subvert testing, such as obtaining an adulterant to bring to the collection site or drinking large amounts of liquid so that his or her urine is dilute, perhaps enough to reduce the concentration of drug(s) below the cutoff. For specimens other than hair, delays may cause concentrations of drugs or alcohol to decrease due to metabolism and potentially drop below the cutoff. Employers can mitigate the opportunity to cheat on a drug test by having on-site collections and limiting the opportunity employees have to retrieve adulterants or substitutes or to dilute their specimen. Each employer should establish a policy that each donor must proceed immediately to the collection site upon notification for testing. *Immediately* means that after notification, all the donor's actions must lead to an immediate specimen collection. The employer's policy should define a refusal to test as the donor's failure to arrive for a test within the defined grace period, for example, within 2 hours of notification or of the scheduled appointment. An employer may choose a longer grace period for reporting to the collection site for preemployment testing—for example, 24 hours—since applicants may have jobs or other obligations that prevent them from getting tested immediately. The employer could even go so far as to write the allowed time interval—e.g., 1–3 pm—for testing on the CCF or on another document that the donor brings to the collection site for his or her test.

If the donor arrives late for a scheduled drug test, the collection site needs to know if it is too late. The collector should ask the DER or C/TPA for the permitted time frame. If the donor fails to arrive in time or leaves the collection site prior to starting the test within the permitted time frame, the collector documents the no-show, sends the documentation to the MRO, and notifies the DER. Under the DOT rule, the MRO reports the no-show as a cancelled test if it is preemployment, no job offer has yet been extended, and the testing process has not started. The MRO reports the no-show as a "refusal to test" in all other situations.

After arriving, the donor can leave the collection site (e.g., to get his or her photo ID from his car) but must be available at the site within the authorized time limit to start the collection. The collector should start the collection without delay unless the donor requires urgent medical attention. If the donor is getting both drug and alcohol tests, the alcohol test should be conducted first if possible. If the donor says that he or she cannot provide a urine specimen, the collector should tell the donor that most people can provide enough urine, even when they think they cannot, and tell the donor they must try (and a refusal to do so is considered a refusal to test). Once the donor has received a urine collection kit or container and unsuccessfully tried to provide a specimen, he or she is supposed to stay at the collection site until he or she provides a sufficient specimen or until 3 hours elapse after the unsuccessful attempt.

DOT and Non-DOT Tests at the Same Visit ■

An employer with a regulated (DOT) testing program may also have a nonregulated (non-DOT) testing program. The nonregulated test may look for additional drugs or use a specimen other than urine or test employees who are not covered by DOT. The two tests are performed on separate specimens (e.g., separate urine voids) and are processed with different chain of custody forms. If someone is scheduled for both a DOT and a non-DOT test at the same visit, the DOT test should be conducted first, if practicable. If someone is scheduled for both a DOT alcohol test and DOT urine drug test, the alcohol test should be conducted first, if practicable. The collector conducts only one collection at a time to avoid any specimen mix-up.

Donor Identification ■

The collector identifies the donor by name using a current photo identification, for example, a driver's license, employee badge issued by the employer, or another photo ID issued by a government agency. The collector looks at both the photo ID and the donor to verify that the donor is actually the person on the photo ID. The photo ID and the donor's signature on the custody and control form establish the identity of whoever presents him- or herself to submit a specimen.

When no photo ID is available, a qualified employer representative may vouch for the donor's identity. This identification is more assured if made in person, but the employer representative may vouch for the donor's identity over the phone if there is some procedure that ensures that the employer representative can truly identify the employee in this manner. Finally, if the donor is self-employed and has no government-issued photo ID, two forms of non-photo ID (e.g., social security card, credit card, union or other membership cards, pay vouchers, voter registration card) can be used. The collector should record in the remarks section that positive (i.e., photo) identification is not available. If the signatures on the identification items do not match the signature on the CCF, the collector makes an additional note in the Remarks section stating "signature identification is unconfirmed."

Faxes or photocopies of identification are not acceptable. It is also not acceptable to identify the donor by taking a photograph of the donor at the collection site and using that photograph as "ID." If someone arrives for a drug test without acceptable identification, the collector should immediately contact the DER.

The collector prints the donor's social security number (SSN) or other identification number in Step 1(c) of the CCF. The identification number is supposed to be the SSN or employee ID number. Given concerns about identity theft, some people do not want to enter their SSNs. Some programs in recent years have started capturing just the last four digits of the SSN. Also, the donor may give a false or incorrect number, not remember or have no number, or refuse to provide it. If the donor gives no SSN or employee ID number, the collector enters a remark in Step 2 and uses an alternative number, e.g., a state-issued driver's license number or a ficticious ID number. It is helpful if the collector writes "fictious ID number" or "driver's license number" or otherwise describes the alternative number in the Remarks section. The donor should know what number was used in case the MRO later calls the donor and tries to confirm his/her identity by this number. Collectors should not reuse the same number for more than one test because this would lead to multiple laboratory reports with the same donor ID, which can be confusing when later trying to retrieve a particular laboratory report by its donor ID.

The collector checks boxes on the CCF to indicate the reason for the test and the type of drug test to be performed, e.g., five-drug/DOT, ten-drug. (The designated employer representative may complete this part of the CCF, instead.)

Federal Agency Identification ■

The collector, based on information provided by the employer or the donor, checks the box in Step 1 that identifies the federal agency under whose authority the test is being conducted. For example, the collector would check the "HHS" box for federal employee testing conducted under the HHS *Mandatory Guidelines*. If the DOT box is checked, the collector must also identify which DOT agency regulation requires the test, e.g., FAA, FMCSA, etc.

Urine Collection Procedure ■

The collector explains the basic collection procedure to the donor. The collector informs the donor that he or she may read the instructions for completing the CCF which are located on the back of the form. The collector answers any reasonable and appropriate questions the donor may have regarding the collection procedure.

REMOVE OUTER CLOTHING, EMPTY POCKETS, WASH HANDS

The collector asks the donor to remove outer clothing, empty his or her pockets, and wash hands. If the donor will not cooperate with the collector's instructions to do these, this is a refusal to test.

Remove Outer Clothing

The collector asks the donor to remove outer clothing to help ensure that the donor is not concealing something that might be used to adulterate a specimen. If the donor refuses to remove his or her head covering based on religious practice, the collector should relent unless the collector observes that the donor is trying to hide, inside the head covering, material that may be used in an attempt to adulterate or substitute a specimen. The DOT rule states the donor must not be asked to remove all clothing and wear a hospital or examination gown unless the donor is also undergoing a physical examination authorized by a DOT agency rule that normally includes wearing a hospital or examination gown. DOT guidelines also state that work boots or cowboy boots do not have to be removed unless the collector has reason to suspect that the donor has something in them that may be used to adulterate or substitute a specimen.

Briefcases, purses, and other such belongings are left with the outer garments. To safeguard the donor's personal belongings, they may be locked in a file cabinet or placed in another secure storage area. Some collection sites give the donor a receipt for the items. If there is no enclosure in which to secure these items, the collector should lock the room containing the donor's belongings when not in use.

Empty Pockets

The donor empties and displays the contents of all pockets including his or her wallet. It is recommended all items from pockets go into the temporary lock box during the collection. The donor can keep his/her wallet, coin purse, money clip, or other item containing money/credit cards; however, the DOT procedures permit the collector to have the donor open his/her wallet/coin purse for inspection to determine if adulterant products, etc., are hidden in the item.

There are products on the market that promise to conceal illicit drug use by substituting a "clean" urine specimen for the drug user's "dirty" one. A donor can even buy a prosthetic penis, in one of a range of skin tones, complete with waistband, fluid reservoir, thermocouple heating device, and externally prepared and yellow-dyed solution marketed as synthetic urine, designed to help evade detection when the collection is performed under direct observation.

If an item is found that appears to have been brought to the collection site with the intent to adulterate or substitute the specimen, a direct observation procedure is used. If the item appears to be inadvertently brought to the collection site, the collector must secure the item and continue with the normal collection procedure. For example, a bottle of eye drops may have been brought inadvertently and would then be secured by the collector while the collection proceeds.

If the donor refuses to show the collector the items in his or her pockets, this is considered a "refusal to test."

Wash Hands

The collector asks the donor to wash his or her hands while the collector watches and to refrain from washing them again until after providing the specimen to the collector. This is a precaution in case the donor has an adulterating substance on his or her hands. Water and liquid soap are preferred over bar soap because a donor could conceal soap shavings under his or her fingernails and use them to adulterate the specimen. In the absence of soap and water, moist towelettes are acceptable.

DONOR RECEIVES COLLECTION CONTAINER

The collector gives the donor or allows the donor to select a specimen collection container. Asking the donor to select reduces the possibility of an accusation that the collector provided a drug-spiked container. This accusation can also be countered by pointing out that, for many drugs, laboratories identify the metabolites and not the parent drugs.

With both present, the collector unwraps or breaks the seal of the collection container. The collector directs the donor to provide a specimen of at least 45 mL, to not flush the toilet, and to return with the specimen as soon as the donor has completed the void. If the donor says he/she cannot urinate yet, the collector advises the donor an attempt must be made (and a failure to try is considered a refusal to test). (If the donor fails to provide an adequate specimen, a 3-hour time limit then starts during which the donor can drink fluids and try again.) The collector ensures the donor takes only the collection container into the room used for urination. The specimen bottles (with seal or wrapping intact) remain with the collector.

DONOR PROVIDES SPECIMEN

The donor enters the prepared urination facility and provides a specimen within a reasonable time. The collector decides what is a reasonable time limit for the donor to be inside the bathroom. If the donor stays in the bathroom more than 4 minutes after urinating into the container, the specimen temperature may fall below 90°, which prompts an immediate observed collection. If the donor flushes the toilet by mistake, this does not invalidate the test; instead, the collector enters a remark in Step 2 and completes the collection procedure.

Donor Cannot Urinate Into Usual Collection Container

If the donor is unable to aim urine directly into the collection container—for example, because the donor is obese or is lying down and undergoing a medical procedure after an accident—the donor can be asked to instead use a clean urinal, bedpan, or other large collection container. The collector will transfer urine from the larger container into a collection cup for temperature and volume measurement. Unusual procedures should be noted in the "Remarks" section of the CCF.

Donor with Catheter

A donor who normally empties his or her bladder by self-catheterization would provide a urine drug test specimen by self-catheterization. An indwelling urine catheter or ileal conduit drains into a bag from which urine can be collected. The bag should first be emptied and both the donor and collector should see and acknowledge that the bag is empty. The donor should drink fluids until enough urine has been collected in the bag. The donor can then pour the freshly produced urine from the bag into the collection container in the privacy of a bathroom. The collector should record whether the temperature is within range, but should also write a remark that the urine was collected from a catheter bag and thus the temperature may be out of range (without prompting a second collection under direct observation). The collector should realize the potential embarrassment that this type of collection can cause the donor and should conduct the collection with appropriate decorum.

COLLECTOR RECEIVES SPECIMEN

The collector should wear disposable gloves. The collector receives the collection container from the donor as he or she exits the bathroom. The collection container and CCF should stay with the collector and in the donor's presence until the specimen is transferred into the specimen bottle(s) and sealed. (If the donor looks or goes elsewhere despite warning(s) by the collector, the collector should document this in the Remarks section of the CCF. The test remains acceptable.)

COLLECTOR CHECKS SPECIMEN INTEGRITY

The collector, upon receiving the specimen, checks its temperature, volume, and physical characteristics.

Temperature
The collector measures the specimen's temperature within 4 minutes of receiving it. The collector reads the temperature strip on the outside of the collection container. (Insertion of a disposable thermometer into the specimen is prohibited.) The strip indicates if the temperature is or is not within the acceptable range. The collector marks the "Temperature between 90° and 100°F?" box as "Yes" or "No" in Step 2 of the CCF accordingly.

i. Urine Temperature Range
The acceptable temperature range is 32°–38°C (90°–100°F) under the federal rules. A few private-sector employers use a more narrow range; for example, the U.S. Postal Service uses 94°–100°F. A temperature within acceptable range helps corroborate that the specimen is freshly voided urine. Urine temperature is about 98.6°F when it leaves the body, cools 1°–2°F as it equilibrates with the specimen container, and cools a total of 4°–8°F within 4 minutes. The permissible temperature range is therefore set far below, but not far above, normal body temperature. A specimen that has been warmed by keeping it in the groin or axillary region may have a temperature a few degrees below body temperature. A specimen kept in the pocket or otherwise further from direct body contact would probably be less warm.

ii. Action Required for Temperature Out of Range
If the specimen temperature is out of range, the collector enters a Remark in Step 2 indicating that a second collection will immediately be done by direct observation and notes the second CCF's specimen ID number. The collector completes the collection procedure including readying the specimen for shipment and then immediately conducting a second collection under direct observation. The collector does not need to first ask the supervisor or DER for permission to conduct the second collection. (The collector should, however, notify the DER later.) The collec-

tor sends both specimens (i.e., from the first and second collections) directly to the laboratory, and skips any on-site screening or instrumented initial test facility. Although the out-of-range specimen is suspicious and perhaps not the donor's own urine, the laboratory analysis is required to help determine if the specimen meets substituted or adulterated criteria. The collector should write "Collection 1 of 2" and "Collection 2 of 2" and print the specimen ID number from the other collection in Step 2 of the CCFs. This will help the MRO recognize that two collections took place at one testing event.

(There is no requirement to take the donor's body temperature if the specimen temperature is out of range. Body temperature measurement was part of the federal procedures in the early 1990s, but has since been removed.)

Volume

The collector ensures the specimen volume is at least 30 mL for a single specimen and at least 45 mL for split specimens. If the volume is acceptable, the collector proceeds with the collection. If the volume is less than required and the temperature registers out of range, the collector finishes that collection procedure, immediately conducts a second collection under direct observation, and sends the first and second specimens to the laboratory. If the volume is less than required and the temperature is within range (or if no temperature at all registers), the collector discards the specimen and tries to collect a new specimen within a 3-hour time frame using a new container. (See also the "Shy Bladder" section of this chapter.)

Unusual Physical Characteristics

The collector inspects the specimen for unusual physical characteristics, e.g., unusual color, presence of foreign objects or material, unusual odor. If it is apparent from this inspection that the donor has adulterated or substituted the specimen (e.g., the specimen is blue, exhibits excessive foaming when shaken, smells of bleach), a second collection using direct observation procedures must be conducted immediately. The collector sends both specimens (i.e., from the first and second collections) directly to the laboratory, and skips any on-site screening or instrumented initial test facility.

The collector checks the Split or Single specimen collection box in Step 2. If the collection is observed, the collector checks the Observed box and enters a remark in Step 2.

IF THE DONOR REFUSES A SECOND COLLECTION

If the donor refuses to undergo a second collection required by the collector (e.g., because of a hot or cold specimen), the collector prints a remark about this refusal to test in Step 2 of the CCF for the second collection and discards the specimen from the first collection. A refusal to test supersedes everything else. (See also the "Refusal to Test" section of this chapter.)

COLLECTOR POURS SPECIMEN INTO BOTTLE(S) AND SEALS THEM

The collector unwraps and opens the specimen bottles. The donor and collector maintain visual contact of the specimen until it is poured into the bottles and labels/seals are placed over the specimen bottle cap(s). The collector pours the specimen from the collection container into the specimen bottle(s). In a single-specimen collection, the collector pours at least 30 mL into one specimen bottle. In a split-specimen collection, the collector pours at least 30 mL into the primary specimen or bottle A, and at least 15 mL into a second bottle, called the split specimen or bottle B. The collector places the cap(s) on the specimen bottle(s), and affixes the label(s)/seal(s) on the specimen bottle(s). Each seal must be centered over the cap and down the sides of the bottle to ensure that the cap cannot be removed without breaking the seal. The collector then writes the date on the seal.

If the collector or donor accidentally breaks a seal that has already been put on the bottle(s), the collector transfers information from the first CCF to a second CCF and applies seal(s) from the second CCF to the bottle(s). The collector places seal(s) from the second CCF perpendicular to the seals from the first CCF to avoid obscuring information from the first seals. The collector draws a line through the specimen ID number and bar code (if present) on the first seal(s) to ensure that the laboratory does not use that number for reporting the results. The first CCF is discarded and the second CCF is sent to the laboratory.

If the collector accidentally reverses the seals (i.e., places the "A" seal on bottle B) and notices this, the collector should print a remark in Step 2 and complete the collection. The laboratory may also redesignate Bottle "B" for "A."

In DOT-mandated testing, leftover urine must be discarded unless it is needed for clinical tests (e.g., protein, glucose) in conjunction with a physical exam required by a DOT agency rule. The DOT rule prohibits the collector from using the leftover urine for drug or specimen validity tests at the collection site.

DONOR INITIALS THE SPECIMEN SEAL(S)

The collector asks the donor to initial the seal(s) after they have been placed on the specimen bottle(s). If the donor fails or refuses to initial the seal(s), the collector notes this on the "Remarks" line of the CCF and completes the collection; this is not considered a refusal to test.

DONOR SIGNS CCF

The collector asks the donor to read and complete the certification statement in Step 5 on CCF Copy 2 (signature, printed name, date, phone numbers, and date of birth). The name and phone numbers should be legible and dark to help ensure that the medical review officer can read them. If the donor refuses to sign the certification statement, the collector prints the donor's name in Step 5, enters a remark in Step 2, and completes the collection.

COLLECTOR COMPLETES CCF

After the donor has signed the CCF, the collector completes Step 4 on Copy 1 (signature, printed name, date, time of collection, and name of delivery service). The collector should ensure that all copies of the CCF are legible and complete. The collector then distributes the copies of the CCF. The collector gives the donor Copy 5 of the CCF and may suggest that the donor list any prescription and over-the-counter medications he or she may be taking on the back of Copy 5. This information may help the donor remember what medications he or she may have taken if a positive result is reported by the laboratory to the MRO.

COLLECTOR PACKAGES SPECIMEN WITH CCF
COPY 1 FOR COURIER PICKUP

The collector places the specimen bottle(s) and Copy 1 of the CCF inside the appropriate pouches of the leak-resistant plastic bag and seals both pouches. The collector gives Copy 5 to the donor and if no other testing is needed tells the donor that he or she may leave the collection site. The collector places the sealed plastic bag in a shipping container (e.g., box, express courier mailer) designed to protect the specimens from damage during shipment. If the collector ships multiple bags of sealed specimens in a single container, the collector may wish to inventory the container's contents in case any specimens get lost between the collection site and laboratory. If a courier from the test facility picks up the specimens from the collection site and brings them to the test facility, the plastic bag may not need to be placed into a shipping container, but still needs to be transported in a manner that protects the specimens from damage.

Under the DOT rule, the collector must send each specimen to the laboratory within 24 hours or on the next business day. If shipment of a urine or oral fluid specimen is delayed, the collection site should refrigerate the specimen if possible until it is shipped. Condition of urine and oral fluid degrades over time, and this may change a result from positive to negative. The federal rules set no maximum time after which collection sites should not ship specimens to laboratories. Specimens for random, post-accident, and reasonable suspicion tests should always be sent to laboratories even if delayed because the events that prompted testing have long since passed by the time any delay is recognized, and there is no sense in collecting another specimen at that point.

Couriers and other personnel involved in the transportation of the sealed shipping container do not sign the CCF. Once the specimen is sealed in the shipping container/package, its security is presumed until it is unsealed. Those who carry the sealed specimens do not have access to the CCF. Entries on the CCF resume when the package is opened at the laboratory.

SPECIMEN SECURITY BEFORE SHIPMENT

If the specimen is not shipped immediately, the collector is responsible for protecting them from any possible damage or theft prior to pick-up by the courier. This is especially important if collections are performed on-site so that donors, if so inclined, can more easily return to take unguarded specimens, e.g., placed outside a door.

COLLECTOR TRANSMITS CCF COPIES 2 AND 4

The flow chart in Figure 6-2 shows how the CCF is distributed after specimen collection. The collector transmits Copy 2 to the MRO and Copy 4 to the DER within 24 hours or on the next business day. Acceptable transmission methods include:

- Faxing to a secure fax machine.
- Scanning the image and sending it to a secure computer.
- Mailing or transporting by courier.

Transmission by fax or electronic image is preferred because it is quicker than mailing or sending by courier. The collector should fax CCFs upright, not upside

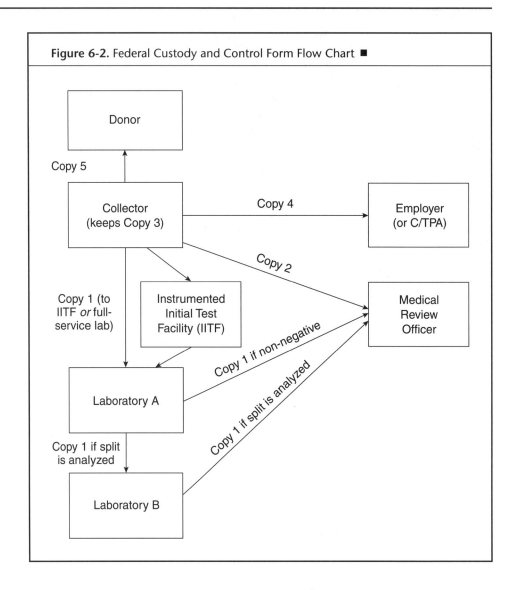

Figure 6-2. Federal Custody and Control Form Flow Chart ■

down. This is because some people receive and store faxes as electronic images, which are easier to view if they have not been rotated. Once the collection site has faxed the DER copy of the CCF, it can discard it. In the case where Copy 2 is faxed or the scanned image is sent securely to the MRO, the collector or collection site should keep Copy 2 with Copy 3 for 30 days. This is in case the MRO asks for retransmittal of Copy 2 and/or asks the collector to read printed entries from the original because the transmitted copy is illegible.

Directly Observed Urine Collection Procedure ■
TRIGGERING EVENTS

Direct observation of the donor urinating into the collection container helps assure that the donor will not adulterate or substitute the specimen. Because direct observation is intrusive, the federal drug testing rules limit its use to situations where there is a clear, heightened risk of cheating. Direct observation is considered too intrusive for workplace tests where there is no individualized suspicion of drug use or cheating. There are many aspects of drug testing procedures, in addition to direct observation, that help reduce the risk of adulteration and substitution and detect it when it occurs.

In DOT-regulated testing, a direct observed collection is conducted *only* when:

- The employer orders direct observation because:
  - The test is follow-up or return-to-duty.
  - The collector learns that a directly observed collection should have been collected but was not, and asks the employer to send the donor back for an immediate recollection under direct observation.
  - The MRO asked for a retest using direct observation because the employee has no legitimate medical reason for certain atypical laboratory results (invalid/dilute with creatinine of 2–5 mg/dL), or the employee's positive, adulterated, or substituted test result had to be cancelled because no suitable split specimen was available. (Note: The HHS rule requires recollection under direct observation if the split specimen fails to reconfirm for any reason.)
- At the collection site, an immediate collection of a second urine specimen is required because:
  - The temperature of the specimen collected during a routine collection is outside the acceptable range.
  - The collector suspects that the donor has tampered with the specimen during a routine collection (e.g., abnormal physical characteristic such as unusual color and/or odor and/or excessive foaming when shaken).
  - The collector finds an item in the employee's pockets or wallet that appears to be brought into the site to contaminate a specimen or the collector notes conduct suggesting tampering.

Laws in some states and cities (e.g., Connecticut, Maine, Oklahoma, Rhode Island, and Boulder, Colorado) prohibit directly observed collections for workplace urine drug tests. (Part 40 supersedes such state restrictions.)

OBSERVER

An observer is someone, not necessarily the collector, who watches the donor urinate into the specimen container. Direct observation serves to reduce opportunities to adulterate or substitute the specimen. The observer for an HHS- or DOT-authorized direct observed collection must be knowledgeable about the direct observed collection procedures. The observer, if different from the collector, is not supposed to handle the urine specimen. The observer must know:

- All steps necessary to perform a direct observed collection correctly.
- The observer's responsibility for maintaining the integrity of the collection process, ensuring the privacy of individuals being tested, ensuring that the observation is done in a professional manner that minimizes the discomfort to the employees so observed, ensuring the security of the specimen by

maintaining visual contact with the collection container until it is delivered to the collector, and avoiding conduct or statements that could be viewed as offensive or inappropriate.

A script may be used to ease the process for both the observer and the donor and to ensure consistent procedures.

The observer must also be of the same gender as the donor. Most donors who undergo directly observed collections are men. Most collectors are women, and thus male physicians or other male staff are often enlisted to serve as observer. If the observer is not also the collector, the collector should print the observer's name on the "Remarks" line of the CCF, e.g., "Joe Citizen—observer." To preclude any potential appearance of collusion or impropriety, the observer should not be a coworker or immediate supervisor unless no one else is available.

DIRECT OBSERVATION PROCEDURES

The collector tells the donor why a directly observed collection is being conducted. The collector completes a new CCF for the directly observed collection and checks off the "Reason to Test." If this collection immediately follows a problem collection (e.g., a specimen that had temperature out of range), the collector checks off the same "Reason to Test" and prints two comments on the "Remarks" line of the CCF: One to help identify it as test 2 of a pair (e.g., "Collection 2 of 2") and another explaining the reason for the second test (e.g., "1st specimen temp out of range)." If the donor refuses to undergo a required second collection under direct observation, the collector notes the "Refusal to Test" in the "Remarks" section, notifies the DER, and discards the first specimen.

Under the DOT rule, the observer, or *witness*, instructs the donor to raise clothing just above the navel; lower clothing and underpants to mid-thigh; then turn around to show the observer he or she does not have a specimen adulteration/substitution device. Some of these devices may include:

1. A long plastic tube connected to a bottle containing heated urine.
2. A short plastic tube attached to a battery-heated plastic bag.
3. A molded (e.g., plastic) penis with a tube in the center connected to a bag or bottle of urine.

If no device is detected, the donor returns his or her clothing to a more normal position for urinating. The observer stays in the bathroom while the donor urinates and watches the urine pass from the body into the collection container. Use of mirrors or video cameras is not permitted. Positioning for direct observation of the urine flow can be difficult in small bathrooms. Many direct observations are performed on men in small bathrooms with the observer standing behind the man and peering over his shoulder.

Although some observers fail to diligently watch the urine pass from the body into the cup, the observer's presence may still deter adulteration or substitution. If the directly observed specimen's temperature is out of range, one may question the observer's diligence but the donor gets the benefit of the doubt and the specimen is assumed to be the donor's fresh urine.

After the donor has urinated into the collection container, the observer and donor leave the toilet stall/restroom and the donor hands the collection container to the collector. The observer must maintain visual contact of the collection container until the donor hands the container to the collector. If the collector is the observer, the collector may receive the collection container from the donor while they are both in the toilet stall/restroom.

Specimens from both collections, observed and nonobserved, are separately packaged with their CCFs and sent to the laboratory. If the collector started the directly observed collection because of suspected tampering, the collector notifies the DER and collection site supervisor that a directly observed collection was performed and why.

Under the DOT rule, if the collector learns that a directly observed collection should have been performed but was not, the collector asks the employer to immediately send the donor for another test, this time collected under direct observation.

Shy Bladder ■

SHY BLADDER EVENT AT COLLECTION SITE

The term *shy bladder* refers to a situation when the donor does not provide a sufficient amount of urine for a drug test. If the donor provides an otherwise normal specimen (i.e., temperature and appearance) but not a sufficient volume of urine, the collector should:

1. Discard the specimen and its container(s).
2. Direct the donor to stay at the site for another collection.
3. Ask the donor to drink up to 40 ounces of fluids.
4. Enter a remark in Step 2 and inform the donor that he/she has up to 3 hours more to provide a specimen. The 3 hours starts the very first time the donor exits the restroom without a sufficient volume of urine.
5. Wait until the donor provides a sufficient specimen, leaves the collection site despite direction to stay (see statement 2), or 3 hours elapses, whichever occurs first. If the donor leaves the collection site before 3 hours or gives up shortly before 3 hours without submitting a sufficient specimen, the collector notes the fact on the "Remarks" line of the CCF and immediately notifies the DER. (See the section "Refusal to Test.")

The donor gets up to 3 hours, even if this goes beyond closing time. The 3-hour clock does not reset with each unsuccessful attempt to provide a urine specimen. Any decision to stop short of the allowed time is made at the discretion of the donor and is considered a refusal to test.

The 3-hour clock does not reset with each unsuccessful attempt to provide a specimen. If, during this 3-hour period, the donor provides a cold/hot specimen or one that shows signs of tampering, the donor still has 3 hours from the first failed attempt, albeit is now subject to direct observation.

The donor must be under the supervision of the collector or other collection site personnel during the 3 hours. This prevents the donor from using a different bathroom or gaining access to adulteration products. The collector should urge, but not demand, that the donor drink up to 40 ounces of fluids. The limit on fluid consumption is intended to avoid water intoxication and specimen dilution. A refusal to drink fluids is not a "refusal to test."

The collector notes any attempts by the donor to provide a specimen. While waiting, the collector may collect specimens from other donors. The collector may also turn the collection procedure over to a different collector and, in so doing, should print a remark on Step 2 of the CCF indicating the handover. The second collector signs the collector statement and is considered the collector of record.

If the donor fails to provide a sufficient volume of urine within 3 hours, the collector checks the "None Provided" box in Step 2 of the CCF and prints a remark, e.g., "9:15 AM insufficient; 10:30 AM insufficient; 12:15 PM insufficient. Consumed 40 oz. Notifying DER," or "Donor left at 2 PM without providing sufficient specimen—Refusal to Test." The collector prints his or her name, signs the CCF, and enters the time that the collection ended in Step 4 of the CCF. The collector immediately notifies the DER and MRO and sends them their CCF copies. DOT does not authorize collection of a non-urine specimen in lieu of urine. Copy 1 of the CCF can be discarded.

The DER (or MRO or other service agent acting on behalf of the employer) should review the adequacy of the documentation. If the documentation is inadequate, the collector should rectify it or the test should be canceled.

DER SENDS DONOR FOR SHY BLADDER EVALUATION

If the documentation is adequate, the DER directs the donor to get a medical ("shy bladder") evaluation by a physician acceptable to the MRO within 5 business days of notification by the DER. The 5-day time frame should be extended if the donor makes a good-faith effort, but fails, to get the evaluation within 5 days. DOT authorizes the employer to remove the employee from work, pending completion of the shy bladder evaluation, only if the shy bladder situation occurred during an observed collection and the employer has a stand-down waiver from DOT authorizing such removal. Figure 6-3 illustrates the shy bladder evaluation process.

If the donor fails to obtain the evaluation, under DOT regulations the outcome is "Test Cancelled" if the test was performed prior to a job offer and is "Refusal to Test" if it was performed after a job offer was extended. This distinction is based on an assumption that some applicants skip shy bladder evaluations for innocent reasons, for example, because they decide not to take the job. DOT does not want to burden any donor who skips the evaluation for an innocent reason with the consequences of a refusal, i.e., having to complete the return-to-duty process and certificate actions under some DOT agency regulations. Either the employer or MRO can document the final outcome, but it is important that the outcome be documented. It can be documented in Step 5 of the federal CCF.

ARRANGING THE SHY BLADDER EVALUATION

The physician who performs the evaluation must have sufficient expertise to deal effectively with the medical issues associated with urination problems, should have some knowledge of workplace drug testing procedures, and should be neutral and objective. The physician should not delegate this exam to an advanced practitioner; the issues are too complex and the stakes are too high. The physician need not be a urologist, but this level of expertise can prove important later if the case is challenged, as many of these are. It can be hard to get timely appointments with urologists, and some urologists are not interested in this kind of

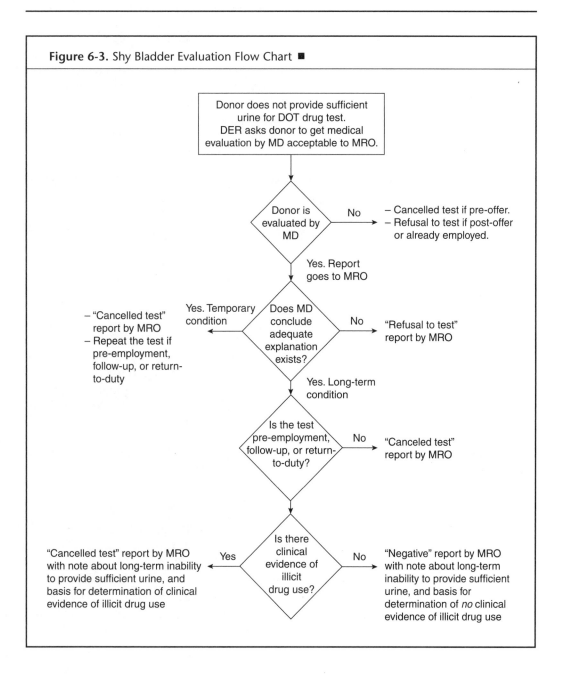

Figure 6-3. Shy Bladder Evaluation Flow Chart ■

Donor does not provide sufficient urine for DOT drug test. DER asks donor to get medical evaluation by MD acceptable to MRO.

Donor is evaluated by MD

No
— Cancelled test if pre-offer.
— Refusal to test if post-offer or already employed.

Yes. Report goes to MRO

Does MD conclude adequate explanation exists?

Yes. Temporary condition
— "Cancelled test" report by MRO
— Repeat the test if pre-employment, follow-up, or return-to-duty

No
"Refusal to test" report by MRO

Yes. Long-term condition

Is the test pre-employment, follow-up, or return-to-duty?

No
"Canceled test" report by MRO

Is there clinical evidence of illicit drug use?

Yes
"Cancelled test" report by MRO with note about long-term inability to provide sufficient urine, and basis for determination of clinical evidence of illicit drug use

No
"Negative" report by MRO with note about long-term inability to provide sufficient urine, and basis for determination of no clinical evidence of illicit drug use

work. Shy bladder evaluations are often performed by MROs who understand the clinical issues, and appreciate and make time for the service. However, the MRO also reviews the shy bladder evaluation report, and objectivity is best served if a different MRO or other physician writes the report than the one who reviews it. The MRO informs that physician of the donor's inability to provide a 45 mL urine specimen and the consequences of a refusal to test. The MRO asks the examiner to determine if there is adequate basis for determining that a medical condition has, or probably has, precluded the donor from providing enough urine. A medical condition includes an ascertainable physiological condition or a medically documented pre-existing psychological disorder, but does not include unsupported assertions of "situational anxiety" or "dehydration." After completing the examination, the referral physician provides the MRO with a written statement of his or her findings and the basis for them. If the referral physician determines that the donor has a long-term condition that precludes providing enough urine, the physician should explain this in the report, too.

The donor's personal physician is unlikely to have the necessary objectivity and is thus a bad choice to conduct a shy bladder evaluation. Donors sometimes go to their own doctors for proof of their "shy bladder" explanations and present their doctors' notes to substantiate their claims. If the MRO chooses to consider information from a physician he or she has not selected, the MRO should insist on reviewing the complete record of that evaluation so that the MRO can better understand the basis for the opinion.

The federal rules do not specify who arranges or pays for the evaluation. Practices vary. Some employers ask the donor to pay for the evaluation and agree to reimburse the donor if the evaluation reveals a shy bladder medical explanation acceptable to the MRO.

SHY BLADDER EXAMINATION PROTOCOL

A medical history, such as that outlined in Figure 6-4, should be included. Simple lab tests—urinalysis, BUN, creatinine—may be included, but a drug test may not. Performing cystoscopy, retrograde urethrography, or formal urodynamic testing is unusual in the context of a shy bladder evaluation. The examining physician is not prohibited from conducting a drug test using a non-urine speci-

---

Figure 6-4. Sample Questions to Ask a Patient with Shy Bladder ■

1. How would you describe your urinary stream? Strong, weak, or variable?
2. Is there any history of infection (gonorrhea or chlamydia) or trauma to the urethra?
3. Have you ever had a bladder infection?
4. Have you had urologic surgery or an instrumented, diagnostic procedure?
5. Have you seen blood in your urine?
6. Do you have trouble postponing urination when the feeling arises?
7. Do you consistently strain to start your urine stream?
8. How many times do you get up at night to urinate?
9. Is there a family history of prostate cancer?
10. Are you on any medication, including over-the-counter medications?
11. Is there any activity or foods that worsen or improve your urinary symptoms?
12. Have you ever suffered neurologic trauma or had abdominal or back surgery during which your nerves could have been traumatized?
13. Do you have any diseases that affect your nerves (e.g., multiple sclerosis, diabetes, stroke)?

---

men. This could be viewed as a legitimate test for assessing the validity of certain medical conditions or the credibility of the donor.

Dehydration and situational anxiety are acceptable explanations for a shy bladder only if supported by medical documentation. For example, dehydration is an acceptable explanation if there is medical documentation of the donor's dehydration at the time of the drug test. Situational anxiety is an acceptable explanation only if the symptoms—and, in some cases, the diagnosis—have been medically documented prior to the test. For example, a donor may have brought urination problems to the attention of his or her personal physician over a period of time, and the personal physician made notes about these problems but entered no specific diagnosis in the medical records. The physician conducting the shy bladder evaluation is responsible for reviewing any medical records provided by the donor and determining if they adequately document the shy bladder condition.

EXAMINING PHYSICIAN'S REPORT

The examining physician provides the MRO with a written report of the exam and his or her determination and the basis for it. The MRO reviews the examining physician's report and determines if the evaluation was properly conducted and, if so, if the donor's medical condition precluded production of a sufficient volume of urine, in one void, in the 3-hour time period. The MRO then notifies the employer, in writing, of the MRO's conclusion: *Either* the shy bladder incident has no adequate medical explanation and thus represents a refusal to test *or* there is a medical condition that explains it and thus the test should be canceled. On the federal CCF, the MRO can check the "Refusal to Test" because box and write a remark, for example, "no medical explanation for shy bladder."

PERMANENT SHY BLADDER

In DOT-regulated testing, if the donor has a long-term shy bladder condition and a negative result is required—i.e., for preemployment, return-to-duty, or follow-up purposes—the MRO determines if there is clinical evidence that the donor is currently an illicit drug user. The MRO determines this by conducting, or having someone else conduct, a clinical examination for drug abuse and, if appropriate, consulting with the donor's personal physician. The clinical examination for drug abuse may include a drug test using an alternative specimen, such as blood. Any drug test result would be incorporated into the clinical assessment and would not be reported to the employer like a standard drug test. If the clinical examination finds no evidence of drug abuse, the MRO reports this as a negative test result with written notations regarding the medical examination required because of permanent shy bladder. However, if the clinical examination does find evidence of drug abuse, the MRO reports this as "Test Cancelled" with written notations regarding the medical examination required because of permanent shy bladder. The donor has not had a positive result nor is the donor able to perform safety-sensitive duties without a negative result.

The NRC rule merely authorizes the MRO to conduct an alternative specimen test if the donor has a long-term shy bladder condition. The NRC rule authorizes this every time, without regard to whether a negative result is required for return to the workplace.

The donor with a long-term shy bladder condition remains subject to drug testing, at least in federally regulated testing. If selected, he or she must report for testing exactly like any other employee and must sit out the 3-hour shy bladder time period exactly like any other employee. However inconvenient, DOT requires this procedure because no DOT agency currently has a regulatory waiver for an employee to be exempted from random testing for any reason. The employer, through the MRO, must verify at each test event that the donor remains physically unable to produce a sufficient specimen. The prudent MRO might require an updated examination if a period of time, like a year, has passed or the previous examination revealed that the disability was not necessarily long term. Otherwise, the MRO might contact the treating physician to determine if the medical disability still exists.

Refusal to Test ■

A donor has refused to take a drug or alcohol test if he or she fails to cooperate with a significant aspect of the testing process or is caught cheating or otherwise overtly obstructing the test. The regulatory definition of a refusal to test includes the following collection or alcohol test site events:

1. Failure to appear for any test (except a pre-employment test) within a reasonable time, as defined by the employer, after being directed to do so by the employer. This includes the failure of an owner-operator to appear for a test when called by a C/TPA. (If the donor is an applicant who has not yet been offered a job, the skipped test is not declared a "refusal to test." This exception exists so that any person who turns down a job offer and skips the test will not be burdened with a drug testing violation on his or her record.)

2. Failure to remain at the site until the collection or alcohol test is complete (with the exception of a donor for a preemployment test who leaves the site before the collection or alcohol test begins. A urine drug test collection begins when the donor is given a collection kit or cup.

3. In the case of a directly observed or monitored urine collection, failure to permit the observation or monitoring.

4. Failure to cooperate with the testing process, e.g.,
   a. Refusal to empty pockets when instructed to do so.
   b. Refusal to wash hands after being directed to do so by the collector.
   c. The donor admits to the collector that he or she adulterated or substituted the specimen.
   d. The donor is found to have a device—such as a prosthetic appliance—the purpose of which is to interfere with providing a real specimen.
   e. Confrontational behavior that disrupts testing.
   f. For alcohol tests, failure to sign the certification at Step 2 of the Alcohol Testing Form.

5. Refusal to take a second test at the direction of the collector or employer.

6. Failure to provide an adequate specimen and:
   a. Failure to undergo a medical evaluation directed by the MRO or employer, or
   b. The medical evaluation was conducted and identified no basis for the failure to provide an adequate specimen.

7. Failure to undergo a medical evaluation directed by the employer because of failure to provide an adequate specimen. (Exception: In the case of a pre-employment drug test, the donor is deemed to have refused to test on this basis only if the pre-employment test is conducted following a contingent offer of employment [49 *CFR* 40.191(a)(7)].)
8. Submission of a specimen that is adulterated or substituted and for which the MRO determines there is no legitimate explanation.

These events do *not* constitute a refusal to test:

1. Refusal to drink fluids.
2. Refusal to sign the CCF or provide one's SSN or sign a release and consent form.
3. Observed behavior suggesting (but not proving) an attempt to adulterate or substitute the specimen. (This triggers a second collection under direct observation.)
4. Noncompliance with procedures if they were not clearly explained to the donor—for example, failure to remain at the collection site when no one has told the donor to remain there.
5. Under the DOT rule, any refusal to take a *non-DOT* test is of no consequence.

When the donor refuses to follow instructions or is confrontational, the collector or alcohol test technician warns the donor of the potential consequences of a failure to cooperate, and, if practical, seeks help from the DER or supervisor to ensure that the donor understands. (No such warning is required when the donor is caught cheating.) If the behavior continues, the collector or technician stops the testing process, documents the refusal on the CCF or Alcohol Test Form (ATF), and discards any specimen that has already been collected from this particular test event. (If a specimen was successfully collected immediately before this test event, that previous specimen should go to the lab.) If the collector or technician runs out of space documenting the refusal on the form, he or she can add another sheet of paper for notes. The collector or technician immediately notifies the DER of the refusal and sends the DER the corresponding documentation. Based on this documentation, the DER decides whether to classify the situation as a refusal to test.

A refusal to test is different from a positive result. DOT-covered programs must distinguish between refusals and positives in their summary reports to DOT. Substance abuse professionals need to know if the result was a refusal to test or was positive for a specific drug, so that they can tailor their treatment recommendations accordingly. The Federal Aviation Administration (FAA) permanently bans workers with two positive drug tests from performing the safety-sensitive duties they performed prior to their second test, but does not permanently ban workers who refuse to take tests. A refusal to test, including an adulterated or substituted result, is cause for a permanent bar from working in the nuclear industry, while a positive result is not.

Collection Site Recordkeeping ■

The HHS *Guidelines* require the collector or the collector's employer to store collection site records (e.g., Collector Copy 3 of the CCF) for at least 2 years. DOT requires that the collector should have ready access to the CCF in its original hard copy format for at least 30 days. This helps in responding to MROs, DERs, and employers who often ask for (re)faxing of CCFs. Copies of the CCFs can also help substantiate charges to clients who may question charges for tests they do not recognize.

Collector Errors ■

The laboratory, MRO, or third-party administrator (TPA) may ask the collector to correct an error identified in the chain of custody after it was completed and sent to the laboratory. They will ask for this correction in writing, often by faxing a form to the collector explaining the correctable error and asking the collector to sign a statement acknowledging the error. (See Table 8-1 for a list of correctable flaws.) Once contacted by the laboratory or the MRO, the collector should respond the same or next business day by fax or courier to the request for a corrective statement. Corrections serve to salvage the tests in which the errors are made. There is no option to start the test over—i.e., collect another specimen—to correct an error.

Laboratories keep specimens for at least 5 business days before discarding them. If a fatal error exists in the collection process or the collector does not provide a timely corrective statement, the laboratory will discard the specimen, report "Rejected for Testing" to the MRO, and add a comment explaining why the specimen was not tested. If the collector was at fault, he or she must undergo error correction training as described earlier in this chapter.

After Hours Collections ■

An employer with second- or third-shift operations may need to conduct tests when the usual collection site is closed. Without planning, it is hard to arrange off-hours tests. However, it is also hard to find reliable service providers for off-hours tests. Employers should keep in mind that DOT-mandated urine drug and breath alcohol tests can be conducted up to 32 and 8 hours after an accident or incident. Thus, many off-hours post-accident and reasonable suspicion incidents can be covered—albeit without the desired immediacy—by tests during regular business hours.

Most service providers that offer off-hours testing are in large metropolitan areas and are already open 24 hours, 7 days a week, or have assigned staff to be on call for after-hours testing. Hospital emergency rooms are rarely reliable for conducting after-hours tests. Service providers that specialize in off-hours tests send medical technicians or other trained persons to accident scenes and other designated locations to perform tests.

Urine Collection Procedures for Alcohol Testing ■

Some nonregulated programs test urine alcohol. A proper urine collection for alcohol testing requires a two-step collection procedure, which collects *recently produced* urine for alcohol testing. In a two-step collection, the collector asks the donor to void completely and then discards this urine. This urine is discarded because it was produced over a potentially long period of time and does not necessarily reflect current levels of alcohol in the body. The donor is instructed to wait and drink no alcohol. After 20–30 minutes, the collector obtains a second specimen and sends it to the laboratory. The container should include a preservative such as sodium fluoride to inhibit ethanol production by microorganisms. The alcohol concentration in the second specimen more closely reflects the blood ethanol concentration in the body during the 20–30 minute time period during which fresh urine was produced.

Hair Collection ∎

Hair is best collected from the vertex, or crown, of the scalp. Compared with other areas of the head, the vertex has less variability in hair growth rate. If the person has sparse hair, the collector may cut from two or three separate locations and combine these. If the person is bald or has a very short hair (e.g., less than 1 cm in length), other types of hair (arm hair or axillary hair) can be collected or the collection site can, with the client's permission, collect a specimen other than hair, e.g., urine. Collection of body hair rather than scalp hair has several problems, including:

∎ It is more intrusive.
∎ It can also be difficult to collect enough.
∎ It cannot be aligned nor can it be cut to represent an approximate period of growth.
∎ It is more porous than scalp hair and thus more susceptible to positive results from passive exposure.

The collector should never mix body and head hair during the same collection, because hair from these different sites offers information about use over different periods of time. The possible sites for a body hair collection in order of preference are chest, underarm, leg, facial hair. As a last resort, one may collect pubic hair. Some service agents resist or refuse to collect body hair, especially pubic hair, because of its invasiveness.

Scalp hair is cut using scissors. If the scissors are nondisposable, they should be cleaned in the presence of the donor with an alcohol wipe just before use. The hair should not be collected with an electric razor or other nondisposable cutting instrument that cannot be readily cleaned. Reuse of an unclean cutting instrument can raise concerns about cross-contamination of the specimen with hair from a different donor.

The collector wears gloves to mitigate against allegations of contamination. (Unfortunately, it is difficult to handle hair and the packaging materials with gloves.) If the donor has lice in his or her hair or if the donor has insufficient accessible hair, the collector stops, notifies the employer, and with the employer's permission, collects urine or another specimen.

The collector cuts the donor's hair close to the scalp. If the hair is braided or twisted, it should be undone to help ensure that the hair can be cut close to the scalp and that the collector can see that the hair is real and not from a nylon foundation, from artificial hair, or from someone else's hair woven in. When hair from the skin is pulled slightly, the skin is pulled up slightly, too. When hair from a hairpiece is pulled, the nylon foundation is pulled and should be visible to the collector. A hair clip can be used to gather and flip forward a section of hair, exposing a section underneath, from which the specimen may be cut. The collector collects a bundle of hair about the diameter of a shoelace tip, or enough so that it is approximately 1 cm in length when laid flat across the finger. If the hair is less than 1½-inch long, a wider specimen should be cut.

The cut hair is placed within a small square of aluminum foil folded in a "V" shape, with the root ends extending out approximately ¼ inch from one end of the foil. If there is excess hair length, it should be wrapped around the foil rather than cut. The laboratory, and not the collector, trims long specimens to a 1.5 inch length, which corresponds to approximately 90 days of hair growth and possible drug use. The foil containing the hair is pinched close and placed in a specimen card or envelope. A security seal from the CCF is placed on the bottom of the specimen card. Both the donor and collector initial and date the seal and specimen card. The collector then completes the chain of custody form and places the form and specimen card in a plastic bag. The donor initials the bag. The collector then seals and places the bag in a mailer for transport to the laboratory.

When body hair specimens are collected, a single-use razor is used and the shavings are placed in the foil without trying to align the ends. The collector should write a remark on the CCF identifying the site on the body from which the hair was collected.

A split specimen hair test can, in theory, be performed by subdividing one collection of hair into two approximately equal specimens. This offers a true second opinion about the first lab result, because the second lab analyzes hair from the same collection. In practice, any retest usually involves the prompt submission of a second specimen. It usually takes a week or two after collection for a positive result to be reported to the employer and a retest agreed upon. Because hair grows relatively slowly, the hair collected 1 to 2 weeks later represents approximately the same window of detection as the first hair specimen. As with split specimen testing, the second specimen is submitted for reconfirmation testing to the limit of detection for only the drug/metabolite(s) detected in the first specimens.

Nail Collection ■

The nails are clipped with clean clippers. If the clippers are nondisposable, they should be cleaned in the presence of the donor with an alcohol wipe just before use. The nails should be clean of all polish, dirt, and debris. The collector clips nails from the fingers and/or toes onto a clean paper. The collector should collect about 100 mg of nail, which corresponds to a 2–3 mm clipping from each of ten fingers. The nail clippings are placed in a bag which is sealed and labeled with identifiers that match it to the chain of custody form.

Oral Fluid Collection ■

Most workplace oral fluid testing programs use absorbent pad collection devices, each of which consists of a pad attached to a small plastic stick. Some pads are treated with salt or otherwise designed to stimulate salivation and collect the oral fluid by saturation. The volume of oral fluid collected varies widely depending on device design and other factors. Another method of specimen collection is to have the donor spit into a container. This offers a more reliable way to measure specimen volume. Some collection sites try to stimulate saliva production by asking donors to chew on citric acid crystals, Teflon pieces, or something else. Stimulation of saliva has the unintended consequence of reducing drug concentrations by increasing saliva flow and is thus not recommended.

The collector tells the donor to remove any foreign material (e.g., food, gum, tobacco products, lozenges, etc.) from his or her mouth. The donor may not eat, drink, smoke, or put anything inside his or her mouth during an observed waiting period of about 10 minutes. This waiting period is intended to preclude marijuana-positive results from passive exposure.

In the presence of the collector, the donor opens a sealed oral fluid collection device. The donor places the pad between the lower cheek and gum of his or her mouth and keeps it there for about 3 minutes. The donor then removes it and puts the pad in a small vial with a preservative solution. Oral fluids and/or drugs seep out into this solution and are stabilized until extraction and analysis by the laboratory. The donor may need to snap off the stick, leaving the pad in the vial. The donor caps the vial and the collector places a seal from the CCF over the top of the vial. The donor dates and initials the seal. The collector and donor sign the CCF. The collector ensures that the specimen ID number on the vial is recorded on the CCF prior to placing the vial and CCF copy in a plastic bag for transit to the laboratory.

Split specimens are collected by using two collection devices, both of the same make and model. The specimens can be collected simultaneously or sequentially.

If the donor has a dry mouth, the collector should offer the donor water and wait 10 minutes before trying again. If the problem persists, an alternate specimen should be collected.

Blood Collection ■

Blood collection (venipuncture) is a medical procedure performed by qualified professionals at clinics or other health care facilities. The blood specimen is collected using chain of custody forms and procedures similar to those used for urine collection. A fluoride/oxalate tube should be used if testing for ethanol, cocaine, nitrazapem, or clonazapem, i.e., for most workplace panels. Tubes and containers containing gel separators or soft rubber stoppers are not recommended. For blood alcohol tests, the collector should clean the skin with a non-alcohol cleanser. Ethanol applied on the skin has been reported to produce false-positive results. This does not occur when using isopropanol-containing antiseptics. Nevertheless, it seems reasonable to use a non-alcohol antiseptic to avoid perceptions of contamination. The blood collection site should be remote from any infusion site.

The donor must stay with the specimen tube until it is labeled with a unique, individualized identification number and sealed. Security tape, initialed and dated, is put over the top and sides of the tube. If blood and non-DOT urine specimens are collected at the same encounter, a single CCF form can be used for both specimens. The specimen should be stored in a secure container or refrigerator if left unattended before shipment to the laboratory.

Point-of-Collection Tests ■

Point-of-collection tests (POCTs) are assays for drugs and specimen validity that can be performed at the collection site. POCT devices for drug tests use an immunoassay technology and provide results within minutes. POCT tests are also called on-site tests, quick tests, and rapid tests.

POCT DEVICE

Most POCT devices are designed to test urine, but some are designed to test oral fluid. Almost all of these devices have an "on-board quality control system" that indicates that the device is functioning.

Most POCT devices are disposable plastic "cards," "cassettes," or "cups" of various shapes and sizes. The actual test component is an absorbent strip, impregnated with an antibody-dye complex, specific for the drug or drugs to which the test is designated. The strips are also available as "dipsticks." The results from all of these POCT devices are visually interpreted.

There are also POCT devices that provide instrument-read (digital) results. These devices initially cost more than disposable devices but are reusable.

POCT COLLECTION AND ANALYSIS

The POCT tester collects the specimen using chain of custody procedures. The tester can document the collection on a standard chain of custody form, which captures donor and employer identifiers, donor and tester signatures, and other important items. The donor and tester can sign a log or some other document instead of the chain of custody form, but the tester must then start a form for each specimen that is sent out for laboratory-based testing. If the donor refuses to sign the chain of custody form, the tester indicates this with a comment on the "Remarks" section of the form.

Most POCTs are conducted on urine. The urine is obtained by the usual procedure, except the specimen volume needs to exceed the laboratory's minimum volume requirement. The collector pours that volume (or more) into the specimen bottle and seals it in the donor's presence. The collector uses the remaining urine for the POCT.

POCT devices are also available for screening drugs in oral fluid. These devices use an absorbent pad to obtain the oral fluid specimen. With one of the more common oral fluid POCTs, the pad is pressed against a receptacle on a small tray, and oral fluid is squeezed out and absorbed along a line. The length of color change along that line can be correlated with the analyte concentration. If the oral fluid specimen is completely used in the analysis—typical of some devices—and if the result is non-negative, the collector must obtain a second specimen to send to the laboratory. In some programs, the collector obtains urine instead of oral fluid for the second specimen.

If the result is negative for drugs and is within range for any validity tests that have been performed, the collector discards the specimen(s). If the result is presumed positive for drugs or out of range for any validity tests, the collector sends the specimen(s) to the laboratory for testing. If the test site must keep a specimen overnight, the specimen should be refrigerated. Before separating the CCF and enclosing a copy with the specimens, the collector should print the presumptive result on the chain of custody form, for example, "Positive for [*drug name*], please confirm."

If the POCT is out of range for any validity tests, the collector should promptly conduct a second test using directly observed collection procedures and send specimens from both the first and second collections to the laboratory.

Most urine POCT devices use cutoffs that are similar to the initial cutoffs that federally certified urine drug testing laboratories use. Cutoffs for oral fluid POCT devices are less standardized.

POCT SPECIMEN VALIDITY

Specimen validity can be tested with quick assays on dipsticks or integrated into the POCT device. Specimen validity tests usually include creatinine, specific gravity, nitrite, and pH. Some products include additional validity tests, such as oxidants, pyridine chlorochromate, and glutaraldehyde. POCT test sites should include specimen validity testing lest donors pass their POCT tests by submitting adulterated or substituted specimens that full-service laboratories could have identified.

POCT RESULT REPORTING

Most POCT sites report negative results directly to employers. Figure 6-5 presents an example of a negative POCT report form. It is prechecked "negative" to reinforce the importance of NOT reporting presumptive positives to employers. POCT test sites should report presumptive positive results to employers only if there are overriding safety concerns. For example, under the Nuclear Regulatory Commission rule, the POCT site reports presumptive positives ONLY for cocaine and marijuana and ONLY if there are protections in place to assure quality control of the testing and job security and income for the donor, pending the final outcome (10 *CFR* 26.24). Otherwise, POCTs should not report presumptive positive results and instead let the laboratory complete its analysis and let the MRO determine and report the final result.

Any presumptive positive reports provided to employers should include a disclaimer. The following disclaimer comes from the Food and Drug Administration's Labeling Recommendations for Drugs of Abuse Screening Tests [1]:

> This assay provides only a preliminary result. Clinical considerations and professional judgement should be applied to any drug of abuse test result, particularly in evaluating a preliminary positive result. To obtain a confirmed analytical result, a more specific alternate chemical method is needed. Gas chromatography/mass spectroscopy (GC/MS) is the recommended confirmatory method.

Employers should not take disciplinary action based on POCT positive results. Some POCT results are false-positive because of cross-reactivity. Some POCT results represent legitimately prescribed medications or over-the-counter medications. This latter concern is not correctable by MRO review because most good MROs will refuse to review non-confirmed, POCT-positive results.

An employer may infer that the screening result was presumptive positive when the employer does not receive a prompt negative result from the POCT site. While this same problem exists to a lesser extent in laboratory-based testing, it is magnified in POCT testing where employers expect same-day results rather than waiting several days. Some POCT sites report all results to MROs or TPAs. With this routing, the employer gets all negative results from a single source, the MRO or TPA. This conceals from employers those results that are non-negative by POCT but negative by laboratory analysis. This routing also gives the MRO or TPA an opportunity to check the paperwork for all POCT tests.

POCT RECORDKEEPING

The POCT test site should keep confidential and secure records of its tests for at least 1 year. This parallels DOT's 1-year requirement for MROs to keep negative test records. The POCT test records can prove important if clients question invoices or if test results are later challenged. If the POCT test site does not send non-negative specimens to a laboratory for further testing, the POCT test site

Figure 6-5. On-Site Test Report ■

Urine Drug Test Report Form for Negative POCT Results

Occupational Health Services
100 Main Street
Springfield, TX
800-123-4567 ph; 800-123-7890 fax

Employee's name: _____   SSN or Emp. ID: _____

Employer's name: _____   Specimen ID number: _____

Reason for test: ❑ Pre-employment   ❑ Random   ❑ Post-accident
❑ Return to duty   ❑ Periodic   ❑ Reasonable suspicion   ❑ Follow-up

Collection date: ___/___/___ Time:

Test kit lot no.: _____ Exp date: ___/___/___

On-site Validity Test Results:

Temp (°F)	Creat.	Nitrite	Glutarald.	pH	Spec Grav.	Bleach	Pyridium Chloro.
❑ <90 *or* >100	❑ 0–10	❑ ≥50	❑ brown	❑ <4 *or* >11	❑ <1.005 *or* >1.020	❑ aqua/green	❑ aqua/grey
❑ 90–100	❑ 20–100	❑ 0–10	❑ light beige	❑ 4–10	❑ 1.005–1.015	❑ white	❑ white

Note to collector: If any of the validity test results fall within the grey zone on this form, send the urine specimen to the laboratory. Otherwise, discard the urine and send this report to the designated employer representative.

Result: ☑ Negative   Tested for: 1. Amphetamines (amphetamine, methamphetamine)
2. Cocaine metabolite
3. Marijuana metabolite
4. Opiates (codeine, morphine, 6-AM)
5. Phencyclidine
... and the validity tests listed above.

(If the result is positive, adulterated, substituted, or invalid, write the presumptive result on the chain of custody and send the specimen to the laboratory for further analysis. Do not report a non-negative screening result to the employer.)

Collector's name: _____

Collector's signature: _____

To: _____
Secure fax no.: _____
Initials: _____ Date: _____

If this transmission is incomplete or illegible, please call us at 123-456-7890. This communication is of a confidential nature. If it has been misdirected to you, or if this fax machine is not in a secure access area, please call us immediately.

should keep records of non-negative results for at least 5 years. This also parallels DOT recordkeeping requirements for non-negative results.

POCT PERFORMANCE TESTING

The more diligent POCT sites monitor their own accuracy by performance testing (PT). The POCT site tests specimen of known type—negative, positive, abnormal validity—on a periodic (e.g., monthly or quarterly) basis and compares actual results against expected results. Sets of performance testing samples should contain the drugs and drug metabolites tested for in the donor specimens and also should contain samples with no drugs or metabolites, i.e., true negatives. Corrective action should be taken when results from any PT samples significantly differ from the expected results. As an extra precaution, some POCT sites test a positive PT sample for the identified drug (or an out-of-range QC sample for the validity test) immediately after any abnormal POCT result. Finally, a fraction of real specimens—for example, one of every 20 real specimens—that test negative should be submitted to a forensic urine drug testing laboratory for purposes of quality control.

POCT ACCURACY

POCT immunoassays should, in theory, be about as sensitive and specific as laboratory-based immunoassays. Process differences may, however, reduce the accuracy of POCT tests, thus increasing the rates of false-negative and false-positive results. Some process differences include:

1. POCTs are usually performed in clinics by technicians who have many other responsibilities and varying degrees of training. Laboratory screens are performed by sophisticated, automated devices run by analysts who only perform drug tests.
2. POCTs are interpreted by change in color or other appearance, i.e., subjectively. By contrast, laboratory screens are interpreted by instruments, i.e., objectively. Potential problems with POCT interpretation include:
   a. A POCT technician might be inclined to call a borderline result "negative," especially if the technician feels pressured by the donor, by time, or by not having enough specimen to send to the laboratory for confirmation testing.
   b. A POCT technician may have poor color vision that interferes with reading the results.
   c. Results from some POCT devices are counterintuitive, e.g., the absence of color means "positive."
3. Few clinics monitor the accuracy of their POCTs. By contrast, laboratories are subject to multiple quality control monitors. There are extensive checks and balances for laboratory-based testing but few, if any, for POCT tests.
4. Laboratories have extensive capabilities to test for substitution and adulteration. Some POCT sites do "dipstick" validity tests. These cover a relatively limited set of parameters, are subject to bias or subjectivity (see the second bullet of this list), and are subject to analytical error caused by reagent bleeding between pads and mistiming of the readings.

Many oral fluid POCTs do not claim, and cannot reach, the low cutoffs that laboratories use for screening oral fluid. Many oral fluid POCT devices are targeted at the delta-9-tetrahydrocannabinol (THC) metabolite (THCA), which is not present at significant concentrations in oral fluid. Reliable detection of marijuana use requires that the POCT oral fluid device be targeted at the parent drug THC. False negative results are relatively prevalent and of particular concern for POCT tests in comparison to laboratory-based tests.

POCT tests are less analytically specific than laboratory-based tests that include confirmation. In other words, immunoassays can produce false-positive results. This is particularly so for the opiates, amphetamines, phencyclidine, barbiturates, and benzodiazepines, as illustrated in Table 8-6. Because POCT tests are liable to false-positive results, each POCT-positive result should be sent to a laboratory for confirmation testing. Confirmation testing does not produce false-positive results.

WHEN TO CONDUCT POCTS

The rapid turnaround in getting negative results is an advantage in pre-employment, reasonable suspicion, and post-accident settings, where employers want quick negative results so that they can quickly put people to work. The ability to test on-site is an advantage in situations where specimens cannot be promptly shipped to laboratories, e.g., on boats and overseas. POCTs are used in many non-workplace settings, including emergency rooms and many criminal justice and drug treatment settings.

The NRC rule is strongly focused on "fitness for duty" and allows POCT testing. The HHS and DOT rules are more focused on deterrence and place less emphasis on the immediacy of results. Thus, neither HHS nor DOT authorize use of POCTs, except that DOT allows use of a few oral fluid POCT tests for alcohol screening tests. The allowed devices appear on the conforming products list published periodically by the National Highway Traffic Safety Administration. Some states have drug testing laws that address POCTs. Those state laws that allow their use generally do so contingent on laboratory-based confirmatory testing of POCT positive results.

Some service agents encourage employers to use POCT tests by promoting the immediacy of results. If an employer is asked, "Do you want your results immediately or in 2 days?," the employer will no doubt respond "immediately." If the employer was instead asked, "Do you want your tests very sensitive or less sensitive?," the employer would no doubt respond "very sensitive." Employers should understand that use of POCT is a tradeoff between immediacy of results and sensitivity at detection.

Reference ■

1. Center for Devices and Radiological Health. Premarket Submission and Labeling Recommendations for Drugs of Abuse Screening Tests; Draft Guidance. Rockville, MD: Food and Drug Administration. December 2, 2003.

Adulterants, Substitution Dilution ■

Many products and techniques have been developed to avoid testing positive on urine drug tests. These products and techniques target drug tests of urine, as opposed to tests of other specimens, because urine specimens are collected in privacy (with limited exceptions) and because drug tests are most commonly performed on urine. This chapter primarily addresses tampering with urine specimens. The following sections describe adulteration and substitution of urine drug test specimens. This chapter also discusses dilute urine specimens, which may result from overhydration by the donor in an attempt to reduce drug/metabolite concentrations.

Adulterants ■

An *adulterant* is a substance that is added to a specimen and is not normally found in that type of specimen or at that high a concentration. Around 1990, one of the first commercially marketed chemical adulterants, Urine Luck (containing glutaraldehyde), appeared on the market. After laboratories started testing specimens for glutaraldehyde, nitrite adulterants appeared on the market. Since then, other urine additive products have been introduced. Most adulterants are purchased over the Internet with next-day delivery options and are packaged in small, easily concealed containers.

ACIDS AND BASES

Extremes in pH can interfere with the drug assays. Several commercially available adulterants contain hydrochloric acid, which lowers pH. Adulteration with bleach or other bases can increase pH.

OXIDANTS

An *oxidizing adulterant* is a substance that acts alone or in combination with other substances to react with and change reagents or drugs/metabolites to prevent their detection. Oxidizing adulterants are most effective in destroying THC metabolites, have some effect on morphine, and have little or no effect on other analytes. Examples of oxidizing adulterants include nitrite, pyridinium chlorochromate, chromate (VI), bleach, halogens, and peroxide. Some agents work longer than others. Some adulterants are only active for a day or two. Peroxidase is an adulterant that dissipates without a trace within hours or days after it has been added to urine. Some adulterant products contain several oxidizing agents.

The following sections describe oxidizing adulterants that are used in urine. While formulations are accurately presented for the time at which this book was written, producers of adulterants often change them as laboratories improve at identifying existing products.

Nitrite

Nitrite is an oxidizing agent that has been identified in Clean X, Clear Choice Instant Clean, Whizzies, and Urine Luck 6.4. Laboratories identify nitrite by a nitrite-specific or general colorimetric test for the initial test on the first aliquot, and a different confirmatory test (e.g., multi-wavelength spectrophotometry, ion chromatography, capillary electrophoresis) on the second aliquot.

Nitrite may be present in urine from a variety of sources, as listed in Table 7-1. Urinary tract infections can cause nitrite in urine, but at a concentration no higher than 150 µg/mL. Use of certain medications—e.g., nitroglycerine, isosorbide dinitrate, nitroprusside, and ranitidine—can lead to nitrite in urine, but at concentrations no higher than 25 µg/mL. The estimated maximum that can arise from all sources (other than adulteration) combined is approximately 300 µg/mL. This is lower than the 500 µg/mL cutoff that laboratories use to define a nitrite-adulterated specimen and much lower than the several thousand ng/mL typically found in nitrite-adulterated specimens. HHS has defined any nitrite concentration at or above 500 µg/mL as *adulterated*. HHS has defined any nitrite concentration of 200–499 µg/mL as *invalid* because this result is suspicious but not proof of adulteration.

Table 7-1. Urine Nitrite Sources and Approximate Peak Achievable Concentrations* ■

Source	Approximate Nitrite Concentration (µg/mL)
Internal sources	
Urinary tract infection	150
Pathological conditions	100
Normal biochemistry	trace
External sources	
Medications	25
All other natural sources	
Food, water, air, occupational exposure, induction by medications	<25
Adulteration after voiding	1,900–15,000

*Not including poisoning.

Source: Urry F, Komaromy-Hiller G, Staley B, et al. Nitrite adulteration of workplace urine drug-testing specimens: I. Sources and associated concentrations of nitrite in urine and distinction between natural sources and adulteration. J Anal Toxicol, 1998;22:89–95.

Nitrite (NO_2) and nitrate (NO_3) are different substances. Like nitrite, nitrate can be normally found in urine. Its presence does not interfere with drug assays.

Chromium (VI)

Chromium (VI) is a strong oxidizing agent and is found in several adulterants. Chromium (VI) is the active agent in Pyridium chlorochromate, a compound that has been found in the adulterants LL418, Randy's Clear II, Sweet Pea Spoiler, and older formulations of Urine Luck. HHS has defined any chromium (VI) concentration at or above 50 µg/mL as *adulterated*. Certain manufacturing workers may be potentially exposed to chromium (VI). However, even if they absorb chromium (VI) from their workplace, it is reduced in their bodies to chromium (III) and is *not* identified as chromium (VI) in their urine.

Halogens

Certain halogenated compounds (e.g., periodate) will cause a positive initial test for general oxidants. Iodine is a halogen that is sometimes used to adulterate specimens. When iodine has been added to urine, the urine is red-brown in color and has a medicinal smell. Normal dietary iodine (I_2) is excreted as iodide (I^-), with an average urinary concentration of 0.16 µg/mL [1]. Adulteration of a specimen with iodine would be expected to produce concentrations of iodide above 100 µg/mL, which are inconsistent with dietary or medicinal iodine intake.

Urine Luck 6.5 contains a mixture of iodate (IO_3, an oxidizing agent) and hydrofluoric acid. Low concentrations of iodate can also be found in unadulterated urine through dietary intake.

Peroxidase, Hydrogen Peroxide

A combination of hydrogen peroxide and the enzyme horseradish peroxidase is available as a product known as Stealth. Peroxide is an oxidizing agent. Peroxidase catalyzes the reaction. The reaction is complete within a few hours, after which peroxidase cannot be detected. Normal urine has no peroxidase activity, but urine contaminated with blood or certain bacteria shows some pseudoperoxidase activity [2].

Surfactant

Surfactants, including ordinary detergents, have been used to adulterate urine specimens. Mary Jane SuperClean 13, a product sold in past years, was similar to Joy lemon-scented dish-washing detergent. Whizzer is an adulterant with a selenium-containing surfactant. When added to urine, surfactant can cause an apparent decrease in concentrations (especially of marijuana metabolites) when tested by immunoassay, especially by EIA. The lyphophilic nature of the marijuana metabolites may cause these compounds to migrate inside of the "bubbles" (micelles) formed within the fluid by surfactants and prevent them from reacting with water-soluble antibodies. A methylene blue procedure can be used to identify and quantitate anionic surfactants. The presence of surfactant is established by surfactant test results greater than or equal to 100 µg/mL dodecylbenzene sulfonate-equivalent concentration. The surfactant test is performed twice, using different assays and on different aliquots. Both results must be greater than or equal to 100 µg/mL to confirm the presence of surfactant adulterant.

Glutaraldehyde

Glutaraldehyde is a clear, colorless liquid contained in the adulterant product D9D. Glutaraldehyde smells like rotten apples. It is used as a sterilizing agent in some hospitals and clinics, as a tanning agent for leather, and as an embalming fluid. A 10% solution can also be purchased over the counter for treating warts. Glutaraldehyde causes unusual readings in the EIA and KIMS immunoassays, for example, negative absorbance changes in the enzyme assays. Glutaraldehyde is never found in unadulterated urine. Any detectable concentration of glutaraldehyde in urine is evidence of adulteration.

Visine

Addition of Visine eyedrops to urine samples can cause false-negative results for THC. Chemical analysis of Visine eyedrops has shown that the ingredients benzalkonium chloride and borate buffer can interfere with the immunoassay test. However, 9-carboxy-THC can still be detected by GC-MS.

Salt

Salt (NaCl) is a normal constituent of urine. When added as an adulterant, it is found at very high concentrations. High concentrations of salt can cause a decrease in the apparent concentrations of several drugs when tested by immunoassay, particularly EIA [3].

Substitution ■

Substitution refers to the donor's submission of a specimen that the donor did not produce. It may be urine from someone else or a non-biological specimen, e.g., apple juice. There are anecdotal reports in sports testing of self-catheterization with drug-free urine to escape detection during an observed collection.

Dilution ■

Dilution of a specimen lowers the concentration of drugs and metabolites. A urine specimen can be diluted by drinking excessive fluids before the collection or by adding fluids to the specimen at the time of collection. More extreme measures include the use of diuretics to dilute urine specimens. Diuretics are tested for in sports drug testing for this reason, but not in workplace drug testing.

WATER LOADING

Some people drink a great deal of liquid before their tests to dilute their urine, thereby lowering any concentrations of drugs or metabolites. This technique, known as water loading, can succeed if the concentration(s) are already close to the cutoffs. It can lower a urine concentration from just above the cutoff to just below the cutoff. Use of diuretics, especially fast-acting prescription diuretics, can likewise reduce drug concentrations below cutoff concentrations. Although the collection site can limit how much water it offers to the donor, it cannot limit water consumption before arrival. This is why employers should, when possible, minimize the advance notice given to donors about their urine drug test appointments.

Pills and Potions ■

Some products that are sold to beat drug tests are meant to be consumed with large volumes of water. Some of these products contain vitamin B_2 or vitamin B complex to make the urine darker yellow. These products are effective only to the extent that they are consumed with large volumes of fluid, thereby diluting the urine. The ingredients of these products are ineffective at destroying or masking drugs or metabolites. Ingestion of large volumes of acidic fluids—for example vitamin C, vinegar, and some fruit juices—may lead to acidification of urine and enhanced excretion of basic drugs, for example, amphetamines and phencyclidine. An urban myth purports that consumption of large quantities of niacin can thwart drug tests, but this actually can just make the user sick [4].

Oral Fluid Test Subversion ■

Several products are marketed for evading detection by oral fluid drug tests. They act by rinsing drug residues from the oral cavity. They do not directly destroy the drugs or interfere with the assays by changing the oral fluid pH.

References ■

1. Hollowell JE, Staehling N, Hannon W, et al. Iodine nutrition in the United States. Trends and public health implications: iodine excretion data from National Health and Nutrition Examination Surveys I and III (1971–74 and 1988–94). *J Clin Endocrinol Metab*, 1998;83:3401–08.
2. Valtier S, Cody JT. Characterization of the effects of stealth adulterant on drugs-of-abuse testing. *J Anal Toxicol* 2001;25:369.
3. Kim H, Cerceo E. Interference by NaCl with the EMIT method of analysis for drugs of abuse. *Clin Chem* 1976;22:1935–36.
4. Mittal M, Florin T, Perrone J, et al. Toxicity from the use of niacin to beat urine drug screening. *Ann Emergency Med* 2007;50:587–90.

Laboratory Analysis ■

A forensic urine drug-testing laboratory must reliably and in a legally defensible manner test specimen validity and distinguish specimens that contain drugs or drug metabolites at or above the cutoff values from those that do not. In regulated drug testing, certified laboratories screen specimens and subject specimens that screen positive to confirmation testing. Screening and confirmation analyses are performed on different aliquots from the specimen. Each confirmation analysis is performed using a definitive technique that is specific for the drug or metabolite and, when properly performed, produces no false-positive results. In addition, a portion split from the original specimen at the time of collection may be analyzed by a second certified laboratory to corroborate the results from the first laboratory. These provisions, together with the use of chain of custody procedures, quality control procedures, and medical review of non-negative results assure that results are accurate.

Laboratory Certification ■

Regulated programs and many nonregulated programs use laboratories that are certified by the U.S. Department of Health and Human Services (HHS) National Laboratory Certification Program (NLCP). HHS certification applies only to laboratories in the United States. Because the U.S. Department of Transportation (DOT) rule also covers certain testing in Canada and Mexico, DOT has authorized use of laboratories certified by Canadian and Mexican organizations that are formally recognized by HHS as having equivalent laboratory certification standards. This recognition has been granted to a few Canadian laboratories but, to date, no Mexican laboratories.

HHS's certification authority is limited to Drug Enforcement Administration (DEA) Schedule I and II drugs. A laboratory becomes and remains HHS certified by satisfactory performance in quarterly proficiency testing and by passing site audits every 6 months. Site audits take 2–3 days and are conducted by two to eight HHS-trained inspectors, depending on the laboratory's size. A list of HHS-certified laboratories is published in the *Federal Register* during the first week of each month. The list is also directly available from the Substance Abuse and Mental Health Services Administration (SAMHSA), a division of HHS (see Appendix A). As of 2009, about 40 laboratories were HHS certified. Two large corporations,

Laboratory Corporation of America and Quest Diagnostics, each own several laboratories that are individually certified.

Most workplace testing is nonregulated, and much of this includes drugs or cutoffs that differ from the HHS panel. Laboratories that are HHS certified can conduct nonregulated tests but do so in operations that are maintained somewhat separate from the certified laboratory operations. Laboratories that are not HHS certified only conduct nonregulated testing. Employers with nonregulated programs should insist on a two-step laboratory analysis—screening followed by confirmation testing—because it is accurate and is the best practice.

The College of American Pathologists Forensic Drug Testing Accreditation Program (CAP-FDT) accredits forensic drug testing laboratories that conform to its standards [1]. Most HHS-certified labs are also CAP-FDT accredited. A few states have their own licensure processes for workplace drug testing laboratories.

Initial Instrumented Test Facility ■

In 2010, HHS planned to implement a certification program for screen-only laboratories that are physically separated from "confirmation" laboratories. HHS calls this type of laboratory an initial instrumented test facility (IITF). An IITF conducts accessioning, initial screening, and validity tests, but does not conduct confirmatory tests. The IITF reports results for specimens that are negative, negative-dilute with creatinine levels between 5 and 20 mg/dL, or rejected for testing directly to the MRO. The IITF sends all other specimens to a full-service laboratory where they are processed like other specimens. IITFs are intended to offload negative specimens from full-service laboratories and shorten turnaround time for negative results.

Accessioning ■

Accessioning is the laboratory's process for receipt, inspection, and labeling of specimens before analysis (see Figure 8-1). The accessioner:

- Inspects the specimen's outer plastic pack for leakage and signs of tampering.
- May (but is not required to) sign the external chain of custody that arrived with the specimen.
- Starts an internal chain of custody form to track the specimen within the laboratory.
- Removes the specimen(s) and CCF from the plastic pack and inspects them for sufficient volume and to verify that numbers on the specimen(s) match those on the CCF.
- Inspects the CCF to ensure the correct form was used, the specimen's temperature range has been recorded, and all necessary collector information and signatures have been entered.

These steps of accessioning are designed to identify significant flaws in the paperwork and packaging. The HHS *Guidelines* and Part 40 distinguish between flaws that are fatal versus correctable versus insignificant. While the federal regulations categorize some of the most common flaws, most laboratories have developed their own acceptance criteria, based on the federal rules and expanded with additional flaws and clarification. Table 8-1 presents flaws that laboratories and MROs

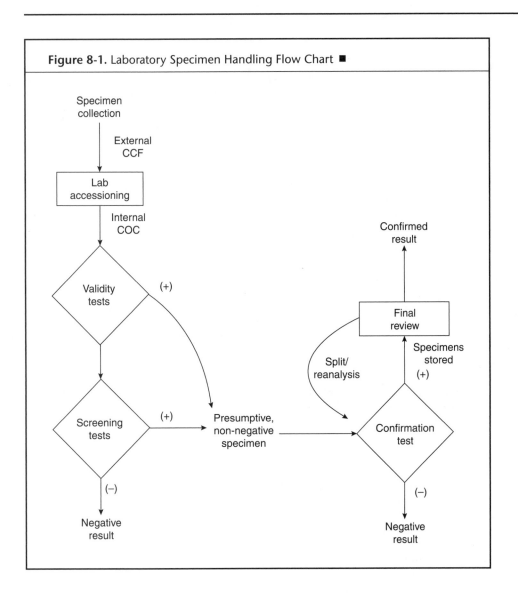

Figure 8-1. Laboratory Specimen Handling Flow Chart ■

may identify in urine tests, and lists the phrases that laboratories use on the "Remarks" section of the CCF to explain why specimens are rejected for testing.

FATAL FLAWS

Fatal flaws cannot be corrected and require rejection of the specimen for testing. For example, if the specimen arrives at the laboratory without a chain of custody form, this is a fatal flaw and the laboratory rejects the specimen for testing.

CORRECTABLE FLAWS

Correctable flaws are fatal if left uncorrected. For example, if the collector prints his or her name on the CCF but neglects to sign it, he or she can later correct this by providing a signed statement acknowledging the omission and indicating steps

Table 8-1. Urine Drug Test Flaws ■

Fatal Flaws	Lab Comment on CCF
1. Specimen ID number on the CCF and bottle label/seal do not match, or the number is missing or illegible on either the CCF or the specimen bottle/seal	Specimen ID number mismatch/missing
2. Collector's signature and printed name are omitted on the CCF	No printed name of collector and no signature
3. Specimen bottle label/seal is missing or broken on the primary specimen (Bottle A) unless the split (Bottle B) can be re-designated as the primary specimen.[a]	Tamper-evident seal broken
4. Insufficient volume for testing of the primary specimen (Bottle A) unless the split (Bottle B) can be re-designated as the primary specimen.[a]	Insufficient specimen volume
5. Specimen unaccompanied by CCF	
6. Specimens spilled at laboratory	

Correctable Flaws	Lab Comment on CCF (if unrecovered flaw)

— The laboratory may identify flaws 1–4

1. Collector's printed name is present, but collector failed to sign the certification statement on the CCF.	Collector signature not recovered
2. Use of a non-federal form or an expired version of the federal CCF for a federally regulated test.	Wrong CCF used
3. Testing for more than the federal five-drug panel, provided that the collection and testing procedures for the federal five-panel drugs and metabolites is otherwise consistent with federal requirements. The collector should provide a statement acknowledging use of the wrong form but stating that the collection otherwise followed federal procedures. The laboratory should also provide a statement that the federal cutoffs were used for the five-drug panel and that the federal requirements for internal and external controls and other procedural requirements were met.	
4. Temperature block not checked on CCF and no explanatory remark. (Corrective statement is sought from the collector; but if no corrective statement obtained, result may be reported after 5 days.)	

— The MRO may identify flaws listed here and some listed previously

5. No accessioner's signature on the CCF.
6. Donor's signature is missing and no comment provided on the "Remarks" line indicating that the donor refused to sign the CCF.
7. No certifying scientist's signature is on the CCF.

Table 8-1. continued ■

Insignificant Flaws

– The laboratory may identify flaws 1–15. –

1. Nothing checked in "Specimen collection" box, i.e., "Split, Single, or None Provided."
2. Observed box is not marked (if applicable).
3. Time and/or date of collection is not indicated.
4. Incorrect or incomplete name, address, or phone or fax number of the collector, laboratory, MRO, and/or employer on the CCF.
5. Wrong or no "Reason to Test" checked on the CCF.
6. "Drug tests to be performed" box not marked.
7. Courier's specific name is omited or incorrectly entered.
8. A minor printed mistake by the collector, for example, the omission of the donor's middle initial, a transposition of numbers in the donor's social security number, entering the wrong date by mistake, or a misspelled word on the CCF.
9. Collector changed or corrected information by crossing out the original information on either the CCF or specimen label/seal without dating and initialing the change.
10. Collector's signature is present but collector's printed name is missing.
11. Failure of the donor to put his/her initials on the tamper-evident bottle seals.
12. Donor name included on the laboratory copy of the CCF or on the tamper-evidence labels used to seal the specimens.
13. Entry of donor's medication information on CCF copy other than the back of Copy 5.
14. Use of collection materials that do not conform with federal standards.
15. Broken seal on the outer shipping container.

– The MRO may identify flaws listed here and some listed previously –

16. Claims that the donor was improperly selected for testing.
17. A minor data entry error by the lab, for example, a transposition of numbers on the printed laboratory result.
18. The accessioner fails to print his or her name.
19. The certifying scientist or certifying technician accidentally initials the CCF rather than signing for a specimen reported as rejected for testing.
20. The accessioner fails to mark one of the "primary (Bottle A) specimen bottle seal intact" boxes, but the laboratory reported a "rejected for testing" result with an appropriate comment on the "Remarks" line.
21. Donor's failure to sign a consent form, waiver, or release form or other form other than the CCF.
22. Use of a chain of custody form preprinted with the wrong account data.
23. Delay in the collection process.
24. Collection of a specimen by a collector who has not completed the required training.
25. Failure to directly observe or monitor a collection when warranted or the unauthorized use of direct observation or monitoring when unwarranted.
26. Review of the result by a physician who has the basic credentials to be qualified as an MRO but who has not met training and/or documentation requirements.
27. Any other procedural flaw during collection that does not undermine donor protections, for example, the collector's failure to add bluing agent to the toilet bowl or the employee's flushing of the toilet after providing the specimen.

[a]If no split was collected, this remains a fatal flaw and the test is cancelled.
Laboratory flaws that the MRO may identify.

that he or she will take to avoid repeating this flaw. Without correction, the laboratory will reject the specimen for testing.

Laboratories identify most correctable flaws during accesssioning. Three types of correctable flaws—missing signatures from laboratory certifying scientists, accessioners, and donors—are identifiable only by the MRO, and thus are the MRO's responsibility to identify and seek correction. For collection-site flaws, the laboratory faxes a fill-in-the-blank corrective statement to the collector. This form has the laboratory's logo and demographic information and a statement like that in Figure 8-2. The federal rules call this form a *memorandum for record*. Some service agents call it an *affidavit*, although this term can mislead people into thinking it must be notarized or otherwise certified by third parties when in fact this is not required. The collector completes the form, faxes it to the laboratory, and keeps it with the CCF. The collector should correct flaws on the same business day on which he or she is notified. If the collector who made the flaw is unavailable

---

Figure 8-2. Example of Memorandum to Correct/Recover Flaw ■

<Use an appropriate letterhead>

Date: <date>

From: <collector's printed name>

To: Drug Testing Laboratory   Medical Review Officer
          1234 Main Street   or   5678 Central Street
          City, State, Zip Code   City, State, Zip Code

Subject: Memorandum to Recover Missing Information (or insert an appropriate
          phrase that describes the issue)

Re: <specimen ID number>
          <donor SSN or other ID number>

On <collection date>, I served as the collector for the above specimen. While completing the custody and control form, I forgot to <appropriate phrase that describes the omission, e.g., mark the box in Step 2 on the CCF to indicate that the specimen temperature was within the acceptable range>. I have reviewed the collection procedure and am certain that I followed all other parts of the procedure <e.g., I looked at the temperature strip on the collection container/specimen bottle> as required.

To ensure that this omission will not happen again, I am planning in future tests to review the entire CCF before I separate the copies and seal the specimen bottle(s) and CCF in the plastic bag.

_____
Collector's Signature

cc: <medical review officer or drug testing laboratory>

to sign the corrective statement, the collector's supervisor can sign it if the flaw is use of a non-DOT CCF for a DOT test or the flaw is missing a collector's signature but the collector's name *was* printed.

The laboratory waits for at least five business days from the date of asking for a corrective statement. If a corrective statement is received within five business days, the laboratory sends the drug test result and a copy of the corrective statement to the MRO. If no corrective statement is received, the laboratory discards the specimen, reports "Rejected" to the MRO, and informs the MRO why the specimen was rejected. The MRO does not have to inform the employer about flaws that have been satisfactorily corrected. However, if a correctable flaw remains uncorrected, the MRO reports the result as "Test Cancelled."

A failure to collect a required split specimen is a flaw that the laboratory does not try to identify. Instead, the laboratory analyzes the single specimen. If the result is verified positive by the MRO *and* the donor asks for the split analysis, the MRO would ask the laboratory for the split analysis, would learn that no split is available, and would cancel the test.

INSIGNIFICANT FLAWS

The third set of flaws in Table 8-1 refers to flaws that are considered insignificant because they do not detract from the test's validity and do not undermine the donor's rights. If a laboratory or MRO observes frequent (e.g., more than once a month) insignificant flaws by a particular collector, it should notify the collector or collector's supervisor who should then take appropriate corrective action, e.g., focused retraining. It should also be noted that an out-of-range temperature is not a specimen flaw. That is, the laboratory does not reject a specimen based on an out-of-range temperature indication.

ALIQUOTING

If the specimen's packaging and documentation meet the acceptance criteria, the laboratory transfers an aliquot into a labeled vial and starts an internal chain of custody document for tracking the aliquot through screening and validity tests. An *aliquot* is a fractional part of a specimen used for testing. Most laboratories process specimens as batches (groups) of aliquots. The number of aliquots in a batch depends on the laboratory's size and workload. Each batch includes internal quality control samples, constituting at least 10% of the total number of specimens in the batch. Each aliquot undergoes initial drug and validity tests. Many laboratories use automated samplers that draw off small volumes as each aliquot is individually conveyed. The sampling device draws in water between aliquots; this rinse is designed to avoid carryover contamination between aliquots.

When split (paired) specimens have been submitted, Bottles A and B are kept together during testing at most laboratories. Bottle A is tested, and Bottle B is kept unopened. If the Bottle A result is negative, the laboratory discards both Bottles A and B.

Specimen Validity Testing ■

Validity tests are analyses intended to determine if adulterants were added to the specimen, if the specimen was substituted, or if the specimen is diluted. Not every attempt to adulterate or substitute a specimen will be detected when the specimen is collected. This is particularly true for urine collected without direct observation. The validity of hair, oral fluid, and certain other alternative specimens is assured primarily by the directly observed collection procedure. Nevertheless, laboratories sometimes receive specimens that, although reputedly collected under direct observation, are not real. Regulated urine testing laboratories check validity by specimen appearance and by tests of creatinine, specific gravity, pH, and oxidizing adulterants. Laboratories vary in their practices with regard to checking validity of nonurine specimens. The following sections describe specimen validity testing in urine, oral fluid, and hair.

URINE VALIDITY TESTING

In regulated testing, laboratories test specimens for:

1. creatinine and specific gravity
2. pH
3. oxidizing adulterants

A laboratory may perform additional specimen validity tests, but few do. The following sections give brief descriptions of the tests just listed.

Creatinine and Specific Gravity
The laboratory measures the creatinine concentration of each specimen and, for specimens with creatinine less than 20 mg/dL, specific gravity. If the results are out of range, the laboratory performs confirmatory tests for creatinine and specific gravity on a separate aliquot from the specimen.

pH
The laboratory measures pH using either a colorimetric pH test or pH meter for the initial test. If the initial pH measurement is too low or too high, the laboratory performs a confirmatory pH test using a pH meter on a separate aliquot from the specimen.

Oxidizing Adulterants
The laboratory screens the specimen for general oxidizing agents by using a colorimetric test with a greater than or equal to 200 µg/mL nitrite-equivalent cutoff, a greater than or equal to 50 µg/mL chromium (VI)-equivalent cutoff, or a halogen concentration greater than or equal to the limit of detection. For a laboratory to report that a specimen contains an oxidizing adulterant, it must confirm the identity of the adulterant by a test specific for that adulterant.

Identifying an unknown adulterant can be difficult. There are many possible adulterants and the array of adulterants in use is constantly shifting. In recent years, an increasing proportion of adulterant products have contained mixtures of nitrite, chromium, and other oxidants. These mixtures cause invalid results without necessarily raising the concentration of any one component high enough to meet adulteration criteria. Some laboratories have faced costly litigation associated with specimens they reported as adulterated. Now, few laboratories routinely test for specific adulterants. Instead, if the general oxidizing agents screen is positive, the laboratory typically does not test for specific adulterants and thus reports the result as invalid.

HHS allows a certified laboratory to run specific adulterant tests in-house or send an aliquot of the specimen to another certified laboratory for adulterant testing. Many HHS-certified laboratories can detect nitrite and chromate and have limited testing capabilities for detecting other oxidizing agents. As previously noted, most laboratories do not routinely test for specific adulterants and instead perform just the required specimen validity tests—creatinine, specific gravity, and pH.

HAIR VALIDITY TESTING

Some, but not all, hair testing laboratories test the specimens for validity. Hair validity tests may include:

- Observing the sheen, texture, or color of the specimen, and noting unnatural findings.
- Movement test: Real hair with intact cuticles (overlapping scales pointed toward the distal end), when rubbed between the thumb and forefinger, will move toward the root end. If the fibers do not move, they are probably not real hair. Cuticles can also be observed microscopically in real hair but not synthetic fibers.
- Chemical tests: Artificial hair does not dissolve in potassium hydroxide but does soften in methylene dichloride and some other solvents. Real hair responds in an opposite manner.

Real hair, if used in a hair piece, often has a plastic coating that can be identified using the aforementioned techniques.

ORAL FLUID VALIDITY TESTING

Laboratories can verify that oral fluid specimens came from humans by measuring human immunoglobulin (IgG). The concentration of IgG in physiologic oral fluid is, on average, 12 µg/mL and ranges from 1.8–48 µg/mL. Any cutoff used to identify an oral fluid specimen as substituted must be much lower. There is as yet no consensus on the appropriate cutoff for IgG, or even whether this is the best approach to test validity of oral fluid specimens. As with urine specimens, laboratories may declare oral fluid specimens invalid if they have unusual physical attributes or give abnormal screening results, or if there is inadequate recovery of the internal standard during confirmation.

Drugs and Cutoff Values ■

The HHS *Guidelines* establish a standard panel of drugs and cutoffs presented in Table 8-2. This panel covers five drugs or categories of drugs: marijuana, cocaine, phencyclidine, amphetamines, and opiates. DOT limits testing to this panel. The HHS *Guidelines* authorize tests with this panel and, in post-accident and

Table 8-2. Urine: Federal Drug Testing Cutoff Concentrations (ng/mL)[1] ∎

Drug or Metabolite	Initial Test	Confirmation Test
Marijuana metabolites	50	
THCA[2]		15
Cocaine metabolites	150	
Benzoylecgonine		100
Phencyclidine (PCP)	25	25
Amphetamines		
Amphetamine/Methamphetamine[3]	500	
Amphetamine		250
Methamphetamine[4]		250
MDMA[5]	500	
MDMA		250
MDA[6]		250
MDEA[7]		250
Opiate metabolites		
Codeine/Morphine[8]	2000	
Codeine		2000
Morphine		2000
6-Acetylmorphine (6-AM)	10	10

[1]This panel was supposed to take effect May 1, 2010. Prior to then, the federal panel did not include MDMA, MDA, or MDEA; had higher cutoffs for amphetamine, methamphetamine, cocaine metabolites, and benzoylecognine; and, required
6-AM tests only for specimens with morphine concentrations greater than or equal to 2000 ng/mL.
[2]Delta-9-tetrahydrocannabinol-9-carboxylic acid (THCA).
[3]Methamphetamine is the target analyte for amphetamine/methamphetamine testing.
[4]To be reported positive for methamphetamine, a specimen must also contain amphetamine at a concentration greater than or equal to 100 ng/mL.
[5]Methylenedioxymethamphetamine (MDMA).
[6]Methylenedioxyamphetamine (MDA).
[7]Methylenedioxyethylamphetamine (MDEA).
[8]Morphine is the target analyte for codeine/morphine testing.

Source: U.S. Department of Health and Human Services. Mandatory guidelines for federal workplace drug testing programs. Federal Register 2008;73(Nov 25):71,858–907.

reasonable suspicion settings where justified, allow employers to include tests for additional drugs listed in Schedule I or II of the Controlled Substances Act.

Some employers conduct testing with panels that are like the federal five-drug panel. Some employers conduct testing with panels that include additional drugs or that use different (typically lower) cutoffs. For almost every drug, a laboratory test exists. However, not every laboratory performs every drug test. A program that wishes to perform less-common drug tests may have to check with several laboratories to find one that can accommodate. Specialty laboratories, or *reference* laboratories, perform the tests that are particularly esoteric.

For each drug/metabolite assay, the cutoff value is used to determine if the result is negative or positive. If the concentration is below the cutoff, the result is negative. If the concentration is at or above the cutoff, the result is positive. *Negative* does not mean "not present" or "undetected" but rather that the apparent concentration of analyte was less than the cutoff concentration for that assay. Cutoff values are based primarily on three considerations:

1. Laboratory capability—Laboratories can reliably test at the cutoffs.
2. Passive exposure—Cutoffs should exceed concentrations achievable by passive exposure.
3. Targeting heroin, not poppy seeds and codeine—Cutoffs for morphine and codeine should strike a balance that limits the proportion of positive results due to poppy seed ingestion and use of prescribed codeine without unduly sacrificing sensitivity at identifying heroin use.

Cutoff values for certain drugs are set higher for the immunoassays than the confirmatory cutoffs. The immunoassays for these drugs may be targeted at a specific analyte but react with multiple analytes. Confirmatory tests are specific for single analytes. For example, the marijuana immunoassay is targeted at delta-9-tetrahydrocannabinol but measures multiple cannabinoids. The marijuana confirmatory test measures only delta-9-tetrahydrocannabinol-9-carboxylic acid. Thus, for marijuana, the immunoassay test is set higher than the confirmatory test cutoff.

Besides the cutoff value, each assay has two additional thresholds as determined by the laboratory:

- Limit of detection—The lowest concentration at which an analyte can be identified, but (for quantitative assays) the concentration cannot be accurately calculated.
- Limit of quantitation—The lowest concentration at which the identify and concentration of the analyte can be accurately established.

The usual sequence, from lowest to highest, is: (1) limit of detection, (2) limit of quantitation, and (3) cutoff.

Tables 8-3 and 8-4 present examples of panels for testing hair and oral fluid, respectively, for drugs. Unlike the Table 8-2 panel used for federally regulated urine tests, there is no industry-standard panel for workplace testing of hair and oral fluid. Instead, the selection of drugs and cutoffs varies by laboratory and by client preferences.

Drug/metabolite concentrations are commonly presented in units of pg/mg (hair) and ng/mL (oral fluid, urine). A picogram is one trillionth (10^{-12}) of a gram. A nanogram is one billionth (10^{-9}) of a gram. A milliliter is one thousandth (10^{-3}) of a liter. The unit of measurement ng/mL is equivalent to parts per billion.

Immunoassays ■

In regulated testing, each specimen is initially tested for drugs using an FDA-approved immunoassay. An *immunoassay* measures the concentration of a substance in a liquid (a portion of a specimen) using the reaction of an antibody or antibodies to its antigen, i.e., drug. With some immunoassay tests, an indicator (tag) is first bound to the target drug, and the antibody binds with that tagged drug target. Table 8-5 lists the more widely used types of commercial immunoassays.

Table 8-3. Hair Drug Testing Cutoff Concentrations (pg/mg)[a] ■

Drug or Metabolite	Initial Test	Confirmation Test
Marijuana metabolites	1	
Delta-9-THC-9-carboxylic acid (THC-COOH)		0.05
Cocaine metabolites	500	
Cocaine[a]		500
Cocaine metabolites[a]		50
Opiate metabolites[b]	200	
Morphine		200
Codeine		200
6-Acetylmorphine[c]		200
Phencyclidine	300	300
Amphetamines[d]	500	
Amphetamine		300
Methamphetamine[e]		300
MDMA	500	300
MDEA		300

Source: HHS proposed alternative specimen procedures [69 FR 19,673].
[a]Cocaine concentration is greater than or equal to confirmatory cutoff *and* benzoylecgonine/cocaine ratio is greater than or equal to 0.05 *or* cocaethylene greater than or equal to 50 pg/mg *or* norcocaine greater than or equal to 50 pg/mg.
[b]Laboratories are permitted to initial test all specimens for 6-acetylmorphine using a 200 pg/mg cutoff.
[c]Specimen must also contain morphine at a concentration greater than or equal to 200 pg/mg.
[d]Methamphetamine is the target analyte.
[e]Specimen must also contain amphetamine at a concentration greater than or equal to 50 pg/mg.

Table 8-4. Oral Fluid Drug Testing Cutoff Concentrations (ng/mL) ■

Drug or Metabolite	Initial Test	Confirmation Test
THC parent drug and metabolite	4	
THC parent drug		2
Cocaine metabolites	20	
Cocaine[a]		8
Opiate metabolites[b]	40	
Morphine		40
Codeine		40
6-Acetylmorphine		4
Phencyclidine	10	2
Amphetamines[c]	50	
Amphetamine		50
Methamphetamine		50
MDMA		50
MDEA		50

Source: Private Sector Oral Fluid Testing Advisory Board. Draft Guidelines for Laboratory-Based Oral Fluid Workplace Drug Testing. K Street Associates, LLC. Flemington, NJ: 2007.
[a]Cocaine or benzoylecgonine.
[b]Labs are permitted to initial test all specimens for 6-AM using a 4 ng/mL cutoff.
[c]Methamphetamine is the target metabolite.

Table 8-5. Common Immunoassays ■

Immunoassay	Brand Name(s)	Manufacturer	Description	Comments
Enzyme (EIA)	EMIT, CEDIA, Abbott, DRI	Abbott Diagnostics, Syva, Microgenics	An immunoassay based on competition for antibody binding sites between drug in the specimen and drug labeled with an enzyme. Enzyme activity decreases upon binding to the antibody, so the drug concentration in the specimen can be measured in terms of enzyme activity.	Inexpensive. Concentration ranges based on changes in absorbance. Equipment is available for automated, high-volume rapid screening by EIA. Sensitive to some adulterants.
Fluorescence polarization (FPIA)	ADx, TDx	Abbott Diagnostics	An immunoassay based on competition between drug in the specimen and drug labeled with a fluorophore. Light emitted by the fluorescently labeled drug/antibody complex will be more polarized. The specimens' fluorescence polarization value is inversely related to the drug concentration. The FPIA test offers a better quantitative response for the class of drug of interest than EIA.	Resistant to a number of adulterants. Gives reasonably good quantitative estimates of concentrations. Slower and more expensive than EIA and KIMS.
Kinetic interaction of microparticles in a solution (KIMS)	OnLine	Roche Diagnostic	An immunoassay based on the principle of the kinetic interaction of microparticles in a solution where the drug content of the urine is directly proportional to the inhibition of the microparticle aggregation.	Equipment is available for automated, high-volume rapid screening by KIMS.

Initial testing of the specimens serves to quickly eliminate the majority of specimens that are "negative" from further consideration and identify the presumptive non-negative specimens. The immunoassays used in drug testing generally have a limited dynamic range and are semi-quantitative. They are designed to have a steep dose-response relationship at the cutoff concentration. The development of monoclonal antibodies allowed for the optimization of some of the immunoassays. Depending to some degree on how the antibodies have been generated, the immunoassays have different degrees of cross-reactivity toward drugs or metabolites with chemical structures similar to the target analytes. For this reason, specimens testing positive by immunoassay are then tested with a more sensitive and specific confirmatory test. Table 8-6 presents overall data from a large study that measured the rates at which urine specimens that screened positive went on to confirm as positive at federally certified laboratories. The lowest confirmation rates (i.e., the highest false-positive rates) occurred with immunoassays for opiates. This is in part due to the wide use of prescription opioids other than morphine and codeine.

If the initial drug test results are below the cutoff values and the validity test results do not meet adulterated, substituted or invalid criteria, the laboratory reports the negative result and discards the specimen. If an initial drug test result is at or above the cutoff for one or more drug classes, the specimen goes on for confirmation testing. If the initial test has been performed by a full-service laboratory, the staff will then take a new aliquot from the specimen, start a new internal chain of custody document for that aliquot, and perform a confirmatory drug test for each identified drug class. If the initial test has been performed by an IITF, staff will make entries in the CCF, package the specimen, and release it to a courier for transport to the full-service laboratory for confirmation testing.

Confirmatory Assays ■

A confirmatory drug test is an independent analytic procedure that uses a different technique or chemical principle from that used in the initial drug test. Confirmatory tests typically consist of an inlet system to separate components of the specimen and mass spectrometry to identify those components. A variety of inlet systems are used; most commonly gas chromatography for urine specimens and liquid chromatography (also known as electrospray) for nonurine specimens. Gas chromatography/mass spectrometry (GC/MS) has been the accepted standard in confirmatory analytical technologies for urine drug testing and, pending a rule change expected to take place in 2010, was the only confirmatory method au-

Table 8-6. Immunoassay Confirmation Rates at HHS-Certified Laboratories, 2006 ■

	Amphetamines	Cocaine Metabolite	Opiates	PCP	Marijuana Metabolite
Overall rate	66.3%	99.3%	25.7%	56.1%	97.3%

Source: Bush DM, Baylor M, Mitchell J, Sutheimer C. Comparison of confirmation rates for initial drug assays of regulated specimens tested in a group of SAMHSA certified laboratories: 2003 and 2006. Rockville, MD: SAMHSA, and Research Triangle Park, NC. RTI. 2006.

thorized under the federal drug testing procedures. In an update to the *Guidelines*, expected to be implemented in 2010, HHS allows the use of either liquid chromatography or gas chromatography for separation, and mass spectrometry (MS) or tandem MS (MS/MS) for identification in confirmatory analyses (73 *FR* 71,858). MS/MS methods are generally more sensitive and therefore require less specimen volume than MS methods. Confirmatory assays, in comparison to immunoassays, take more time, require a higher level of expertise to perform, and cost more.

An aliquot from the specimen is prepared for GC/MS by extracting the drug or drug metabolite and, in most cases, chemically combining it with another compound to form a derivative. Deuterium-labeled drug analogs are added to the aliquot as internal standards to provide relative retention time data for identifying and quantifying drug(s)/metabolite(s) from the real specimen. Chemicals in the real specimen are volatilized within the GC and travel through a GC column. The chemicals separate based on their physical and chemical properties. The identification of the drug is based on both the retention time in the GC and the mass spectrum produced. Mass spectrometry is accomplished by fragmenting the molecules into charged particles (ions) and separating these fragments according to their mass-to-charge ratios. A record of the ions formed and their relative abundance provides a unique mass spectrum that is used to identify the drug or metabolite. The ratios of these ions are compared to ratios of ions from standards for particular drugs/metabolites. If the ratios meet laboratory acceptance criteria for a drug or metabolite, the result is positive. The drug/metabolite concentration is calculated using either peak areas or heights for mass ions compared to the calibration.

Laboratories may batch certain tests and perform them every other day or on some other non-daily schedule. This is more typical of smaller laboratories and of tests that are performed less often, for example, *d* and *l* methamphetamine isomers and some adulterants.

Hair Analysis ■

The laboratory receives and accessions the hair specimen. If the specimen's packaging passes inspection and the information on the chain of custody form matches the specimen card, the accessioner starts an internal chain of custody document, cuts a proximal section of the hair (e.g., 3 cm) if it has been submitted as aligned strands (as opposed to loose hair or shavings), and weighs it. The laboratory verifies that it has enough hair for the requested immunoassay tests and at least one confirmatory test, if needed.

Most laboratories wash hair specimens. Among the agents used in washing are detergents (e.g., shampoo, surgical scrubbing solutions) and organic solvents (e.g., acetone, methanol, ethanol). Generally, a single washing step is used, but sometimes a second identical wash is performed. The washing procedure is intended to remove surface contaminants such as oils, lotions, and drug residues that may be present from environmental exposure.

After washing, a portion of the hair specimen is taken and may be pulverized or cut into segments. It is dissolved in solution, e.g., dissolved in sodium hydroxide. The technician extracts the analytes of interest. Aliquots of the extract are submitted for screening assays, for example, by radioimmunoassay or enzyme-linked immunoabsorbent assay. If an aliquot from the specimen screens positive, the remainder of the specimen is pulled from temporary storage, and another portion of hair is removed, weighed, and washed. This second portion undergoes confirmation analysis. In recent years, tandem mass spectrometry with gas chromatography (GC/MS/MS) or liquid chromatography (LC/MS/MS) separation, have emerged as the confirmation methods of choice for identification of drugs at very low cutoffs, for example, at a 0.05 pg/mg cutoff for marijuana metabolite. Laboratory cutoffs for hair are set much lower than those for urine. The marijuana metabolite cutoff is especially low because marijuana metabolite is identifiable in hair only at very low concentrations. Most laboratory panels used in workplace hair testing programs include reporting requirements whereby certain drugs, such as cocaine, are reported only if one or more metabolite(s) are also present in significant concentrations or ratios relative to the parent drug. This helps reduce the likelihood that a positive result could be caused solely by environmental exposure to parent drug(s).

Oral Fluid Analysis ■

A portion of the specimen is screened using an immunoassay. If the screening result is positive, another portion of the specimen undergoes confirmation analysis by GC/MS or liquid chromatography and mass spectrometry (LC/MS). GC/MS/MS or LC/MS/MS may be necessary because of small specimen volume and very low cutoff concentrations. Some collection processes cause the oral fluid specimen to be diluted—for example, by mixing it with preservative solution—which means the cutoffs that are actually achieved are somewhat higher than those used by the laboratory.

Laboratory Review ■

The laboratory conducts a final review of each result before reporting it to the MRO. Each negative result is reviewed by a certifying technician/scientist, who verifies the chain of custody and scientific reliability of the result. The certifying technician/scientist checks the appropriate result box(es) (i.e., negative, dilute) and either initials or signs their name on Step 5A of Copy 1 of the CCF, and stamps their name, if required. Each non-negative result is reviewed by a certifying scientist who verifies the chain of custody and reviews the initial and confirmatory test data. The certifying technician/scientist checks the appropriate result box(es) and signs and stamps their name in Step 5A of Copy 1 of the CCF. If the result is adulterated, invalid, or rejected for testing, the laboratory prints a comment describing the reason for this determination. If the result is substituted, the printed comment includes the creatinine and specific-gravity values. If additional space is needed for remarks, the laboratory can attach a separate sheet describing the problem and reference that sheet on the "Remarks" line.

Reporting Laboratory Results ■

WHEN

HHS-certified laboratories must report results within an average of 5 working days after specimen receipt. In practice, laboratories usually report negative results within 24 hours and non-negative results within 72 hours. Laboratories are prohibited from providing any information about a specimen's result prior to completion of testing.

TO WHOM

In federally regulated testing, the laboratory reports results only to the MRO's office. In nonregulated testing, laboratory accounts are sometimes set up so that results are sent directly to the employer or to a third-party administrator (TPA). Some accounts are set up with dual reporting, whereby results are sent to both the MRO and either the TPA or the MRO. This speeds the employer's access to negative results, while continuing to give MROs immediate access to non-negative results.

REPORT CONTENT

An HHS-certified laboratory reports the results for each primary specimen tested as *one* or more of the following:

- Negative
- Negative—dilute, with creatinine and specific gravity numeric values
- Rejected for testing, with standard explanatory remarks
- Positive, with drug(s)/metabolite(s) noted
- Positive, with drug(s)/metabolite(s) noted—dilute, with creatinine and specific gravity numeric values
- Adulterated, with remark(s)
- Substituted, with creatinine and specific gravity values
- Invalid result, with remark(s)

The laboratory reports each assay's result. Panels include multiple assays and specimen validity tests. Therefore, reports can list multiple results. For any drug/metabolite positive result, the laboratory names the drug/metabolite and its concentration. The laboratory report also includes this information:

- Testing laboratory name and address
- Employer/third-party administrator's name
- MRO's name
- Specimen identification number
- Donor SSN or employee identification number (if provided)
- Reason for test (if provided)
- Collector's name and telephone number
- Date of collection
- Date specimen received by laboratory
- Date certifying scientist released test result
- Certifying scientist's name
- CCF result(s) annotated
- Remarks if required

All of this information should be printed on the CCF. If the laboratory sends an electronic report instead of the CCF, this information must appear on the electronic report.

STANDING ORDERS

The laboratory may have account-specific standing orders asking for automatic reporting of certain details. Examples of standing orders include:

- Drug/metabolite concentrations. HHS certified laboratories report concentrations of all positive results, nonregulated laboratories may or may not. An MRO can submit a blanket request to the nonregulated laboratory for concentrations for all positive results *or* for all results of a particular type, e.g., all opiate-positive results.
- *d* and *l* isomers. The MRO may ask the laboratory to perform *d* and *l* isomer ratios for all methamphetamine-positive results prior to reporting those results. This adds cost and delays reporting of some methamphetamine-positive results, but it also gets the isomer ratios to the MRO before starting the review.

REPORT FORMAT

In regulated testing, if the result is positive, adulterated, substituted, or invalid, the laboratory sends the CCF to the MRO with the result checked off in Step 5a and a remark entered, if appropriate. Laboratories report negative results to MROs in a variety of formats including computer-generated electronic reports, faxed CCFs or standalone reports, and data posted to secure websites. Laboratories must ensure that transmissions and access to data are reasonably confidential and secure. For example, laboratories that fax results must ask MROs for assurance that their fax machines are in secure-access areas. Laboratories must have on file letters from MRO attesting to the security of off-site faxes and printers.

Because verbal reports are prone to misunderstanding, misdirection, and misrepresentation, certified laboratories are prohibited from reporting results by phone. The MRO can, however, call the laboratory to discuss any result after it has been received.

INVALID RESULTS

HHS laboratories are directed to contact the MRO about each invalid result to discuss the likely cause(s) and options for further testing, *unless* the invalid is due to inconsistent creatinine and specific gravity values, abnormal pH, or a nitrite of 200–499 µg/mL. In practice, laboratories often merely print a comment on the electronic report to the MRO highlighting the invalid result and inviting the MRO to call if any questions.

Storage of Specimens and Records ■

Laboratories promptly discard negative and rejected specimens. They freeze and save non-negative specimens for at least 12 months. For split specimen tests, if Bottle A tests negative, the laboratory immediately discards Bottle B. If Bottle A tests non-negative, the laboratory saves Bottle B for at least 12 months or until it is sent to a second laboratory for analysis. In the latter case, the second laboratory stores Bottle B for at least 12 months. Because of the potential for drugs and metabolites to deteriorate at room temperature in urine, the laboratory retains urine specimens in a frozen state. Laboratories will store specimen and their documentation longer if asked to do so in writing by an MRO, donor, employer, or a federal agency—for example, because of a legal challenge. Laboratories store test records for 2 years.

Semi-Annual Laboratory Reports ∎

Laboratories provide clients with semi-annual summary reports of account-specific data. The HHS *Guidelines* require them to send summaries within 14 days of the end of each semiannual period, either January through June, or July through December. The DOT *Procedures* have a similar requirement except laboratories have 20 days in which to issue reports and must not issue a report for less than five tests. Each summary report includes the number of:

1. Specimens reported by test type.
2. Specimens reported as negative and negative dilute.
3. Specimens reported as rejected for testing, by reason for rejection (i.e., fatal flaw or uncorrected flaw).
4. Specimens reported positive by drug.
5. Adulterated specimens.
6. Substituted specimens.
7. Invalid specimens.

If an MRO or C/TPA pays the laboratory account on the employer's behalf, the MRO or C/TPA will likely receive the semi-annual laboratory reports and is then responsible for providing reports to the employer. MROs and C/TPAs often use a single laboratory account for multiple employers. If so, the laboratory's summary reports then contain data from multiple employers. Thus, the account holder who receives the lab reports needs to produce employer-specific summaries from the aggregate data and distribute each summary to the respective employer.

The DOT *Procedures* require laboratories to send DOT semiannual reports of aggregate DOT data, similar to the employer-specific reports.

Data Package ∎

A data package—also known as a full documentation package or litigation package—is a complete set of documents associated with the testing of a particular specimen. A standard data package provided by an HHS-certified laboratory includes the following items:

- A cover sheet that provides a brief description of the drug testing procedures and specimen validity tests performed on the donor's specimen.
- A table of contents page that lists, by page number, all documents and materials in the package.
- A copy of the federal CCF along with any attachments and a copy of the electronic report (if any) generated by the laboratory.
- A brief description of the initial drug tests and initial specimen validity tests (e.g., instrumentation, batch quality control, and test data format).

- A brief description of confirmatory drug tests and confirmatory validity tests (e.g., instrumentation, batch quality control, and test data format).
- A copy of the curriculum vitae for the certifying scientist that certified the test result.
- A copy of the curriculum vitae for the laboratory's responsible person(s).
- Donor-specific information, including:
  - Internal chain of custody records for the specimen.
  - Memoranda (if any) generated by the laboratory.
  - Copies of the initial drug and specimen validity test data for the donor's specimen, with all calibrators and controls identified and copies of all internal chain of custody documents related to the initial tests.
  - Copies of the confirmatory drug and specimen validity test data for the donor's specimen, with all calibrators and controls identified and copies of all internal documents related to the confirmatory tests.

A data package is usually requested because a test has been legally challenged. An MRO who is going to testify about a specific test may be perceived as more credible if he or she has reviewed the data package. The laboratory must provide the documentation package within 10 business days of receipt of a written request from an authorized recipient—this means the employer, donor, or MRO. The employer or donor typically route their requests through the MRO. The cost for a data package is variable, but has been known to be as high as $200–$300. The MRO may be able to get additional documents from the laboratory upon request—for example, a description of the laboratory's chain of custody procedures or a description of the laboratory's quality assurance program. Each laboratory also offers experts who, for a fee, will testify about specific drug test results.

Reference ■

1. *Standards for Forensic Drug Testing Laboratory Accreditation*. Northfield, IL: College of American Pathologists. 2009.

Laboratory Results ■

This chapter describes what laboratory results mean. A summary of this information as it applies to regulated testing appears in Table 9-1.

Negative Result ■

A negative result means the specimen and its custody and control form (CCF) met forensic criteria, specimen validity results were in the acceptable range, the analyses were completed, and no drug or drug metabolite was identified at or above the cutoff concentrations. A negative result does not mean the donor does not use drugs. The donor may have used drug(s) that went undetected for various reasons, including elimination of the drug(s) from the body (either eliminated or reduced below the cutoffs), selection of a specimen (hair, urine, oral fluid, etc.) in which the drug(s) do not appear, selection of a test panel that does not target the drug(s), and substitution of the specimen.

Positive Result ■

A positive result means the specimen and its CCF met forensic criteria, the analyses were completed, and the drug or drug metabolite *was* identified at or above the cutoff concentration.

Invalid Result ■

An invalid result means that one or more analyses were not completed because of the specimen's abnormal condition but the specimen does not meet adulterated or substituted criteria. HHS developed the following general criteria for declaring a specimen invalid:

- Interference occurs during the immunoassay drug tests on two separate aliquots.
- Interference occurs during the confirmatory drug test on at least two separate aliquots.
- The physical appearance of the specimen is such that testing the specimen may damage the laboratory's instruments.
- The physical appearances of paired, split specimens are clearly different, and the primary specimen screened negative for drugs.

Table 9-1. Laboratory Results ■

Lab A Result	Additional Result	Check Box(es) on Federal CCF (Step 5a) or Result Indicated on Electronic Report	Remarks Line on CCF (Step 5a) and on Electronic Report	Note
Negative	<None>	Negative	For DOT-regulated specimens, provide creatinine and specific gravity values.	All drug tests are negative and all specimen validity test results are acceptable
	Dilute	Negative and Dilute		All drug tests are negative; the creatinine is less than 20 mg/dL and the specific gravity is less than 1.003; and the substituted criteria are not met
Positive, specific drug	Specimen Validity Test Acceptable	Positive and specific drug	<no comment required>	The drug/drug metabolite was detected at or above the cutoff concentration on both the screening and confirmatory assays
	Dilute	Positive, specific drug, and dilute	<no comment required>	
	Adulterated	Positive, specific drug, and adulterated	State reason for adulterated result (see below)	Positive (see above) and Adulterated, Substituted, or Invalid (see below)
	Substituted	Positive, specific drug, and substituted	Provide creatinine and specific gravity values	
	Invalid Result	Positive, specific drug, and Invalid Result	State reason for invalid result (see below)	
Adulterated	Negative	Adulterated	State reason for adulterated result (see below)	
	Invalid Result	Adulterated and invalid result	State reason for adulterated & invalid results (see below)	
	Substituted	Adulterated and substituted	State reason for adulterated result (see below) and provide creatinine and specific gravity values	
Substituted	<None>	Substituted	Provide creatinine and specific gravity values	Cr <2 mg/dL and sp. gr. ≤ 1.0010 or ≥ 1.0200
	Invalid Result	Substituted and Invalid Result	Provide creatinine and specific gravity values and state reason for invalid result (see below)	
Invalid Result	<None>	Invalid Result	State reason for invalid result (see below)	Valid initial drug test results could not be obtained, or an unknown substance interfered with the confirmatory test.
Rejected for Testing	<None>	Rejected for Testing	State reason for rejecting specimen (see below)	

Comments Required on Remarks Line (Step 5a) of the CCF and on Electronic Report

Test Result(s) on a Single Specimen or Bottle A Specimen	Comment	Note
Substituted	Creatinine = (conf. test numeric value) mg/dL and specific gravity = (conf. test numeric value)	Specific gravity ≤ 1.001 and creatinine < 2
Adulterated	pH = (conf. test numeric value)	1. pH < 3 or ≥ 11
	Nitrite = (conf. test numeric value) µg/mL	2. Nitrite ≥ 500 µg/mL
	Chromium (VI) = (conf. test numeric value) µg/mL	3. Presence of chromium, halogen, glutaraldehyde, pyridine, surfactant, or any other adulterant
	(Specify Halogen) Present	
	Glutaraldehyde = (conf. test numeric value) µg/mL	
	Pyridine = (conf. test numeric value) µg/mL	
	Surfactant Present	
	(Specify Adulterant) Present	
Invalid Result	Abnormal pH	
	Creatinine < 2 mg/dL; Sp. Gr. Acceptable	Sp. Gr. > 1.0010 & < 1.0200
	Specific Gravity ≤ 1.0010; Creatinine ≥ 2 mg/dL	
	Bottle A and Bottle B—Different Physical Appearance	Alerts MRO to a problem with the split specimens
	Possible (characterize as oxidant, halogen, aldehyde, or surfactant) Activity	
	Immunoassay Interference	
	GC/MS Interference	
	Abnormal Physical Characteristic (Specify)	
Rejected for Testing	Fatal Flaw: Specimen ID number mismatch/missing	The specimen was received with a fatal flaw or correctable but significant flaw that remained uncorrected.
	Fatal Flaw: No collector printed name & no signature	
	Fatal Flaw: Tamper-evident seal broken (or missing)	If redesignation is not possible
	Fatal Flaw: Insufficient specimen volume	
	Uncorrected Flaw: Wrong CCF used	Wait 5 business days before reporting flaw if uncorrected
	Uncorrected Flaw: Collector signature not recovered	

Adapted from U.S. Department of Health and Human Services. NLCP: Reporting Table. Rockville, MD, January 14, 2003.

An invalid result may be caused by adulteration. Some adulterants are formulated to produce specimens that meet invalid, but not adulterated, laboratory criteria, e.g., formulated to produce urine nitrite concentrations of 200–500 µg/mL. A laboratory will also report a result as invalid if it detects an adulterant but does not perform a confirmatory test to verify that adulterant. Other potential causes of invalid results include medicine use, imprecision in the specimen validity tests so that a true-normal result is reported as out of range, and specimen degradation due to time, heat, or other physical conditions. Prior to reporting an invalid result, the federal rules direct the laboratory to contact the MRO to discuss whether sending the specimen to another laboratory for testing would be useful to being able to report a positive or adulterated result.

The laboratory reports a specimen as invalid by checking the "Invalid Result" box in Step 5a of the CCF and printing a comment on the "Remarks" line. If a regulated urine specimen is invalid and a negative drug test result is needed (e.g., for pre-employment purposes), another urine specimen must be collected.

A specimen can be positive for one or more assays and invalid for the others. The laboratory will report this type of result as "positive" for the drug(s) or metabolite(s) that are identified, and "invalid" or "no test" for the other assays. The positive result(s) are valid and the other results are not.

Criteria for defining specimens as invalid have been well developed for urine. Criteria for defining specimens as invalid are less well developed for hair and oral fluid and vary among laboratories.

INVALID URINE

The following sections describe the laboratory criteria for different types of invalid urine specimens.

Possible Adulterant Activity, Immunoassay Interference, or GC/MS Interference

If the immunoassay or GC/MS confirmatory test cannot be completed and the laboratory suspects the presence of an adulterant or use of an interfering medication, the laboratory reports the result as invalid. This usually involves the immunoassay test. For example, the Tolectin metabolite absorbs ultraviolet light at the same wavelength as the NADH/NAD reaction used in some enzyme immunoassays (EIAs) and may interfere with the detection of drugs and drug metabolites. For this particular kind of invalid result, the laboratory may try an alternative, non-enzyme-based immunoassay. Some invalid urine results are caused by nitrite at concentrations greater than or equal to 200 µg/mL but less than the 500 µg/mL threshold for establishing adulteration.

Perhaps one in every few hundred invalid results caused by adulterants or medications involve failure of the confirmatory assay as opposed to failure of the immunoassay. Most confirmatory failures are for opiates or for cocaine metabolite. This can be caused by adulterants or medications that specifically interfere with the ability to get a reliable GC/MS result. This can also be caused by use of an adulterant that destroys the deuterated drug standards that are added to specimens as part of the analysis. For example, if the initial test result is presumptive positive for THC metabolite and the laboratory cannot find the deuterated internal standard during GC/MS, it declares the specimen invalid. In this case, the unidentified oxidizing agent did not destroy all the THC metabolite before the initial test, but did oxidize the deuterated analog during confirmation. A second example is the presence of a sufficient quantity of fluconazole to "scavenge" the derivatizing reagent used in some of the benzoylecgonine GC/MS assays. The laboratory would also report this result as invalid.

Abnormal pH

The laboratory reports the result as invalid and reports the pH value if it is ≥ 3.0 and < 4.5 or ≥ 9.0 and < 11.0. At these pH values, the ability to identify certain drugs is compromised. These pH values are not extreme enough to definitively establish adulteration.

Low Creatinine Value or Low Specific Gravity Value

If one value is normal and the other value is too low, the laboratory reports both values and reports the result as invalid. "Too low" means a creatinine of less than 2 mg/dL or a specific gravity less than or equal to 1.0010.

Bottle A and Bottle B: Different Physical Characteristics, or Abnormal Physical Characteristics

If the contents of bottles A and B look clearly different and the drug testing results are negative, the laboratory reports the specimen as invalid. In this case, the contents of Bottles A and B appear not to represent a single void or something was added to one bottle but not the other. If the urine has an unusual odor (e.g., bleach) or appearance (e.g., blue or green), the laboratory may report it as invalid. Laboratories are especially likely to report such a specimen as invalid if their physical characteristics may affect the analytic techniques or damage the equipment.

INVALID HAIR

Heavily Contaminated Specimen or Specimen Does Not Meet Metabolite Criteria

A hair testing laboratory may report a specimen as invalid if the specimen is so heavily externally contaminated with drug residue that it is unclear if the drug detected represents use of the drug or absorption into the outer layers of the hair shaft from contact with external residues. Laboratories that invalidate specimens on this basis do so by setting upper limits on the acceptable ratios between the concentrations of drug residue in washes of the hair and the concentrations in the hair shaft. If the ratios do not meet these limits, the test cannot reliably distinguish internal from external exposure. An invalid result based on external contamination with drug residue most often involves analysis for cocaine and its (metabolites benzoylecgonine, cocaethylene, and norcocaine).

INVALID ORAL FLUID

Specific criteria for identification of invalid results for oral fluid specimens have not yet been established.

Adulterated Specimen ■

An *adulterated specimen* is a specimen that has been altered, as evidenced by test results showing either a substance that is not a normal constituent for that type of specimen or showing an abnormal concentration of an endogenous substance. An HHS-certified laboratory reports a urine specimen as adulterated when [69 *FR* 19,641]:

1. pH < 3 or ≥ 11;
2. Nitrite ≥ 500 µg/mL;
3. Chromium (VI) at ≥ 50 µg/mL on screening and at a concentration at or above the laboratory's limit of detection using a different, confirmatory test;
4. Surfactant ≥ 100 µg/mL dodecylbenzene sulfonate-equivalent; or,
5. Presence of halogen (e.g., bleach, iodine, fluoride), glutaraldehyde, pyridine, surfactant, or any other adulterant verified by using an initial test on the first aliquot and a different confirmatory test on a second aliquot.

No physiologic conditions, disease states, or workplace or environmental exposures are known to cause these results.

The laboratory notes the adulterated result by checking the "Adulterated" box in Step 5a of the CCF and printing the reason on the "Remarks" line. The laboratory also prints "adulterated" and the reason on the electronic form.

The laboratory is not authorized to neutralize an adulterant so that the drug assays can be completed. Nevertheless, some drug assays can be completed despite the presence of an adulterant. Thus, a laboratory may report that a specimen is both adulterated and drug-positive.

Dilute Specimen ■

A *dilute specimen* is a specimen that contains physiologic constituents at concentrations that are lower than expected but are still within the physiologically producible ranges. If a specimen meets dilute criteria, the laboratory reports it as "dilute" and reports the drug assay findings, i.e., positive or negative. A laboratory reports a dilute result only in conjunction with a negative or positive drug test result. If the result is negative or lab-positive/MRO-negative, the dilute finding has potential consequences because the employer may retest the donor. If the result is adulterated or invalid, the specimen has probably been tampered with and, if it also happens to satisfy the dilute criteria, the dilute result would actually be meaningless.

CRITERIA FOR DILUTE URINE

A dilute urine specimen is one with creatinine and specific gravity values less than expected but which does not meet substituted criteria (see Table 9-2 and Figure 9-1). The laboratory checks the "Dilute Specimen" box in Step 5A of the CCF and prints the numerical values for creatinine and specific gravity on the "Remarks" line. The laboratory prints "dilute specimen" and the creatinine and specific gravity values on the electronic report, also.

Table 9-2. Urine Creatinine and Specific Gravity ■

Lab Report	Creatinine	Specific Gravity	MRO Report (per DOT)
Substituted	< 2 mg/dL	≤ 1.0010 *or* ≥ 1.0200	Refusal to test unless donor has an acceptable medical reason for the substituted finding.
Invalid	< 2 mg/dL	≥ 1.0010 *and* < 1.0200	Test cancelled—invalid result.
	OR		— If the donor has no acceptable explanation for the finding, ask the employer to retest under direct observation.
	≥ 2 mg/dL	≤ 1.0010	
			— If the donor has an acceptable explanation for the finding, cancel the test. Employer retests if a negative result is needed.
Positive and Invalid	(See above)		Positive for <drug>. (Do not report the invalid information.)
Negative Dilute	≥ 2 and < 5 mg/dL	> 1.0010 and < 1.0030	Negative dilute. Ask the employer to retest under direct observation.
	≥ 5 and < 20 mg/dL	> 1.0010 and < 1.0030	Negative dilute. Employer has option of one immediate retest, not under direct observation.
Positive Dilute	≥ 2 and < 20 mg/dL	> 1.0010 and < 1.0030	Positive for <drug>.

Urine specific gravity is a measurement of the density of urine relative to the density of water. Water is assigned a specific gravity of 1.000. Urine specific gravity is normally 1.0030–1.0300. Glucose, protein, or dyes used in diagnostic tests increase specific gravity. Certain disease states, such as diabetes insipidus, glomerulonephritis, and renal failure, can reduce specific gravity. Creatinine is a by-product of protein metabolism and is excreted in urine. There is no standard reference range for random urine creatinine values. The values are rarely less than 5 mg/dL and never less than 2 mg/dL [1]. Women have in general lower muscle mass and thus lower urinary creatinine concentrations compared with men. Ingestion of creatine supplements has no significant effect on urine creatinine measurements [2]. Creatinine concentration in urine is increased by exercise and the presence of cooked meat in the diet and is age, weight, and sex dependent.

The proportion of dilute specimens was reported as 4% in one publication and 7.6% in another [3,4]. That second publication also noted that 10% of the dilute specimens had drugs/metabolites present at below cutoff concentrations [4]. In DOT-regulated testing, the laboratory is not permitted to report any drug or drug metabolite concentration detected below the designated cutoff(s), and is not permitted to estimate these concentrations by "normalizing" (adjusting) them upward based on low creatinine and specific gravity values. By contrast, the NRC rule allows the laboratory to test to the limit of detection if the urine is dilute and the concentration appears to be at or above 50% of the cutoff value.

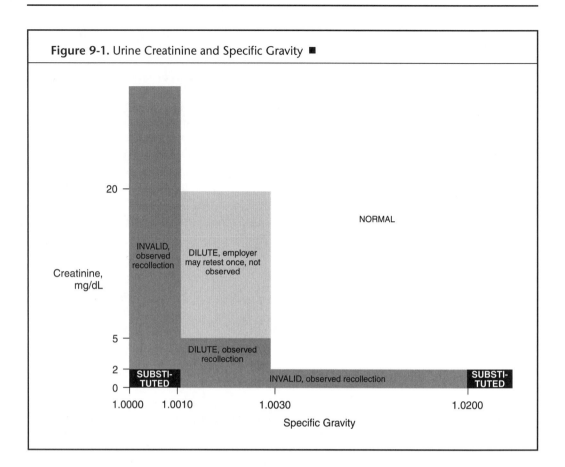

Figure 9-1. Urine Creatinine and Specific Gravity ■

CRITERIA FOR DILUTE ORAL FLUID

No definitive criteria have been established for identifying dilute oral fluid specimens.

CRITERIA FOR DILUTE HAIR

Hair specimens are not subject to dilution.

Substituted Specimen ■

A *substituted specimen* is identified by the laboratory as one that has been submitted in place of the donor's urine as evidenced by creatinine and specific gravity values that are outside the physiologically producible ranges of human urine. Substitution can also mean having someone other than the professed donor provide the specimen. However, the laboratory would identify that specimen as real and not as "substituted."

CRITERIA FOR SUBSTITUTED URINE

Criteria for declaring urine specimens as substituted are standardized and supported by extensive scientific literature. The criteria for declaring urine specimens as substituted are based on creatinine and specific gravity values that are clearly inconsistent with human urine. A urine specimen is identified as "substituted" if its creatinine concentration is less than 2 mg/dL and its specific gravity is less than or equal to 1.0010 or greater than or equal to 1.0200. These values are considered to be outside of physiologic ranges. If the specimen meets *both* the specific gravity and creatinine criteria for substituted, the laboratory checks the "Substituted" box in Step 5A of the CCF and prints the creatinine concentration and specific gravity values. If the creatinine concentration is below the laboratory's minimum detection limit, the laboratory reports this finding as "creatinine not detected."

CRITERIA FOR SUBSTITUTED ORAL FLUID, HAIR

There are no widely accepted criteria for identifying non-urine specimens as substituted.

Specimen Rejected for Testing ■

If the laboratory has identified a fatal flaw or an unrecovered correctable flaw, the laboratory checks "Rejected for Testing" in Step 5A of the CCF and prints a comment on the "Remarks" line, explaining the reason for the rejection. The electronic report states "rejected for testing" or something similar, such as "no test," and explains the basis for the rejection.

References ■

1. U.S. Federal Aviation Administration. Workplace Urine Specimen Validity Testing Colloquium. Tampa, FL, February 4–6, 2003.
2. Ropero-Miller J, Paget-Wilkes H, Doering P, et al. Effect of oral creatine supplementation on random urine creatinine, pH, and specific gravity measurements. *Clin Chem* 2000;46:295–97.
3. Peat M. *A Brief Introduction to Oral Fluid Drug Testing.* Lenexa, KS: LabOne. March 27, 2000.
4. Substance Abuse and Mental Health Services Administration. *PD 025; Notice to Laboratory Inspectors and Laboratory Directors.* Rockville, MD: May 3, 1993. Department of Health and Human Services.

MRO Review of Drug Test Results ■

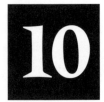

This chapter describes how MROs receive, interpret, and report test results. As described in the "MRO Assistant" section of Chapter 1, some of these tasks can be performed by an MRO assistant under the MRO's direction.

Documents Required for Review ■

In federally (e.g., U.S. Department of Transportation, or DOT) regulated testing, the MRO must have certain copies of the custody and control form (CCF) to properly complete the review prior to reporting to the employer (see Table 10-1). The result cannot be reported, not even as an interim report, until the CCFs have been reviewed. To emphasize this point, DOT requires each drug test report from the MRO's office to include the date on which the MRO received CCF Copy 2. The MRO's office should date-stamp each CCF as it is received by mail or courier. CCFs received by fax are (or can be) automatically date stamped by the fax machine. Original copies, photocopies, and electronic images of CCFs are equivalent for purposes of the review.

In regulated testing, the MRO reviews Copy 2 of the CCF for each non-negative result to verify the donor's signature. If Copy 2 is unavailable, Copies 3, 4, or 5 will suffice because they also have the donor's signature. If the result is non-negative, the MRO also reviews Copy 1 of the CCF to verify that the laboratory certifying scientist has signed it.

In nonregulated testing, chain of custody forms are usually designed so that all copies have the same information. Thus, in nonregulated testing the MRO usually needs to review only one copy of the chain of custody form.

The MRO also receives a computer-generated test report from the laboratory. Typically, the MRO assistant matches laboratory reports with CCFs and gives the non-negative files to the MRO for review. This collating of files takes time and is among the reasons why MROs charge for the handling and reporting of both negative and non-negative results.

Table 10-1. MRO Review of Documents in Regulated Testing ■

Lab Result	MRO Must Have These Documents[a]	Elements of the Review
Negative	1. The electronic report or Copy 1 of the CCF *and* 2. A CCF copy with the donor's signature, i.e., Copy 2, 3, 4, or 5	■ The MRO or the MRO assistant performs the review ■ If the laboratory electronic report is used instead of Copy 1, verify that the donor ID and specimen ID on the electronic report match the IDs on the CCF with the donor's signature ■ Verify that the donor has signed the certification statement or that the form includes a remark about the donor's refusal to sign, and that the current version of the federal CCF has been used
Positive, adulterated, substituted, invalid, or rejected for testing	1. Copy 1 of the CCF with the certifying scientist's signature *and* 2. A CCF copy with the donor's signature, i.e., Copy 2, 3, 4, or 5	■ The MRO or MRO assistant reviews the forms for flaws. This includes verifying that the donor has signed Step 5 of Copy 2 of the CCF or that the form has a remark about the donor's refusal to sign. ■ The MRO reviews Copy 1 of the CCF and ensures that it is consistent with the information contained on Copy 2, that the test result is legible, and that the certifying scientist signed the form.

[a]The original CCF or a legible copy (fax, photocopy, image) of the CCF can be used.

The MRO does not receive the laboratory's internal chain of custody documents unless he or she asks for them, nor is the MRO expected to review those documents.

The collector sends Copy 2 of the CCF directly to the MRO. Delays in receiving Copy 2 can delay review and reporting of positive results. The collection site is not supposed to send the Copy 2 of the CCF (with the donor's name) to the laboratory because the donor's identity is supposed to be hidden from laboratory personnel. However, the accidental routing of Copy 2 form to the laboratory is not grounds for cancelling a test. Within the accessioning area of a HHS-certified laboratory, each aliquot is labeled with a number, not a name, before it is transferred to those who perform the analyses. Even if accessioning staff know the donor's name, it is extremely unlikely that the donor's name would be available to those who perform the analyses.

Review of Test Documents ■

The laboratory reviews the CCF and packaging of each specimen during accessioning. Laboratories identify most CCF flaws and, where applicable, gets statements to correct them, as described in the "Accessioning" section of the laboratory chapter of this book. The MRO (or MRO assistant) also reviews CCFs, may identify uncorrected flaws, and may obtain statements to correct them. The

MRO or MRO assistant review of the forms provides a final check of the CCF and verifies the donor's signature, which the laboratory does not get. The MRO is an advocate for quality; if the MRO identifies repeated collection flaws that do not require corrective statements but nevertheless suggest a problem, the MRO should notify the collection site.

DOT directs laboratories to wait 5 days for each corrective statement that it requests. Likewise, although not specifically stated in the DOT rule, the MRO should wait 5 days for each requested corrective statement. If no corrective statement is received, the MRO cancels the test. The following sections describe several correctable flaws that MROs and their assistants typically identify.

MISSING DONOR'S SIGNATURE

A missing donor's signature with no comment about the omission (i.e., no collector's remark about a refusal to sign) is a correctable flaw. In regulated testing, the donor's signature would not appear on the laboratory copy of the CCF, so it falls to the MRO to identify and correct any missing donor's signature. The collector (and not the collector's supervisor) can provide a corrective statement to correct this flaw. Alternatively, the MRO could ask the donor for a corrective statement that the donor refused or failed to sign the form.

USE OF THE WRONG CHAIN OF CUSTODY FORM

DOT Test Performed with Non-DOT Form

Use of a non-DOT CCF for a DOT-authorized test is usually correctable. The DER may identify this error upon receipt of the MRO's report. The MRO can reclassify the test as "DOT" if the MRO establishes that the laboratory is HHS certified and a DOT-like panel (including cutoff levels) and procedures were followed. The MRO can ask the laboratory to also reclassify the test as DOT so that the laboratory counts it as DOT in its statistical reports. However, DOT does not require that laboratories reclassify, and some laboratories will not do this.

If the MRO reclassifies a non-DOT single specimen test to a DOT test after the MRO interview and verification of a positive, adulterated, or substituted result, the MRO will need to inform the donor of his or her right to a split test. If the donor asks for the split test and no split is available, the MRO cancels the test.

If the collector knew the test was DOT but used a non-DOT form by mistake or because no federal form was available, the collector should provide a statement describing how he/she will avoid this error in the future. Sometimes collectors do not have adequate or correct information about which tests are DOT and which are non-DOT.

Non-DOT Test Performed with DOT Form

A test mistakenly performed with a DOT CCF may suffice for a non-DOT program. However, the test may not have the drugs or cutoffs particular to that non-DOT program. If the MRO is going to verify the result as positive, the employer will take action based on that outcome and there is no immediate need to test the specimen for any missing drugs/metabolites. If the laboratory result is negative, the laboratory will usually have already discarded the specimen, so there is no opportunity to test for additional drugs/metabolites. In this latter situation, the MRO should report the negative result and list the drugs/metabolites that were tested. For completeness, the MRO may also list which drugs/metabolites were omitted.

FAILURE TO COLLECT UNDER DIRECT OBSERVATION

If the MRO discovers that a urine specimen with a negative result should have been collected under direct observation but was not, the MRO does not report the result. The MRO instead directs the DER to send the donor for another test, this time collected under direct observation.

REVIEW OF MRO ASSISTANT'S WORK

The MRO is responsible for his or her assistant's work. In DOT-regulated testing, this responsibility includes the MRO's personal review of at least 5% of all CCFs reviewed by his or her assistant(s) (i.e., the laboratory-negative results) each quarter, including all CCFs with correctable flaws [49 CFR §40.127(g)(2)]. This requirement is capped at 500 negative results per quarter. The MRO's review must include CCFs, electronic laboratory reports (if available), corrective documents, and reports sent to employers. The MRO must correct any mistakes that are discovered and document the corrective action. The MRO must document the reviews by initialing the CCFs that he or she reviews, and must make these CCFs easily identifiable and retrievable for audit by regulatory agencies.

Cancelled Drug Test ∎

Only MROs cancel drug tests. Under the DOT rule, the MRO reports a cancelled test if:

1. A suitable specimen was not collected because the donor:
   a. Was not given 3 hours;
   b. Had a "shy bladder" *and* the MRO accepted the donor's medical explanation for this. (Exception: If the shy bladder is permanent and the test is pre-employment, return-to-duty, or follow-up, the donor needs a negative result to perform safety-sensitive duties. In these situations, the MRO arranges for a clinical evaluation for illicit drug use and, if the evaluation is negative, reports "Negative" instead of "Test Cancelled.")
   c. The donor declined to undergo an exam required by the MRO (e.g., for opiate abuse) or by the DER (e.g., for shy bladder), *and* the test was conducted pre-offer, i.e., with no contingent offer of employment.
2. The laboratory reports that the specimen is rejected for testing or the MRO identifies a fatal flaw or uncorrected flaw. (For more information about fatal flaws and correctable flaws, see Table 8-1.)
3. The laboratory reports the result to the MRO as invalid *and* the donor has no medical explanation. (Exception: If the donor admits to adulterating or substituting the specimen, the MRO reports a "Refusal to Test.")
4. A split specimen fails to reconfirm.
5. The laboratory reports the result to the MRO as adulterated or substituted *and* the MRO determines there is a legitimate medical explanation for it. (This occurs rarely, if ever.)

An MRO does not cancel a test based on a mistake in the process that does not have a significant adverse effect on the right of the donor to a fair and accurate test. Insignificant flaws, such as those listed in the second half of Table 8-1, are not cause for cancelling a test.

A cancelled test is neither negative nor positive. In DOT-regulated programs, it is not cause for the employer to order a non-DOT test or a reasonable suspicion DOT test, or to take disciplinary action. It does not satisfy any requirement to have a negative result prior to starting work. It does not count toward any required random rate or number of follow-up tests.

The MRO checks the "Test Cancelled" box (Step 6) on Copy 2 of the CCF, and prints a remark about why the test was cancelled, for example, "Fatal flaw, _____" (with the flaw stated) or "Uncorrected flaw, _____" (with the flaw stated). If the cancellation is because of a collector error, the remark should indicate this as a prompt to the employer or service agent (e.g., C/TPA) responsible for ensuring that error-correction training takes place.

If the test was cancelled because of a result that is invalid for unknown reasons, or because the split was unavailable or produced an invalid result, the donor is retested using a directly observed collection. Otherwise, if a negative result is required, i.e., for pre-employment, return-to-duty, or follow-up purposes, the donor is retested without direct observation.

Negative Result Review ■

If the laboratory result is negative, the record undergoes an administrative review, typically by the MRO's assistant. If the reviewer identifies no fatal flaws or correctable flaws that remain uncorrected, the reviewer checks the "Negative" box in Step 6 of Copy 2 of the CCF and signs and dates the report. An MRO assistant can sign Step 6 with the MRO's name and initial it or stamp Step 6 with the MRO's signature stamp. If the reviewer identifies a fatal flaw or a correctable flaw that remains uncorrected, the MRO personally reviews the record to verify that the test should be cancelled.

Dilute Result ■

If the laboratory reports that the specimen is dilute and either negative or positive, the MRO reports to the employer that the specimen, in addition to being negative or positive, was dilute. (The MRO does not report dilute findings for specimens that are also invalid or adulterated.) The MRO also reminds the employer about retesting options, as described in the "Reporting MRO Results" section of this chapter. The federal rules do not authorize any disciplinary action for a dilute result other than retesting the donor if the drug results are negative. MROs do not interview donors for legitimate explanations for dilute findings. A "dilute" finding is not proof of tampering.

CONCENTRATIONS

Certified laboratories routinely report drug/metabolite concentrations to MROs. An MRO can get concentrations from non-certified laboratories, too—on a test-by-test basis as needed or (with submission of a written "blanket request") routinely for all tests or all tests of certain types, e.g., opiate-positive results. Only the MRO is authorized to ask for and receive drug/metabolite concentrations directly from a certified laboratory. The donor and the substance abuse professional (SAP) are authorized to receive drug/metabolite concentrations, too, but must route their requests through MROs.

The laboratory may report that the concentration is higher than it can reliably measure, i.e., is higher than the limit of quantitation. In nonregulated testing, the MRO can ask the laboratory to dilute an aliquot from the specimen, test it, and then extrapolate and report the concentration of drug/metabolite(s) in the original specimen.

Concentrations matter to the MRO in limited circumstances.

- In regulated testing, if the opiate concentrations exceed 15,000 ng/mL, the results cannot be attributed to poppy seed ingestion.
- In NRC-regulated testing, the MRO decides if the concentration of a positive return-to-duty test is consistent with new use or residual excretion, and changes the result to negative if it is from residual excretion.

MROs should be wary of trying to interpret concentrations. Extremely high values may suggest misuse of a prescribed drug and thus a safety issue. However, correlation of urine concentration to dose is difficult because the scientific literature on this is scant and many patient variables affect concentrations. Also, medication use by workers is often short-term or "as needed," so steady state elimination kinetics cannot be assumed.

The Interview ■

The MRO gives the donor an opportunity to speak directly and confidentially with him or her about the test result if it is positive, adulterated, substituted, or invalid. This is true even for results for which there are no medical explanations, for example, phencyclidine (PCP). The discussion between the MRO and donor informs the donor of the result and gives the donor an opportunity to ask questions about the test. It gives the donor an opportunity to present the MRO with medical explanations for the result or admit to misuse of the drug. The interview is an opportunity for the MRO to inform the donor of the opportunity for the split test to be tested, if applicable.

The federal rules refer to the "interview" in the singular, like a one-time event. In fact, some interviews are concluded in one conversation but others require multiple communications, e.g., if the donor does not have his or her medical information immediately available.

HOW INTERVIEWS TAKE PLACE

The MRO interview process is intended to take place by telephone. It can take place in person, but this would be atypical. Telephone contact is faster, cheaper, and, if the donor and MRO are located far apart, the only viable means of communication. The MRO calls the donor at the telephone number(s) listed on the CCF. These are often cell phone numbers where donors can be reached both day and evening. If the listed phone number(s) fail, the MRO can try other phone numbers that may be available from the collection site (from their copy of a release and consent form or registration form), DER, or other sources.

If someone other than the donor answers the phone, the MRO should leave a brief message requesting that the donor return the call. If asked, the MRO might explain that the call pertains to a recent test result and is for routine follow-up, i.e., is not an emergency. The MRO should be discrete and not mention the drug test.

The MRO must document contact efforts, including the dates and times of each attempt to contact the donor. Most MROs use a checklist, like that presented in Figure 10-1, for documenting the review process. The MRO's comments may include notes about answering machines, messages, and disconnected or wrong telephone numbers. The MRO's comments should reflect the tone and content of the worker's response, for example, "Smoked last year, not since," or "Denies cocaine use; says it's a mistake." This documentation helps establish that the donor was given an opportunity to discuss the results. It also provides a permanent record of the decision-making process for each positive, adulterated, substituted, or invalid result. The MRO's notes are stored with the laboratory test report and CCF. If any legal challenge arises years later, the MRO may recall little of what happened during the review process, but can refer to the contemporaneous notes he or she took.

Some MROs ask their assistants to make initial contact with the donor because this can be time consuming. Some people are hard to reach by phone. Some chain of custody forms have illegible, incorrect, or missing phone numbers. The MRO's assistant can confirm the donor's identity, inform the donor of the consequences of declining to speak with the MRO (i.e., that the MRO will verify the test without input from the donor), ask the donor to have medical information ready to present at the interview with the MRO, and schedule the discussion with the MRO. Reviews should be handled promptly, and thus MROs should want to speak with donors as soon as they are contacted. If the MRO assistant starts the contact, the assistant should promptly transfer the call to the MRO, even if it means interrupting the MRO from other, non-urgent business. If the MRO cannot take the call, the MRO assistant can still help expedite the process by verifying the phone number(s) at which the donor can be reached and asking about the best time for the MRO to reach the donor. The initial contact usually provides enough information for decision making, and the process works best when the MRO gets involved early. The MRO assistant should not disclose the result or ask the donor about legitimate medical explanations. The assistant is not qualified to explore medical explanations, and the donor may think after such discussion that there is no need to speak with the MRO. The MRO assistant also cannot ask the donor if he or she wishes to speak with the MRO. Depending on how it is phrased, this question can be inappropriately used to discourage donors from speaking with MROs. In addition, the question is moot because the MRO is supposed to speak directly to the donor. If the donor expressly refuses to speak with the MRO, the MRO assistant must document the donor's refusal, including the date and time.

If the donor and MRO speak different languages, a translator may be used. Ideally—but infrequently—the MRO has a translator. Certain commercial services offer over-the-phone interpreter services. Sometimes the donor's family member or friend translates, which is unfortunate but may be the only option. Use of a coworker or workplace supervisor is the last resort. If the donor is deaf,

Figure 10-1. MRO Punchlist ∎

Donor's Name: _____   ID No. _____

Review the custody and control form (copies 1 and 2, if regulated) and verify that it is acceptable.

If the employer has a stand-down policy, notify the DER if positive, adulterated, substituted, or invalid: ___/___/___, _____
notified on: (Date)   by: (initials)

Provide the donor with an opportunity to discuss the positive, adulterated, substituted, or invalid test result. Note each attempt.

Date	Time	Phone#	Contact	Comments	Initials
_____	_____	( )___-___	Y/N	_____	_____
_____	_____	( )___-___	Y/N	_____	_____
_____	_____	( )___-___	Y/N	_____	_____

If unable to contact the donor after three attempts/24 hrs, ask the designated employer representative (DER) for help

_____	_____	( )___-___	Y/N	_____	_____
_____	_____	( )___-___	Y/N	_____	_____
_____	_____	( )___-___	Y/N	_____	_____

If the donor has not contacted the MRO within 72 hrs of contact from the DER, verify lab result.

If neither the MRO nor DER can contact the donor within 10 days of the lab report, verify lab result.

✓ Identify yourself as a physician calling on behalf of the employer about a recent exam.
✓ Confirm the individual's identify, e.g., read five digits of their SSN and ask for the last four digits.
✓ Tell the donor the result(s)—the drug(s) or specimen validity test results.
✓ Explain the verification process. Give your name and phone number.
✓ Explain that fitness-for-duty information may be shared with the employer or other responsible authority.
✓ Seek potential sources of the drug(s), e.g., prescribed medications, invasive procedures, poppy seeds, etc.
✓ If the donor claims use of prescribed medication, ask the donor to help with corroboration of the prescription(s).
✓ If amphetamines-positive and the donor reports using Vicks Inhaler or the generic equivalent during the 3 to 4 days before the collection, order d- vs. l-isomers.
✓ If opiates-positive at levels below 15,000 ng/mL and not positive for 6-AM, verify positive only if there is clinical evidence of unauthorized opiate use.

Verification decision:

❏ Negative   ❏ Positive for: _____   ❏ Test cancelled   ❏ Refusal to test because:
                                            ❏ Invalid   ❏ Errored   ❏ Adulterated   ❏ Substituted   ❏ Other

Reason: ❏ No alternative medical explanation(s)

                      MRO's Signature: _____

✓ If regulated test, complete Step 6 of CCF Copy 2. Notify the DER. If also "dilute," notify the DER that it is dilute.
✓ If DOT-regulated test, notify ODAPC if cancelled because of medical explanation for "adulterated" or "substituted" finding.
✓ If positive, adulterated, or substituted, inform the donor that: (1) he/she has 72 hours to ask for split analysis for drug/metabolite/validity parameters, and (if DOT) (2) advance payment is not required. If the donor asks for analysis of the split specimen, complete the following:

Donor's request received at: Date: ____/____/____, time: _____

Send the laboratory a written request for analysis of the split specimen.

✓ Attach this punchlist to the drug test record. Do not routinely send this punchlist to the employer.

the MRO and donor could communicate by a teletype service or through an American Sign Language interpreter. Most interviews are performed by telephone, with the interpreter either connected by conference call or with the MRO or donor. The donor's consent to sharing information with the interpreter is implied because the donor surely knows that the interpreter is participating in the interview.

WHEN

The MRO must try to make contact promptly after receiving the complete drug test record. The DOT rule directs the MRO to make at least three attempts over 24 hours after receipt of the record. HHS has published similar guidance [1]. The MRO may try to make contact upon receipt of the laboratory result. However, in regulated testing, the MRO cannot report the result until both Copy 1 and Copy 2 (or its equivalent) of the CCF have been received and reviewed. The MRO who interviews the donor before both copies are received risks two awkward situations: First, the donor knows he or she has a positive result and the MRO cannot yet tell the employer. Second, the MRO might find a fatal flaw on the CCF(s) after concluding the interview. Therefore, the MRO should wait until both CCFs have been received and reviewed before contacting the donor.

Just as telemarketers most readily reach people in the evenings, MROs can most readily reach donors at the home number in the early evening. Other advantages of calling the donor in the evening include a reduced potential for alerting coworkers and reduced likelihood of a heated confrontation between the donor and the as-yet-uninformed employer. The federal regulations ask MROs to call the donor at least three times in 24 hours, using the donor's daytime and evening phone numbers.

The MRO must be accessible for call-backs. Some large providers of MRO services have MROs on-call after hours. Experienced MROs know they can be more effective by handling at least some MRO work during evenings and weekends. Methods for remaining accessible include a toll-free phone number for drug testing calls, and after-hours access through use of an answering service or a cellular telephone.

DER ASSISTANCE

If the MRO, after making reasonable efforts, has not contacted the donor within a reasonable time, the MRO (or MRO assistant) asks the DER for help reaching the donor. Under DOT rules, the MRO makes at least three attempts, within 24 hours, before asking the DER for help. In practice, there is little advantage to waiting; MROs should get DERs involved sooner, not later, in the process. In addition to helping expedite contact between the donor and MRO, the notification to the DER may stop the employer from mistakenly hiring a drug-positive applicant (should the employer assume no news is good news). It may also prompt the employer to remove a current, drug-positive employee from safety-sensitive duties pending completion of the MRO review, a process called "standing down" the employee (see Chapter 4). If the donor's phone numbers are missing or incorrect (e.g., disconnected, employee not known at that number), the MRO should immediately ask the DER for help, since waiting 24 hours serves no purpose. The

MRO does not tell the DER the test result is positive, adulterated, substituted, or invalid, although this is surely implied. The DER understands the situation and is supposed to keep this information confidential. The MRO documents the dates and times of attempts to contact, and actual contact with, the DER.

Once called, the DER is supposed to immediately try to contact the donor. The DER documents the dates and times of attempts, and actual contact with, the donor. Under DOT rules, the DER must make at least three attempts over 24 hours to reach the donor. If the DER is unable to directly contact the donor within this 24-hour period, the DER must leave a message for the donor by voice mail, e-mail, letter, or other means to contact the MRO. If the DER successfully contacts the donor, the DER tells the donor to call the MRO immediately and tells the donor that the MRO will declare the test positive if the donor fails to call the MRO. The DER also informs the MRO.

NONCONTACT POSITIVES, ADULTERATED, OR SUBSTITUTED RESULTS

The MRO can verify a positive, adulterated, or substituted result without interviewing the donor if reasonable efforts to perform that interview have failed. According to the DOT rules, the MRO can do this in only three circumstances:

1. The donor expressly declines to talk with the MRO.
2. The donor fails to contact the MRO within 72 hours after notification by the DER. These 72 hours should be a time period during which the MRO is accessible. This 72-hour clock starts when the DER establishes contact with the donor and not when the DER leaves a message for the donor. (According to the NRC rule, the MRO can verify a noncontact positive after 24 hours from contact by the DER [10 *CFR* §26.185(d)(3)].)
3. Despite reasonable attempts, neither the employer nor the MRO can contact the donor within 10 days of the date on which the MRO received the positive, adulterated, or substituted result.

In nonregulated testing no law imposes these time frames and some MROs report noncontact positives, adulterated, and substituted results more quickly, particularly for results that are rarely explainable. For example, if the donor has a highly safety-sensitive job (e.g., police officer) and the test is positive for a drug that is rarely explainable (e.g., cocaine), the MRO may report the result if the donor is unreachable after one or two tries. The MRO makes a more extensive effort to reach the donor if the test is positive for a commonly prescribed medication, or if split specimens were collected and the donor needs to be told of his/her right to the split test.

When reporting a verified, noncontact positive, adulterated, or substituted result, the MRO can tell the DER that the donor was not contacted. This should not affect the employer's actions except to make the DER aware in case the donor later contacts the DER. The MRO may re-open the verification process if, within 60 days from the date of verification, the donor presents documentation of a serious illness or injury or other extenuating circumstance that prevented timely contact with the MRO. After 60 days, the MRO cannot change a DOT verification decision without permission from the Office of Drug and Alcohol Policy and

Compliance (ODAPC). (See "Changing the Verification Decision" at the end of this chapter.)

INTERVIEW THE DONOR

"Mr. Perez, this is Dr. Hamilton at Industrial Medical in Springfield. I'm calling about a recent test you had at our clinic. I have your test result in front of me, and need to make sure it is yours. I have your social security number on the form. It reads: 1–3–3–5–5 [pause]. Would you please help me with the last four numbers, so that I know you are the correct Mr. Perez? [pause] 8-7-6-6? Yes, that's the number. I'm calling because the drug test you took on the 23rd came back positive for marijuana. The company doesn't know this yet. I'm telling you first. If there's any medicine you took that could have caused this, I need to know so that we can change the result to negative. I also must tell you that if I learn about any medical information affecting your ability to perform safety-sensitive duties, I will be obliged to notify your employer."

The MRO wants the donor's help in identifying and corroborating alternative medical explanations. A professional, nonconfrontational approach helps sustain dialogue with the donor and reinforces the credibility of the process. The MRO's interview with the donor is not a criminal investigation or a personal crusade. The donor is responsible for presenting alternative medical explanations and the MRO has some responsibility to help guide the donor through this process.

Identifying the Donor

The MRO does not initially know if the "John Citizen" who answers the phone is John Citizen Jr., John Citizen Sr., or someone else. The MRO should try to corroborate, using something other than the name, that the person who is on the phone is, in fact, the donor. For example, the MRO can read the first part of the donor's social security number (SSN) and ask for the latter part. If it turns out the number on the CCF is not the donor's actual SSN, the MRO should try some other item of information, like the donor's birthdate or the name and location of the collection site, to help establish that the correct John Doe is on the phone. This type of interchange also serves to alert the donor that the MRO knows something about him or her and thus helps establish the MRO's authenticity.

The donor's ID number is used as a pseudonym for the donor's name. The donor ID number is usually the donor's SSN, but in some cases is an employee ID number or even a made-up number. If the donor later alleges that the donor's ID number on the form is incorrect, the MRO or MRO assistant can point out that the donor has signed a statement on the CCF, ". . . the information provided on this form and on the label affixed to each specimen bottle is correct." Even if the donor refused to sign the statement and the refusal was documented, the incorrect ID number is still not a fatal flaw because it is the photo ID at the collection site, not the ID number, that is used to positively identify the donor.

Explaining the Process to the Donor

Under the DOT rule, at the start of the interview, the MRO must:

- Tell the donor the laboratory result. After telling the donor the drug(s) or the basis for a finding of adulteration, substitution, or invalid, the MRO should pause and wait for the donor's response. The tone and content of the donor's response may be revealing.

- Explain the interview process. The MRO should tell the donor at each step what will happen next and should give time frames. For example, "I will wait for you to call me back within 24 hours," or "My assistant will report this to the employer tomorrow morning."
- Explain that further medical evaluation may be required, and if the donor refuses such evaluation, it will lead to an adverse determination. The DOT rule directs the MRO to say this at the start of the interview. In practice many MROs reserve this only for the few cases where it applies, e.g., if the MRO requires an exam for an opiate-positive result.
- Explain that test result and medical information affecting the donor's medical qualification or performance of safety-sensitive duties will be reported to third parties, e.g., the employer, without the donor's consent. This process has been compared to reading the *Miranda* rights: "Anything you say can and will be used against you. . . ." The MRO is not expected to tell the donor precisely what information would trigger a medical qualification or safety issue.
- Explain that, if the donor is taking a legally prescribed medication that poses qualification or safety concerns, the MRO will allow the donor up to 5 days to have the prescribing physician contact the MRO to determine if another medication that does not pose qualification or safety concerns can be substituted.
- If the test is FAA regulated, the MRO asks the donor if he or she holds or would be required to hold an airman medical certificate. (If "yes," special reporting requirements apply, as described in the "Reporting MRO Results" section of this chapter.)

At this point in the interview, the MRO should give his or her name and phone number to the donor in the case the call gets disconnected or the donor chooses to call back for other reasons. Exchanging this information may also help build rapport.

Review the Collection Procedure

An MRO may ask the donor about the collection procedure. If the donor describes a proper collection procedure—the specimen did not leave his or her sight until it was sealed with tape, initialed by the donor, and placed in a box or plastic bag—documentation of this conversation can be helpful if the test is later challenged. If a significant issue is raised, such as an allegation that the unsealed specimen was left unattended on a counter with other unsealed specimens, the MRO may choose but is not obliged to check with the collector. If the MRO has concerns about the integrity of the specimen, the MRO can ask the laboratory to pull the specimen from the freezer and describe, over the phone, the bottle's appearance—for example, the donor's initials printed on the seal, the label with the accessioning number or some other kind of identification for reassurance that these specimens are intact. The MRO may not cancel or otherwise negate a test based on a significant collection error that is not documented on the CCF unless both the collector and donor acknowledge that the error took place. Otherwise, the MRO must base his or her review on the record as presented. If the donor and collector dispute what took place during the collection, the MRO has no role in resolving the dispute unless the answers can clearly be found in the test record. The MRO likewise does not cancel a test based on claims that the donor was tested in error. Instead, the MRO reviews the test and reports its outcome to the employer.

If the donor insists that the specimen was not his or hers, the MRO can remind the donor that he or she signed a statement on the CCF certifying that the specimen was his or hers.

The following sections describe procedures for review of positive, invalid, adulterated, and substituted results.

Positive Result Review ■

The MRO asks the donor if he or she has a legitimate medical explanation for the positive result. "Legitimate medical explanation" means a medication legally prescribed or given during a medical procedure [2]. This is usually straightforward with a verifiable explanation. For example, the donor tests positive for codeine, presents a prescription for codeine, and the MRO changes the result to negative. If the donor presents no legitimate medical explanation, the MRO reports the result as positive.

There is an important exception for codeine- and/or morphine-positive results. Some of these results are due to poppy seed ingestion. Therefore, a more complex process is required for reviewing these results, as described in the "Codeine/Morphine/6-AM Result Review" section of this chapter.

The NRC rule has this additional provision: The MRO may not change the result for a prescribed or over-the-counter medication to negative if the MRO has identified corroborating clinical evidence of abuse.

The MRO tells the donor what drug(s) were detected. This helps the donor present a legitimate explanation. If the donor presents a false explanation, this will be apparent when the donor cannot provide the MRO with acceptable corroboration of the explanation. The MRO should be nonjudgmental and nonconfrontational. The MRO can ask the donor if he or she used illicit drugs, but that question can make the donor defensive and raise barriers to further discussion. This is a style issue; some MROs ask donors if they used illicit drugs and others do not. The donor's admission to misuse of the drug may expedite the review, but the fundamental issue remains whether the donor has a legitimate medical explanation for the result. If the donor admits to misuse of a drug that was not detected by the test but which poses a likely safety risk or medical disqualification issue, the MRO can alert the employer as described later in this chapter. The MRO cannot, however, turn such an admission into a positive result for the drug if it was not detected by the test.

Donors who test positive for more notorious drugs (e.g., cocaine and methamphetamine) tend to be more confrontational and likely to challenge their results than those who test positive for less-notorious drugs (e.g., marijuana). Current employees are more likely than applicants to challenge positive results.

Table 10-2 presents medications sold in the United States that can cause confirmed positive drug test results for the drugs most often included in workplace drug testing panels. The MRO should ask what medications were taken, and should consider medications taken during the specimen's detection period. In urine testing, this period is typically no more than 2–3 days but can be longer for drugs that are fat-soluble and can accumulate in the body. Most drugs are essentially completely eliminated from the body within five half-lives. However,

Table 10-2. Medications Sold in United States That Can Cause Confirmed Positive Drug Test Results ■

In HHS Five-drug Panel?	Medications	Nonprescription Medications	Prescription Medications
YES	AMPHETAMINES		
	Amphetamine, methamphetamine	*l*-Methamphetamine Vicks Inhaler (and generic equivalents)	*l*-Amphetamine and *l*-methamphetamine Selegiline (Eldepryl, Ensam patch) is metabolized to *l*-methamphetamine and *l*-amphetamine
			l-Amphetamine and *d*-Amphetamine Adderall (approximately 3:1 mixture of *d*- to *l*-amphetamine)
			d-Amphetamine Dexedrine Dextrostat Vyvanse (lisdexamfetamine dimesylate) is metabolized to *d*-amphetamine
			d-Methamphetamine Desoxyn (This drug contains *d*-methamphetamine. It is metabolized to *d*-amphetamine.)
			d-Amphetamine and *d*-methamphetamine Didrex (benzphetamine) is metabolized to *d*-methamphetamine and *d*-amphetamine
NO	BARBITURATES		
	Butabarbital	None	Pyridium Plus
	Butalbital	None	Esgic and Esgic-Plus Fioricet Fiorinal Phrenilin and Phrenilin Forte Zebutal
	Pentobarbital	None	Nembutal
	Phenobarbital	None	Bellamine Bellaspas Bellergal Dilantin with phenobarbital Donnatal Duragal-S Mebaral (mephobarbital) is metabolized to phenobarbital Spastrin

Table 10-2. continued ■

In HHS Five-drug Panel?	Medications	Nonprescription Medications	Prescription Medications
<u>NO</u>	BENZODIAZEPINES		
	Alprazolam	None	Niravan Xanax
	Chlordiazepoxide	None	Librax Librium Limbitrol
	Clonazepam	None	Klonopin
	Clorazepate	None	Tranxene
	Diazepam	None	Diastat Valium
	Estazolam	None	<available as generic>
	Temazepam	None	Restoril
yes	Cocaine	None	Cocaine hydrochloride, solution or viscous, used as a vasoconstrictive anesthetic, e.g., in otolaryngology, ophthalmology, and dentistry TAC (tetracaine, adrenaline, and cocaine mixture used in some emergency rooms as a topical anesthetic, e.g., before suturing) Brompton's Cocktail (contains an opiate—usually morphine—and cocaine and/or a phenothiazine; used for pain control of the terminally ill)
yes	Marijuana	None	Dronabinol Marinol Marijuana Several states allow use of marijuana for certain medical conditions under a physician's direction. These laws do not supersede DOT's position that marijuana is not an acceptable medical explanation for a positive result
no	Methaqualone	None	None

continues

Table 10-2. continued ■

In HHS Five-drug Panel?	Medications	Nonprescription Medications	Prescription Medications
	OPIOIDS		
no	Buprenorphine	None	Burprenex Suboxone Subutex
yes	Codeine	Several states allow over-the-counter sales of codeine-containing cough medicines, such as those listed to the right	Cheratussin with codeine Fioricet with codeine Fiorinal with codeine Halotussin-AC syrup Nucofed Promethazine VC with codeine Robitussin-AC and -DAC syrup Soma with codeine Tylenol with codeine
no	Fentanyl	None	Actiq Duragesic Fentora Ionsys Transdermal System Onsolis Sublimaze
no	Hydrocodone	None	Anexsia CodiCLEAR DH Entex HC Hycodan Hycotuss Hydromet Lorcet Lortab Maxidone Norco Reprexain Tussigon Tussionex Pennkinetic Vicodin Vicoprofen Zydone
no	Hydromorphone	None	Dilaudid
no	Meperidine	None	Demerol Meprozinel
no	Methadone	None	Dolophine Methadose

Table 10-2. continued ■

In HHS Five-drug Panel?	Medications	Nonprescription Medications	Prescription Medications
yes	Morphine	Donnagel-PG Infantol Pink Kaodene with paregoric Quiagel PG	Astramorph PF Avinza Brompton's Cocktail (contains an opiate—usually morphine or heroin—and cocaine and/or a phenothiazine) DepoDur Duramorph Embeda Infumorph Kadian MS Contin Oramorph Roxanol and Roxanol 100
yes	Opium (codeine and morpine)	None	B&O suppositories Paregoric
no	Oxycodone	None	Combunox Endocet Endodan Oxycontin OxyIR Percocet Percodan Roxicet Roxicodone Roxilox Tylox
no	Oxymorphone	None	Opana
no	Propoxyphene	None	Darvocet Darvon

the cutoffs used in workplace testing are higher than the limits of detection, and this has the effect of reducing windows of detection to less than five half-lives. Table 10-3 presents the length of time various drugs can be detected in urine.

The donor may have listed, before the analysis, medications that he or she recently took, but these lists can be incomplete or inaccurate. The MRO may review the list with the donor and use it to help refresh the donor's memory about what drugs he or she may have taken. MROs can help donors by suggesting pertinent, common drugs (Did you take Valium?) or medical conditions (Do you take medication for migraines?). The DOT rule allows the MRO to give the donor up to 5 days to present the MRO with alternative explanation(s) and corroborating evidence. During this time, the donor can check with his or her physician(s) about medication(s) that may have been prescribed. The MRO can conclude the verification process in less than 5 days. MROs should conclude reviews promptly when the positives are for drugs that are rarely or never prescribed (e.g., heroin,

Table 10-3. Detection Periods of Drugs in Urine ▪

Drug(s)	Approximate Detection Period
Alcohol	7–12 hours
Amphetamine, methamphetamine	2–4 days
Barbiturates	
Short-acting (e.g., pentobarbital)	24 hrs
Long-acting (e.g., phenobarbital)	3 wks
Benzodiazepines	
Short-acting (e.g., lorazepam)	3 d
Long-acting (e.g., diazepam)	3 wk (longer after extended use)
Cocaine metabolite (benzoylecognine)	2–4 d
Marijuana (cannabinoids)	
Single use	3 d
Moderate use (four times/wk)	5–7 d
Daily use	10–15 d
Long-term heavy smoker	> 30 d
Opioids	
Codeine, morphine	2–3 d
Hydrocodone	24 hrs
Hydromorphone	48 hrs
Methadone	3 d
Oxycodone	2–4 d
Propoxyphene	6–48 hrs
Phencyclidine	8 d

cocaine, marijuana) and should allow more time for reviews of results for drugs that are commonly prescribed (e.g., codeine).

POSITIVE FOR THE SAME DRUG, AGAIN

The MRO may recognize the donor from a previous test that was positive for the same drug where the MRO changed the result to negative because of a verified medical explanation. While that same explanation may account for the current positive result, the federal rules do not authorize MROs to skip interviews based on information from past reviews. The MRO is obliged to interview the donor again, at least in federally regulated testing.

The federal rules give MROs discretion in how they corroborate the authenticity of prescriptions. If the MRO has recently verified the authenticity of a prescription for a previous test, the MRO could reference that with a comment in the current test file, rather than reverifying the authenticity of the prescription. After some period of time—for example, 12 months—the MRO would no longer rely on the old verification and would want to reverify the authenticity of the prescription.

Unapproved Use of Prescription Medication ▪

People sometimes obtain and take prescription drugs in unconventional ways that fall somewhere between use as prescribed and abuse. This is an issue that arises more often when testing for prescription drugs beyond the HHS five panel.

Few employer policies define when prescription drug use is acceptable and when it is not. If the policy addresses this, or if the employer representative offers an opinion, that policy or opinion typically prohibits anything but use of one's medication as prescribed. More often, the MRO is wholly responsible for deciding if an explanation is acceptable. Employers typically treat all positives the same, whether caused by illegal drug use or unapproved use of prescription drugs. The punishment (loss of employment) may seem out of proportion to the crime (e.g., borrowing someone else's Tylenol with codeine). Should the donor then be referred for treatment, it seems unclear what treatment to offer if the infraction was a judgment error and not addiction or abuse of illicit drugs.

The specimen collection procedure can establish chain of custody. The laboratory analysis can definitively identify the drug. The MRO's decision about a positive result caused by unapproved prescription medication use varies depending on the situation and the MRO. While individual MROs may act consistently, there remains concern among the MRO community about inconsistency among MROs. Inconsistencies are tolerated and expected in clinical practice—for example, when assessing work fitness after a low back strain. By contrast, MROs and other drug testing service providers pride themselves for making precise, rule-driven decisions as part of a process fundamentally designed to detect illicit drug use.

There are limited applicable federal rules and guidelines. In some situations, the decision is left to the MRO's judgment. While there is some solace in any MRO who takes a consistent approach in his or her reviews, the real issue is inconsistency between MROs in handling ambiguous situations. To promote consistency, the following sections offer guidelines for MRO reviews of certain types of unapproved prescription drug use.

BORROWED MEDICATION

About a third of adults and a smaller proportion of adolescents admit to use of medicine borrowed from family members, friends, and other acquaintances, usually for convenience rather than recreational use [3,4,5]. The proper and intended medical purpose of a prescribed drug is that it be used by the person for whom it was prescribed. There is no guarantee that it will be effective or safe for use by someone else. Federal law prohibits sharing of prescribed controlled substances. Prescriptions for controlled substances in Schedules II, III, and IV are labeled "Caution: Federal law prohibits the transfer of this drug to any person other than the patient for whom it was prescribed" [21 *CFR* §290.5]. Federal law also prohibits possession of a controlled substance that has not been legitimately prescribed, i.e., "It shall be unlawful for any person knowingly or intentionally to possess a controlled substance unless such substance was obtained directly, or pursuant to a valid prescription or order, from a practitioner, while acting in the course of his professional practice" [21 U.S.C. §844]. DOT also does not sanction the use of borrowed medication. In its 1990 *Medical Review Officer Guide*, DOT advised MROs, "An employee who acknowledges taking another individual's controlled substance prescribed medication has admitted unauthorized use of a controlled substance and the positive result should be verified positive."

Virtually all MROs reject explanations of borrowed prescription medication. In some reviews, the MRO often has to draw out the "confession" of borrowed medicine during the interview, for example, "Did you borrow anyone else's Tylenol 3?" The MRO then accepts the confession as fact and declares the result positive, often to the donor's surprise. This feels like entrapment. This is especially consequential for results that are morphine/codeine-positive at concentrations below 15,000 ng/mL. As described in the "Codeine/Morphine/6-AM Result Review" section of this chapter, this result is assumed to represent poppy seed ingestion unless the MRO identifies clinical evidence of opiate abuse. Had the donor instead offered no explanation, the MRO would have changed the result to negative based on the assumption of poppy seed ingestion. However if a donor admits use of borrowed medication or, in a panic lies and says he or she borrowed medication, the MRO verifies it as positive because the admission of unauthorized use is considered clinical evidence of abuse.

Any MRO who is willing to consider borrowed medication as a potential legitimate explanation should do so only for nonregulated tests and only if:

1. The MRO obtains written proof that the donor's physician told the donor, prior to the test, to borrow that medication.
2. The donor has an unfilled, recent prescription for the same medication in his/her name but took someone else's medicine for convenience or to save money.
3. The employer asks the MRO to make an exception and the MRO is willing to make that exception. The MRO should first corroborate, with help from the prescription's actual designee, that the prescription was valid for that designee.

INTERNET MEDICATION

According to guidance DOT issued in June 2006, an MRO is authorized to accept a donor's prescription for medication obtained over the Internet only if there is proof that a legitimate doctor-patient relationship was established. This guidance further states that a legitimate doctor-patient relationship has these elements:

- A patient has a medical complaint.
- A medical history was taken.
- A physical examination was performed.
- Some logical connection exists between the complaint, the medical history, the physical examination, and the drug prescribed.

Some Internet pharmacies feign a doctor-patient relationship by asking customers to complete online questionnaires that physicians working for the websites review later. This does not establish a proper doctor-patient relationship. The American Medical Association (AMA) and the Food and Drug Administration have said that physicians who issue prescriptions without personally examining patients are engaging in substandard care. Some state laws can be interpreted as requiring a face-to-face medical evaluation to establish a doctor-patient relationship in which medications can be prescribed.

The MRO should consider the following items when reviewing the validity of a donor's prescription obtained over the Internet:

- The name, physical location, and state(s) of licensure of the prescribing practitioner.

- Whether the donor was professionally evaluated for the current medical complaint by the prescribing practitioner, and the last time the donor was in direct contact with the prescribing practitioner.
- Whether the donor initiated the request to the pharmacy for a particular medication.
- Whether a proper doctor-patient relationship existed.

It is the donor's responsibility to provide sufficient documentation to answer these inquiries. If the donor did not originally get the prescription from a local health care provider, the MRO will typically reject this explanation and report the result as positive.

FOREIGN MEDICATION

If the donor says he or she obtained the medication abroad, the MRO should ask for a copy of the medication label. The label lets the MRO verify the medication's identity and, possibly, the ingredients. The MRO might desire additional input from that provider, but this is often impractical if not impossible because of communication barriers. The MRO should also ask for documentation of travel abroad. The MRO should consider if travel dates are consistent with the claimed use and drug's detection period. MROs should also remember that certain drugs sold by prescription in the United States are dispensed over the counter in some foreign countries.

DOT directs MROs to *not* accept the use of substances that are Controlled Substance Act (CSA) Schedule I, i.e., deemed to have no legitimate medical use in the United States. The MRO must reject any such explanation even if the medication was obtained in a country where it is legal.

Use of Medication Abroad
If a donor says that he or she obtained and used the medication abroad, the MRO should change the result to negative if the MRO corroborates the prescription (or, if over the counter, the travel).

Use in the United States of Medication Obtained Abroad
If a donor says that he or she recently obtained the medication abroad and used it in the United States, the MRO should change the result to negative if the MRO gets corroboration that the donor obtained the medication while recently traveling abroad. This recommendation is consistent with the FDA's "Coverage of Personal Importations" policy, which allows the consumer to import up to a 90-day personal supply of medication if he or she provides evidence that the medication is for the continuation of treatment begun in a foreign country. The MRO should extend the time frame if the medication is one that was prescribed for use on as-needed basis.

The DOT rule asks MROs to consider whether medicines from foreign countries have been obtained legally and used for their intended purposes [49 *CFR* §40.137(d)]. Some foreign medications that are prohibited in the United States nevertheless slip by customs inspectors during reentry screening. The MRO role does not include border enforcement. MROs should apply the same principles as with any other review; if the medicine was obtained legally abroad and the donor can prove this, the MRO should change the result to negative.

Some imported dietary supplements, most notoriously weight-loss products from Brazil and products from China, have been found to illegally contain amphetamine or benzodiazepines [6]. Use of non-prescribed, drug-containing supplements is not considered a legitimate medical explanation for a positive DOT drug test.

OLD MEDICATION

The donor may say he or she took an old prescription, perhaps for a new illness or injury. There is no law that prohibits the use of one's old medication. No law prohibits use of one's medication for a different reason than that for which it was prescribed. Can a medication be too old to explain a drug test result? If so, how old is "too old"? Opinions vary. While medication labels list expiration dates, these dates refer to its shelf life based on the manufacturer's recommendations for chemical and physical stability. In most cases, actual drug stability exceeds the listed expiration date.

From 2006–2009, the FMCSA has posted the following interpretation on its website:

> **91. Can a driver be certified who tests positive for a controlled substance on the urine test, but claims that the prescription was legally prescribed 5 years before?**
>
> No. Controlled substances expire no later than 1 year after the date of the original prescription.

FMCSA took this position because it thought it unwise for commercial motor vehicle drivers to take medicines prescribed to them long ago. FMCSA's position was based in part by safety concerns over use of prescription drugs without a physician's direction and oversight. In addition, February 2007 guidelines from the Office of National Drug Control Policy urge disposal of unused, unneeded, or expired prescription drugs to help combat diversion and abuse. FMCSA removed this interpretation from its website in 2009 without comment and no longer offers an opinion about how old is too old.

Some MROs accept prescriptions older than 1 year as legitimate medical explanations. An argument could be made that drug testing is supposed to identify substance abuse, whereas substance abusers probably use up their drugs instead of storing them for years.

Some MROs worry that if they accept old prescriptions, then one valid prescription for a controlled substance could be a life-long pass to abuse of that drug without risk of failing a drug test. This theory has little credence because donors rarely present MROs with prescriptions that are more than a year or two old. More often, donors who say they took old medications are unable to present MROs with labels or other corroboration of those explanations, and the MROs therefore reject their explanations.

In addition to reporting the result as positive or negative, the MRO has the opportunity to consider a safety warning or other notification to the employer about the use of any medication outside of current treatment and its potential impact on safety.

TOO MUCH MEDICATION

The donor may say he or she took excessive doses of medication, but, if later challenged, might deny this. The MRO may suspect the drug or metabolite concentration is unusually high. Nevertheless, one cannot determine the drug dose based on the urine concentration from a workplace test result. If the donor has a prescription that accounts for the result, the MRO should change the result to negative. If the MRO suspects, after an interview or a clinical evaluation of the donor, overuse of the medication and a likely safety risk, the MRO should notify the employer or other responsible authority.

SELF-PRESCRIBED MEDICATION

Some physicians prescribe or dispense medications for themselves and their family members. Ethical guidelines discourage this. Most state medical licensing boards restrict physicians from treating or prescribing for themselves and family members except in emergencies. Some states restrict prescribing to situations where there is a doctor/patient relationship. DOT directs MROs to accept prescriptions only if they are prescribed within the context of a legitimate doctor-patient relationship and legal. Self-prescribed medication is not within the context of a legitimate doctor-patient relationship and some state laws specifically declare it illegal. MROs should therefore reject it as an explanation for a positive workplace drug test result.

MEDICAL MARIJUANA

As of early 2010, 14 states permit use of marijuana for certain medical reasons. These states are Alaska, California, Colorado, Hawaii, Maine, Michigan, Montana, New Jersey, Nevada, New Mexico, Oregon, Rhode Island, Vermont, and Washington. Marijuana remains illegal under federal law. That is, federal and state laws conflict. Federal drug testing regulators naturally take positions consistent with federal law, i.e., that use of marijuana or any other drug listed in Schedule I of the CSA is not a legitimate medical explanation for a positive drug test. Most MROs follow the federal directive in nonregulated programs, too, unless the employer's policy explicitly allows use of medical marijuana. Figure 10-2 illustrates the MRO's process for reviewing medical marijuana explanations.

Few employers address medical marijuana in their policies. If pressed, few employers will accept medical marijuana, and many defer to the MRO's judgment, which invariably means a positive result. Some states have included in their laws provisions whereby employers do not have to accommodate medical marijuana use. The case law about this issue is scant but supports an employer's decision to reject medical marijuana as an explanation for positive results in their testing programs.

Drugs versus Metabolites ■

Prescription Drug A may be metabolized to prescription Drug B. The presence of Drug B may then be attributable to use of Drug A or use of Drug B. MROs face this issue most often with amphetamines, benzodiazepines, and opioids. For example, hydrocodone (Vicodin) is metabolized to hydromorphone (Dilaudid). If a donor takes hydrocodone and produces a hydromorphone-positive specimen, is this attributable to just hydrocodone use? Because the presence of metabolites can be interpreted as unauthorized use of a prescription drug and may result in penalty, it is essential that MROs be aware of these conversions and correctly

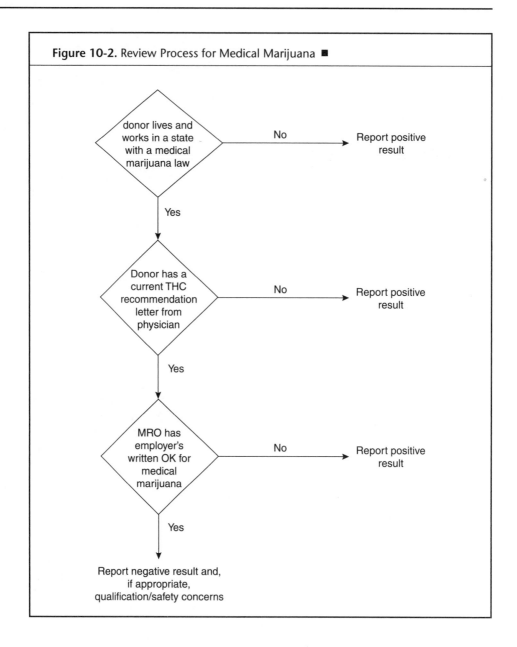

Figure 10-2. Review Process for Medical Marijuana ■

donor lives and works in a state with a medical marijuana law

No → Report positive result

Yes ↓

Donor has a current THC recommendation letter from physician

No → Report positive result

Yes ↓

MRO has employer's written OK for medical marijuana

No → Report positive result

Yes ↓

Report negative result and, if appropriate, qualification/safety concerns

interpret results. The opioid profiles in Chapter 13 offer some guidelines for evaluating positive results for opioid drug/metabolite combinations. Identifying the source can be difficult and sometimes impossible. The MRO should assume that the metabolite is from use of the parent drug unless there is unequivocal evidence otherwise.

Corroboration of Explanations for Positive Results ■

The MRO verifies the authenticity of any prescribed medication that the donor claims use of and which could explain the test result. The MRO needs to confirm that the medication was prescribed or dispensed to the donor prior to the date of the test. The process for verification is largely left to the MRO's judgment. The DOT rule says the MRO must take "reasonable and necessary steps" to verify medical explanations. The donor is responsible for helping the MRO obtain verification of the prescription. MROs should make this clear to donors, lest the donors believe their responsibility ends with giving the MRO the name and phone number of their doctor or pharmacy.

Verification can be made in various ways. If the MRO is located close to the donor, the donor can bring the prescription bottle to the MRO's office. However, most MRO reviews are handled by phone, often from far away. Like the interviews, medication verifications are made from a distance, by phone call or fax.

Forgery or other fakery is always possible, especially for drugs of abuse (e.g., cocaine). The lengths to which an MRO should go, and the time allowed for the donor to present information, to verify a medical explanation is left to the MRO's judgement. If the explanation seems far fetched and the donor's job is highly safety-sensitive, the MRO may tell the donor that he or she must promptly provide information to corroborate the explanation. On the other hand, if the explanation is likely to be true and the donor has a non-safety-sensitive job, the MRO may allow longer to get the corroborating information. The DOT states that MROs can wait up to 5 days for this information. Without the information, the MRO should reject the explanation.

The MRO should remember that last names can change, e.g., with marriage. For example, if an MRO calls a pharmacy to corroborate a medication and the pharmacist does not recognize the donor's name, the MRO should consider whether the donor's last name may have changed.

WRITTEN CORROBORATION

The MRO can use a copy of the medication label, a receipt, or a faxed letter or copy of relevant medical records to corroborate the donor's explanation. While the MRO and donor may discuss "the prescription," a copy of an unfilled prescription obviously cannot account for the presence of a drug in the donor's specimen. If the written documentation is a letter or medical records from the prescribing health care provider, that information should be transmitted directly from the health care provider to the MRO. A letter that is not on office letterhead or a fax that did not come directly from a health care provider's office should prompt a follow-up telephone call to confirm its authenticity. The most reliable corroboration is probably a copy of the actual medical record documenting the prescription and transmitted directly from the treating health care provider to the MRO. Personal physicians may go to great lengths writing letters to help out their patients, but would not falsify their medical records.

PHOTO CORROBORATION

The donor may photograph the label or prescription receipt by cell phone and send that photograph to the MRO's cell phone or e-mail address. The MRO can forward picture messages from a cell phone to an e-mail address so that they can be stored on and printed from a computer. Photographs are usually blurry but legible enough to corroborate the prescription. The blurry pictures may validate their legitimacy because fake (e.g., computer-altered) photos are more clear. The danger of this is that an occasional angry donor will spam the MRO's cell phone number or e-mail address.

TELEPHONE CORROBORATION

Most MROs accept telephonic verification from the dispensing pharmacist or prescribing practitioner to corroborate prescriptions, particularly for drugs that are commonly prescribed and of low-abuse potential, e.g., codeine, Adderall. It is usually easier to get the information from the pharmacist instead of the physician or other prescriber. Telephonic corroboration is usually easier and quicker than written corroboration, but may carry a greater risk of deception. This risk can be reduced by asking the donor for details about his or her prescription—for example, the prescription number, name of the medicine, prescribing physician's name, the name and phone number of the pharmacy, and the date the prescription was filled—and then verifying this information with the pharmacy. Also, the MRO can cross-check the prescribing health care professional's name with listings of licensees posted by state agencies. If an MRO is speaking with the prescribing physician but has doubts about whether the person on the phone is actually a physician, the MRO can ask for that physician's DEA number. The second digit of the number should be the first letter of the physician's last name.

The openness of pharmacists to divulging customers' medications to MROs varies. Some will do this without the customer's consent. Some want the customer's written consent first. The MRO can usually facilitate this by asking the donor to first authorize the pharmacist or prescribing health care provider to divulge the information to the MRO. The MRO would instruct the donor as follows: "I am going to call the pharmacist and corroborate the prescription, but the pharmacist needs your permission to speak with me about this. Please call the pharmacist and explain that you had a positive drug test because of that medicine and that I need to speak with him or her. Ask for the pharmacist's name and give the pharmacist permission to speak with me about the medicine. Then, call me with the pharmacist's name and phone number. As soon as you do, I will call the pharmacist and get corroboration of the medicine." Once the donor has done this and called the MRO, the MRO calls the pharmacist to confirm the prescription. "This is Dr. Smith. I am calling to confirm that Joe Donor received Tylenol 3 last month that had been prescribed by Dr. Welby. Can you confirm this for me, please?"

Passive Exposure ∎

The federal cutoff levels for urine tests are set high enough to prevent positive results caused by passive exposure to drugs, such as may occur by touching drugs or breathing in second-hand smoke. DOT has told MROs that passive exposure is not a legitimate medical explanation and is not cause for changing a positive result to negative. In the absence of unusually intense or recent environmental exposure, and with use of appropriate cutoffs, passive exposure does not appear to cause positive results for hair or oral fluid. This is discussed in greater detail in Chapter 12 and in the amphetamines, cocaine, and marijuana sections of Chapter 13. In any event, passive exposure is not a medical explanation and should be rejected by MROs reviewing positive hair or oral fluid test results.

Illicit Drugs In Foods And Beverages ∎

The DOT rule [49 *CFR* §40.151(d)] and the HHS *Medical Review Officer Manual* instruct the MRO to disregard claims that positive results for marijuana or cocaine metabolite were caused by unknowing consumption of the drugs in food or beverages. MROs and employers are not equipped to determine the truth of any such explanations. Furthermore, consumption of marijuana or cocaine in a food or beverage is not a legitimate medical explanation.

Some workplace testing policies state that ingestion of THC and cocaine in food or beverages *is not* an acceptable explanation for a positive result, but most policies do not address this issue. MROs invariably follow the federal lead and reject such explanations for nonregulated tests. MROs are under no obligation to test a donor's food or beverage product for suspected drug(s). The sections on cocaine and marijuana in Chapter 13 discuss use of these drugs in foods and beverages.

SPIKED DRINKS

The issue of spiked drinks has become notorious in cases of date rape in which a short-acting sedative—for example, flunitrazepam or gamma hydroxybutyrate—has been added to drinks of unsuspecting young women. Some drugs can be added to drinks and consumed by unsuspecting victims. This is not a legitimate medical explanation. The MRO cannot assess the truthfulness of such claims and, if anything, might suggest to the donor that he or she notify law enforcement of the crime.

Codeine/Morphine/6-AM Result Review ∎

The approach to reviewing codeine-, morphine-, and/or 6-AM positive results depends on which of these was detected and, for codeine and morphine, the concentrations.

6-AM Positive
The presence of 6-AM indicates heroin use, without regard to the morphine and codeine concentrations. The MRO allows the donor an opportunity for an interview. The donor will have no legitimate medical explanation. The MRO informs the donor of the result and, if applicable, informs the donor of his or her right to a split test. The MRO then reports the result as positive for 6-AM.

6-AM Negative, Morphine/Codeine-Positive at <15,000 ng/mL
In regulated testing, when the results are morphine/codeine-positive at concentrations below 15,000 ng/mL and 6-AM negative, the MRO can verify these results as positive only if there is corroborating, clinical evidence of opiate misuse. These results are considered consistent with poppy seed ingestion and are insufficient by themselves to establish drug misuse. Poppy seeds contain small amounts of morphine and smaller amounts of codeine. Ingestion of normal dietary amounts of poppy seeds can cause morphine-positive urine drug test results and sometimes detectable amounts of codeine. Typical morphine concentrations after poppy seed ingestion are no higher than several hundred. There are isolated reports of concentrations exceeding 10,000 ng/mL, but never as high as 15,000 ng/mL [7].

Poppy seed ingestion is assumed to be a potential cause for these results even if the donor does not remember eating poppy seeds. Employers cannot reasonably prohibit poppy seed ingestion. MROs cannot rule out poppy seed ingestion based on the donor's recall, because many foods contain poppy seeds and people may not know or remember. The science shows that results where codeine predominates are inconsistent with poppy seed ingestion [8]. Nevertheless, under the federal rules, the MRO is compelled to change a morphine/codeine result below 15,000 ng/mL to negative unless there is corroborating clinical evidence of unauthorized opiate use, even if the concentrations suggest codeine use.

Many MROs follow the regulated approach for nonregulated urine test results with morphine/codeine less than 15,000 ng/mL and change these results to negative unless there is corroborating clinical evidence of opiate misuse. No doubt this has allowed many people who "misuse" codeine to evade detection because their concentrations did not exceed 15,000 ng/mL. On the other hand, codeine is a medication that is more often used unconventionally but without illicit intent, e.g., use of old/borrowed/foreign/etc.

Clinical evidence of unauthorized opiate use often consists of the donor's admission of unauthorized use of a prescription opiate, e.g., use of someone else's medicine. Clinical evidence could come from a physical examination that looks for needle-track marks from heroin abuse, but physical examinations are not required, uncommon, and rarely productive. If the donor offers no clinical evidence of abuse during the interview, the MRO can change the opiate result to negative. There is no requirement that the MRO conduct, or arrange for, a physical examination. The need for a physical examination seems more compelling if the morphine concentration is closer to 15,000 ng/mL and less compelling if the morphine concentration is low, particularly if the donor says he or she ate poppy seeds.

A physical examination for clinical signs of opiate abuse can be conducted by the MRO or by another physician selected by the MRO. The examiner need not be a specialist in addiction medicine. Observations by the employee's supervisors or by nonprofessional staff at the collection site are useful only to the extent that they may supplement clinical evidence of recent use as observed by the examiner. If the MRO directs the donor to undergo a physical exam and the donor fails to follow through, the MRO reports the outcome as a refusal to test. The DOT rule allows an exception for *pre-offer* tests where donors fail to undergo required exams; the MRO reports these as canceled.

If the employee both has a legitimate medical explanation for the result *and* the MRO identifies clinical evidence of unauthorized use that could account for the result, the MRO should report the result as positive only if the clinical evidence is unequivocal.

The preceding paragraphs refer to urine tests. The issue is less well settled for oral fluid and hair tests. There are limited data that suggest that poppy seed ingestion may cause a morphine-positive oral fluid result using a confirmation cutoff of 40 ng/mL, albeit only for up to 1 hour after ingestion [9]. There are limited data that suggest that poppy seed ingestion would not cause a morphine-positive hair result using typical cutoffs [10].

6-AM Negative, Morphine or Codeine ≥ 15,000 ng/mL

Use of a controlled substance is the assumed cause of morphine/codeine-positive urine test results with concentrations at or above 15,000 ng/mL. Poppy seed ingestion does not cause concentrations this high. Table 10.2 lists controlled substances that contain morphine, codeine, or opium. In some states, these drugs can be obtained in small amounts over the counter. The purchaser must sign a bound record book at the pharmacy; thus, there is some record of the purchase that the MRO can use to corroborate this explanation.

Outcome: Positive, Negative, or Cancelled ■

For each lab-positive result, the MRO determines if the outcome is negative, positive, or cancelled. The MRO's verification decision must be consistent with applicable laws, e.g., DOT. The MRO's decision should also be reasonably consistent with the employer's policy. Employer policies do not preempt federal drug testing rules nor should they preempt the MRO's professional judgment and standards of practice, as reflected in MRO training courses and publications. MROs are expected to maintain high standards, even if those standards put them in conflict with donors or employers. The MRO should not be influenced by what action the client may take. The MRO should not be critically influenced by perceptions of the donor's honesty.

Invalid Result Review ■

The MRO asks the donor what medications he or she took and tries to determine if the donor has a medical explanation for the invalid result. If the MRO identifies *no* medical explanation (this is usually the case), the MRO cancels the test and asks the employer to immediately retest the donor under direct observation. If the MRO *does* identify a medical explanation, the MRO merely cancels the test. The employer retests the donor only if the employer needs a negative result, e.g., for preemployment purposes. (Slightly different procedures may apply for the second of two consecutive invalid results, as described later in this chapter.)

The DOT rule directs the laboratory to contact the MRO to determine if further testing is necessary, for example, at another laboratory. In practice, laboratories do not call MROs and instead print comments on the invalid reports inviting MROs to call them. The MRO may learn from the laboratory that it suspects an unidentified adulterant because there was interference with the immunoassay or confirmation assay—or the MRO may learn that the immunoassay interference looked like that seen from use of certain prescription drugs.

The DOT rule directs the MRO to interview the donor and ask about medications. (This contact should follow any discussion with the laboratory, since information from the laboratory may influence the interview.) In doing so, the MRO should explain about potential disclosure of safety-related medical information, as described earlier in this chapter. The MRO tells the donor that the specimen was invalid and why. The MRO can ask the donor if he or she adulterated or substituted the specimen, but some MROs find this too blunt. In the unlikely event that the donor admits to adulteration or substitution of the specimen, the MRO carefully documents what the donor said, adds an explanatory remark (e.g., "Adulterated with a product Mr. Jones says he purchased over the Internet") and reports the outcome as "Refusal to Test" rather than "Test Cancelled." In the unlikely event that the donor admits to using a drug, the MRO carefully documents what the donor said and reports that admission to the employer, but still reports the test result as cancelled and asks the employer to immediately retest the donor under direct observation.

The following sections describe procedures for MRO review of different types of invalid urine drug test results. MRO review procedures for non-urine specimens should parallel those described here.

LOW CREATININE, LOW SPECIFIC GRAVITY, OR POSSIBLE ADULTERANT

If one but not both of the creatinine and specific gravity values are in the substituted range, this suggests but does not prove the specimen was substituted. If an adulterant is suspected but the specimen does not meet criteria for adulteration, this suggests but does not prove adulteration. The MRO's discussions with the laboratory and donor are unlikely to produce a medical explanation for the result. With no medical explanation for this type of result, the MRO reports the result as cancelled and asks the DER to immediately retest the donor under direct observation.

ABNORMAL pH

The invalid pH range is ≥ 3.0 and < 4.5, or ≥ 9.0 and < 11.0. These values are not definitive evidence of adulteration and thus warrant recollection under direct observation. An exception can be made for pH values in the 9.9–9.5 range, as follows.

If more than a day elapsed between collection and laboratory receipt of the specimen, the pH can rise into the 9.0–9.5 range due to the effects of microbial action. This is especially likely if the specimen was left unrefrigerated, but MROs may not know if specimens were refrigerated or not. MROs *do* know how many days elapsed between collection and laboratory receipt; the dates are printed on the lab report and CCF. An interval of more than a day, particularly if the specimen was left unrefrigerated, should be considered a medical explanation for a pH in the 9.0–9.5 range, and thus warrants cancellation without recollection unless a negative test result is required [11].

BOTTLE A AND BOTTLE B: DIFFERENT PHYSICAL CHARACTERISTICS OR ABNORMAL PHYSICAL CHARACTERISTICS

Because split specimens are supposed to come from a single urine void, Bottles A and B should have similar appearance and other physical characteristics. The MRO should notify the donor if the laboratory reports that Bottles A and B have different physical characteristics or if both have abnormal physical characteristics. The MRO should ask the donor if he or she has any explanation. If the abnormality is different characteristics between Bottle A and B, the MRO can ask the donor to describe the collection procedures to ascertain if there were two separate collections or one collection that was split. The federal rules do not allow a separate collection for each bottle in a split specimen test, but this may still happen in error. If the MRO determines that two voids were probably used instead of one void that was split, the MRO cancels the test, a retest under direct observation is not required, and the collector should undergo corrective training (as described in Chapter 6).

Unusual urine color may be due to use of a prescription medication that discolors urine [12]. If the abnormal appearance involves unusual color, the MRO should consider whether the donor's medications may have caused this finding. Blue/green urine color can be caused by use of amitryptilline, doxorubicin, indomethacin, methenamine, and methylene blue. Orange urine color can be caused by use of laxatives, pyridium, rifampin, and warfarin.

Urine Color	Medication(s)
Blue/green	amitriptyline
	doxorubicin
	indomethacin
	methenamine
	methylene blue
Orange	laxatives
	pyridium
	rifampin
	warfarin

Immunoassay Interference or Gas Chromatography/Mass Spectrometry Interference

Use of certain medications can cause interference with immunoassays, particularly the enzyme multiplied immunoassay test (EMIT). Table 10-4 presents examples of these. (Analytic interference from medication use is not observed in confirmatory assays.) If the donor claims use of an interfering medication, the MRO should seek independent corroboration of this claim, as described later in this chapter. The MRO may ask the laboratory to reanalyze the specimen using a different immunoassay to try to get a valid result. Some immunoassays are more susceptible than others to particular types of interference.

OUTCOME: TEST CANCELLED WITH REMARKS

If all of the assay results are invalid and the donor has not admitted to adulterating or substituting the specimen, the MRO checks the "Test Cancelled" box and writes "Invalid Result" on the Remarks line of the Copy 2 of the CCF. The MRO also enters either of two comments on the Remarks line:

- "Direct observation not required" if the donor gave an acceptable explanation for the result, e.g., medication interference. The employer retests the donor if a negative result is needed, e.g., for preemployment purposes. The donor cannot be required to stop taking his or her prescription medicine, but if the donor stops taking it, any retest should be delayed a few days to allow for its elimination.
- "Recollect under direct observation" if no valid explanation for the result has been identified. The employer attaches no consequence to the invalid result other than recollecting immediately under direct observation. The donor is not entitled to a split test for an invalid result.

A specimen can have one or more assays that are positive, adulterated, or substituted and others that are invalid. The MRO reports any positive, adulterated, or

Table 10-4. Medications That Can Interfere with Immunoassays ■

Medication	Drug Class	Assay Affected	Reference
Ciprofloxacin	Antibacterial	EMIT	[13]
Fluorescein	Radiologic dye	FPIA	[14]
Mefenamic acid	Analgesic	EMIT	[15]
Metronidazole	Antifungal and antibacterial	EMIT	[16]
Tolmetin	Nonsteroidal anti-inflammatory	EMIT	[17]

substituted results and does not report the invalid/cancelled results. The MRO would subsequently review and report the invalid result only if the split specimen fails to reconfirm the positive, adulterated, or substituted result(s).

CONSECUTIVE INVALIDS

If two consecutive tests are invalid for different reasons, the MRO asks the DER to immediately send the donor for another test collected under direct observation.

If two consecutive tests are invalid for the same reason, the MRO reviews the second test's CCF to ensure that a directly observed collection was documented.

- If "no," the MRO does not interview the donor, does not report the result, and instead again asks the DER to send the donor for another test collected under direct observation.
- If "yes," the MRO cancels the test and does not ask the DER to retest the donor. If a negative result is required—in DOT-regulated settings, this means a preemployment, return-to-duty, or follow-up situation—the MRO determines if there is clinical evidence that the donor is currently an illicit drug user. The MRO does this by conducting, or having someone else conduct, a clinical examination for drug abuse and, if appropriate, consulting with the donor's personal physician. The clinical examination for drug abuse may include an alternative specimen (e.g., hair) drug test. Any drug test result would be part of the clinical assessment and would not be reported to the employer like a standard drug test. If the clinical examination finds no evidence of drug abuse, the MRO reports this as a "negative test" with written notations about the medical examination required because of consecutive invalid results for the same reason. However, if the clinical examination does find evidence of drug abuse, the MRO reports this as "Test Cancelled" with written notations about the medical examination required because of consecutive invalid results for the same reason. Although the donor has not had a positive result, the donor also cannot perform safety-sensitive duties without a negative result.

Adulterated or Substituted Result Review ■

The MRO asks the donor if he or she has a legitimate medical explanation for the laboratory findings with respect to presence of the adulterant or the nonphysiologic creatinine and specific gravity findings. As with positive results, the DOT rule allows the MRO to give the donor up to 5 days to present a legitimate medical explanation for the adulterated or substituted result.

While some donors admit to unauthorized use of drugs, virtually no one admits to adulterating or substituting their specimens. Few donors offer medical explanations for adulterated specimens. For example, it would be far-fetched for someone to claim, "I drink glutaraldehyde for my arthritis, so that's why it's in my urine." Some donors try to explain substituted findings by claiming over-hydration. *No* medical condition has been identified that can cause a specimen to meet the adulterated or substituted criteria. The federal rules leave open the possibility that such conditions will some day be identified. So far, they have not.

An occasional specimen collected under direct observation is reported as adulterated or substituted. The phenomenon of adulterated, substituted, and invalid specimens collected under direct observation speaks to the lack of rigor in how some observers approach their responsibility.

VERIFICATION OF EXPLANATIONS FOR ADULTERATED AND SUBSTITUTED RESULTS

The MRO decides the legitimacy of any explanation that the donor presents for the adulterated or substituted test result. This is a two-step process: First, the MRO decides if the explanation is plausible. Second, the MRO directs the donor to obtain further evaluation by a physician to determine if the explanation is true. Figure 10-3 outlines this process, as established by DOT.

Is the Explanation Plausible?
The MRO uses his or her judgment to evaluate the plausibility of the donor's explanation for an adulterated or substituted result. The MRO can ask the donor to provide evidence to support the explanation. An assertion that race, gender, or some other personal characteristics explain an adulterated or substituted specimen can be considered plausible only if the donor presents evidence showing that these characteristics actually result in the physiologic production of urine meeting the adulterated or substituted criteria. The MRO must reject any medical explanation for the presence of soap, bleach, glutaraldehyde, or any other substance that cannot be produced physiologically in urine. The MRO must also reject any explanation for the absence of creatinine in the urine; this is also a physiological impossibility.

If the MRO rejects the donor's explanation, the MRO reports a refusal to test, as described later in this section. If the MRO accepts the donor's explanation as plausible, the MRO then directs the donor to obtain further evaluation by a physician to determine if the explanation is true.

Evaluation by Referral Physician
The referral physician evaluates the donor to establish whether there is credible medical/scientific evidence to support the donor's explanation for producing a specimen with the properties that triggered the adulterated or substituted finding. The referral physician is someone who has expertise in the medical issues raised by the donor's explanation and who is acceptable to the MRO. It often falls to the MRO to identify this physician, because the donor may not know who to go to. While the MRO can also be the "referral physician," a different physician can provide a more independent assessment. The MRO informs the referral physician

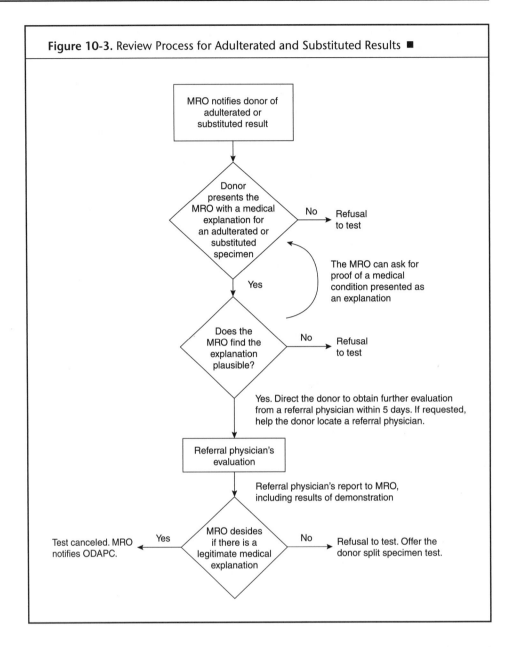

Figure 10-3. Review Process for Adulterated and Substituted Results ■

MRO notifies donor of adulterated or substituted result

Donor presents the MRO with a medical explanation for an adulterated or substituted specimen

No → Refusal to test

The MRO can ask for proof of a medical condition presented as an explanation

Yes

Does the MRO find the explanation plausible?

No → Refusal to test

Yes. Direct the donor to obtain further evaluation from a referral physician within 5 days. If requested, help the donor locate a referral physician.

Referral physician's evaluation

Referral physician's report to MRO, including results of demonstration

MRO desides if there is a legitimate medical explanation

Yes → Test canceled. MRO notifies ODAPC.

No → Refusal to test. Offer the donor split specimen test.

about the test results, the consequences to the donor of submitting an adulterated or substituted specimen, and guidance on what is expected from the evaluation. The MRO should ask the referral physician to promptly provide a signed, written report about whether there is a legitimate medical explanation for the urine finding. DOT states that the donor must obtain the referral evaluation within 5 days of the verification interview by the MRO. DOT also encourages the MRO to extend this time frame if the donor has made good-faith, but unsuccessful, efforts to obtain the evaluation within 5 days. DOT states that neither the MRO nor the employer are responsible for arranging, conducting, or paying for the evaluation.

The donor must be able to demonstrate to the referral physician that he or she did produce or could have produced urine, through physiologic means, that met the adulterated or substituted criteria identified in the drug test specimen. Typically, this demonstration includes recollection or urine under reliable direct observation and submission of the urine for drug and validity tests. The referral physician is authorized to conduct any other tests he or she feels should be included in the evaluation but is restricted to use of a laboratory certified by HHS. This limits the range of urine tests that can be ordered, since HHS-certified laboratories generally conduct tests for just pH, specific gravity, creatinine, and some adulterants. The referral physician reports his or her determination to the MRO in a signed, written report. The MRO reviews this report and makes the final determination of whether there is a legitimate medical explanation for the laboratory finding.

OUTCOME: TEST CANCELLED OR REFUSAL TO TEST: ADULTERATED/SUBSTITUTED

If the MRO *accepts* the donor's explanation, the MRO checks the "Test Cancelled" box (Step 6) on Copy 2 of the CCF, prints on the CCF the reason why the test is cancelled, reports the result to the employer *and* notifies ODAPC. If the MRO *rejects* the donor's explanation, the MRO checks the "Refusal to Test" box and either the "Adulterated" or "Substituted" box (Step 6) on the Copy 2 of the CCF, prints the specific adulterant or specimen validity criteria on the Remarks line, and notifies the donor of his or her right to have the split specimen tested.

Although adulteration and substitution of drug test specimens is illegal in several states, neither the MRO nor other service agent(s) are legally obliged to report such a finding to law enforcement.

Safety Risk and Medical Disqualification ∎

While reviewing a drug test, the MRO may incidentally learn something about the donor that suggests a safety risk or medically disqualifying condition. The "something" could be use of prescription drugs that can cause impairment. It could also be use of an illicit drug not identified by the drug test or a medical condition that can cause impairment.

DOT

The DOT rule authorizes MROs to report likely safety risks and medical disqualification information. The MRO does not need the donor's permission to report. The MRO reports the information to someone who can take appropriate action, which can be one or more of the following: (1) the employer, (2) a health care provider responsible for determining the medical qualification of the donor under an applicable DOT agency safety regulation, (3) a SAP evaluating the employee as part of the return-to-duty process, (4) a DOT agency, or (5) the National Transportation Safety Board when conducting an accident investigation. If the safety risk involves an owner-operator, the MRO should notify both the owner-operator and a third party who can take appropriate action. This third party can be a DOT agency or the C/TPA who administers the owner-operator's program.

If the safety risk or medical disqualification risk involves use of a prescribed medication, the MRO both reports the likely safety risk or medical disqualification *and* notifies the donor that he or she has 5 days to have the prescribing physician contact the MRO to determine if the medication can be changed to one that is compatible with safe job performance. If the prescribing physician informs the MRO that the medication has been so changed, the MRO issues an amended report indicating that the concern has been resolved.

NON-DOT

An MRO may disclose safety risks and disqualification information uncovered while reviewing a non-DOT drug test. When the MRO does this for a non-DOT test, the MRO cannot cite Part 40 as justification for such disclosure nor is the MRO compelled by Part 40 to make such disclosure. However, the MRO could cite the federal HIPAA privacy rule, which includes a provision for reporting safety concerns. The HIPAA privacy rule provides that covered entities may disclose protected health information that they believe is necessary to prevent or lessen a serious and imminent threat to a person or the public, when such disclosure is made to someone they believe can prevent or lessen the threat (including the target of the threat) [45 *CFR* 164.512(j)].

Some state laws include provisions whereby health care professionals are granted immunity from liability for good-faith reporting of impairment in public safety workers to public agencies. Even in the absence of such law, a health care provider could cite a public interest defense if he or she intervenes to prevent a potential adverse event and someone then sues for breach of confidentiality or other infringement of personal rights. Although some MROs may fear lawsuits from employees who are removed from duty because of safety or qualification concerns raised by the MRO, a failure to report such information can leave the MRO liable to suit from someone who is injured due to the donor's unsafe conduct. Both legal theories are largely untested. MROs want to avoid lawsuits and do not want to inconvenience workers and employers over speculative concerns. MROs should therefore disclose information only when there is a relatively strong safety risk or clear medical unqualification.

The following sections discuss the extent to which MROs should or must report information about safety risks and disqualification in certain non-DOT settings.

Drivers, Non-Commercial

The AMA recommends that physicians notify the Department of Motor Vehicles (DMV) if impaired patients they are treating fail to restrict their driving appropriately [18]. Most states provide an opportunity for physicians to voluntarily report unfit drivers—not just commercial drivers—to appropriate governmental agencies [19]. In some states, physicians must, by law, report unsafe drivers to the state's DMV. In other states, physicians are legally required to notify the DMV if a patient has certain medical conditions, such as epilepsy. Massachusetts and Washington, D.C., require a physician's certification that older drivers are physically and mentally fit to drive. Doctors who report under these laws are provided anonymity and immunity from patient lawsuits.

Health Care Workers

Positive test results for illicit drug use by health care professionals suggests a potential risk to patients. Laws about reporting of drug abuse by health care professionals vary from state to state and by job (physician, nurse, etc.). Some states require reporting of chemical dependency of any type; some mandate reporting for dependency on drugs but not alcohol; and some have no laws that address this. Most states have laws that provide immunity from liability to those who report such information, provided they believe the information is true, are not reporting it to be malicious, and report the information only to the applicable authority. Questions about reporting obligations should be directed to the regulatory board and professional society in the state where the health care professional is licensed.

Physicians are rarely drug tested by hospitals because few are employed by hospitals. Physicians are more likely to face preemployment drug tests when they join large non-hospital medical groups.

Employer-Mandated Reporting of Medication Use

An employer can require workers to report the use of medications that may pose a safety risk, but according to at least one court decision cannot require reporting of all medications without regard to safety risk [20]. The FRA rule allows covered employers to require certain employees to report their use of prescription and over-the-counter medications to supervisors. The Federal Transit Administration (FTA) has posted on its website a "Tool Kit" for transit employers regarding policies and procedures for dealing with prescription and over-the-counter medications that may impact safety. Some companies provide their workers with lists of high-risk drugs and ask workers to report use of such drugs. Like most other medical qualification decisions, decisions about medication use are best made on an individualized basis, unless the medication use is an automatic disqualifier, for example, insulin use by a commercial truck driver.

SCOPE OF DISCLOSURE

For confidentiality reasons, the MRO should limit how much detail is disclosed to the employer. Ideally, the MRO can provide details to the employer's occupational health care provider who can follow up on behalf of the employer. However, if the employer has no designated health care professional to evaluate its employees, the MRO will have to disclose at least enough detail to help the employer adequately follow up on the issue.

The following sections describe potentially disqualifying medications and conditions and the duty to report such information.

IDENTIFYING LIKELY SAFETY RISKS AND DISQUALIFICATION

From an MRO's perspective, most qualification concerns are safety related and involve either the use of medications that can impair cognitive function or underlying medical conditions that can cause sudden incapacitation. Several classes of drugs can cause drowsiness and make driving unsafe. More than 700 drugs listed in the *Physicians' Desk Reference* carry warnings about potential impairment. Despite ubiquitous warnings, the appropriate use of most prescription drugs is unlikely to pose a safety risk and may in fact improve performance by reducing pain or otherwise helping to restore the worker's well-being. Many employees take drugs for medical reasons and work safely and without apparent performance problems. This contrasts to recreational users of drugs, who deliberately seek altered mental status.

Unless the safety issue is clear cut—e.g., a truck driver taking Dilantin for seizures—the MRO cannot know if the donor is unsafe or unqualified based just on a phone call and without full knowledge of the job duties. It is unreasonable if not an abrogation of the MRO's responsibility to report every possible safety concern. The DOT rule asks the MRO to report information that "is likely to result in" disqualification or "is likely to pose a significant safety risk" [49 *CFR* 40.327(a)]. Any risk assessment considers both the likelihood of the event and potential magnitude of harm. For example, a risk that is tolerable in a pipeline repair worker may not be tolerable in a commercial airline pilot.

In response to such notification, an employer typically either asks the worker for a note from his/her doctor or sends the worker to the employer's occupational health physician for an independent opinion. For example, the employer may ask the worker to get a note from the prescribing practitioner stating that use of the medication will not pose a safety risk. However, the personal physician may have little knowledge of assessing work fitness, has no responsibility to the employer, and may not recognize his/her responsibility to public safety. This is why many employers turn to an occupational health physician, who offers a more independent opinion of the employee's fitness-for-duty. The MRO, if local, can do this exam at the employer's request, but this is outside the context of the MRO role.

Most fitness-for-duty decisions are made without job-specific standards and are individualized based on the specifics and the judgment of the medical professional. As described by the Americans with Disabilities Act (ADA), someone is unqualified for employment if he or she has a medical condition that poses a direct threat to safety or that makes him or her unable to perform the essential duties of the job. There are a few conditions and drugs that, per statute or authoritative guidelines, are disqualifying from certain jobs. For all other drugs and jobs, there is insufficient scientific or medical evidence to support banning use of the drug for safety or qualification reasons.

The following sections describe nationally recognized medical qualification standards for commercial motor vehicle (CMV) drivers, airplane pilots [21], mass transit operators, and firefighters [22].

Disqualifying Conditions for Commercial Motor Vehicle Drivers

FMCSA has issued regulations [49 *CFR* §391.41(b)], guidelines ("Medical Advisory Criteria") [23] and technical reports ("Medical Conference Reports") about how certain medical conditions effect qualification of CMV operators. With regard to medication use, the FMCSA regulations and guidelines state that an individual is unqualified for CMV operation if he or she takes:

- Insulin to control diabetes, with exceptions allowed for those drivers who have obtained a waiver from this rule.
- Medication to control seizures.
- Methadone.
- Varenicline (Chantix).
- Warfarin (Coumadin) during the first month of use in treatment (Thereafter, it is acceptable if the individual's international normalized ratio [INR] is within range and monitored monthly.).

- Any Schedule I drug, such as marijuana.
- An amphetamine, a narcotic, or any other habit-forming drug, with exceptions allowed if it has been prescribed by a licensed medical practitioner who is familiar with the driver's medical history and assigned duties and has advised the driver that the prescribed drug will not adversely affect the driver's ability to safely operate the vehicle. (If the medication issue is brought to the medical examiner's attention—for example, at a DOT physical—the medical examiner gets to make the final decision about whether the driver's use of this medication is safe.)

Published research on the use of prescription sedatives and driving safety is scant. This does not mean there is no risk, but any employer or MRO who disqualifies a CMV operator because of use of a prescription drug will be doing so without definitive evidence that such use impairs performance or causes accidents. Some studies report that initial use of prescription opiates causes impairment in some psychomotor or cognitive functions [24,25,26] and in simulated driving performance [27], but other studies report no such effect [28,29]. Studies of chronic stable use of prescription opiates report no impairment of cognitive or psychomotor function, mood, behavior, or driving performance [30,31,32,33]. The common knowledge is that use of prescription opiates impairs driving and can cause accidents. Thus, many MROs get concerned when they find out a donor operates a CMV and takes a prescription opioid. An investigation of any accident by an opioid-using driver would no doubt conclude that use of the prescribed opioid was causative. Thus, many MROs alert employers when they learn a driver is taking a prescribed opioid, especially hydrocodone or oxycodone. Many MROs also notify employers of drivers who take benzodiazepines because they cause sedation, which seems inherently dangerous.

Published research on the use of stimulants and driving safety fails to demonstrate impairment. To the contrary, use of stimulant medication as prescribed seems to improve driving among those with attention deficit disorders [34].

A current clinical diagnosis of alcoholism is a disqualifier for CMV operation [49 *CFR* §391.41(b)(12)]. The term *current clinical diagnosis* is intended to include current alcoholic illness and circumstances in which the person's physical condition has not fully stabilized. Because alcoholics often underreport their alcohol use, it seems incumbent on MROs to take any report of excessive drinking seriously and alert the employer to the likely safety concern. The medical examiner or other examining physician can then review the situation and may want to seek information from third parties, including review of recent personal health records with the driver's permission.

Disqualifying Medical Conditions for Pilots
Table 10-5 lists conditions that are specifically disqualifying from medical certification as pilots, unless FAA grants the person a waiver or special certification [21]. FAA guidance also states that a pilot may not use varenicline, disulfiram, cetirizine, guanethidine, lithium, methyldopa, nitroglycerin, "older" (sedating) antihistamines, reserpine, or any psychotropic medication, including antidepressants and sleep aids. If the MRO identifies a condition in a pilot that is likely to be medically disqualifying, the MRO should inform the employer and the FAA Aeromedical Certification Division in Oklahoma City, Oklahoma (405-954-4821).

Table 10-5. Disqualifying Medical Conditions for Pilots ■

1. Angina pectoris.
2. Bipolar disorder.
3. Cardiac valve replacement.
4. Coronary artery disease that has required treatment or, if untreated, that has been symptomatically or clinically significant.
5. Diabetes mellitus requiring insulin or other hypoglycemic medication.
6. Disturbance of consciousness without satisfactory medical explanation of the cause.
7. Epilepsy.
8. Heart replacement.
9. Myocardial infarction.
10. Permanent cardiac pacemaker.
11. Personality disorder that is severe enough to have repeatedly manifested itself by overt acts.
12. Psychosis.
13. Substance abuse and dependence.
14. Transient loss of control of nervous system function(s) without satisfactory medical explanation of cause.

Under the FAA rule, the MRO reports any verified positive FAA drug test conducted on a pilot to the FAA's Drug Abatement Division [14 *CFR* Part 121].

Disqualifying Conditions for Mass Transit Operators

FTA has not established medical standards for qualification of mass transit operators. FTA's drug and alcohol testing rule is sometimes misunderstood as prohibiting mass transit operators from using any drug in the DOT five-drug panel. This misunderstanding is based on the section of FTA's drug testing rule that states, "Consumption of these products is prohibited at all times" [49 *CFR* §655.21]. This prohibition is in the context of positive DOT drug test results. FTA does not prohibit legitimate medical use of these drugs.

DRUG TESTS AND MEDICAL EXAMS

Sometimes the MRO is also the physician who determines if an examinee is medically fit for duty. If the physician performing the medical exam knows the examinee used illicit drugs, the physician cannot help but consider that information in his or her assessment. If the physician performing the medical exam does a drug test as part of that exam, the test is used for clinical purposes and its result should not be disclosed to the employer or used for disciplinary purposes. If the employer wants a drug test result, the employer should order a drug test, which would then be outside the context of a medical exam.

Drug Tests and Impairment ■

While the presence of a drug or metabolite in the urine indicates recent drug use and suggests past pharmacologic effects, it does not necessarily correlate with blood concentrations of the drug and does not prove current or past impairment [35,36,37]. Drug concentrations in urine do not corrrelate very well to drug concentrations in blood [38]. Blood concentrations offer better information about impairment, since blood concentrations are usually indicative of concentrations in the brain. A number of states have passed laws under which a positive drug test or an alcohol test concentration or above a certain level is considered evidence of impairment or *under the influence.* While the scientific consensus is that drug test results are poor measures of impairment (an exception may be made for certain drug tests performed on blood), some state laws nevertheless establish a presumption of impairment and, after an accident, fault.

One Test Event, Two Specimens ■

Two specimens may be collected at one testing event. This could be two different types of specimens, e.g., urine or hair. This could be two urine specimens, e.g., one nonobserved and the other observed. The MRO may receive one result before the other. If the MRO receives and reports a negative result first and a non-negative result second, the employer might put the donor to work upon receipt of the negative result unless the employer knows to wait for the second test result. To avoid this, DOT asks the MRO to report paired urine tests together. This means the MRO needs procedures to identify paired results. They can be identified by tip-offs on the chain of custody form, for example:

- Collector's remarks, e.g., "first of two tests," "second of two tests."
- A checked out-of-range temperature box.
- Receipt of two CCFs with the same donor number but different specimen numbers.

DOT authorizes the MRO to hold the first result received if it is negative until the MRO receives the second result. (If the first result is non-negative, the MRO does not delay reporting.) Table 10-6 lists DOT requirements for MRO reporting of paired specimens. "Non-negative" refers to both to non-negative laboratory results and refusals to test as reported by the collection site. If the MRO reports one result but not the other, there is no requirement for the MRO to sign and send CCF2 to the employer for the non-reported result.

Some collection sites charge for paired collections with just one collection fee. Some MROs who charge by the test charge for paired tests as if they were one, but if the collection site and/or MRO charges for two tests, the client may question receiving two charges and just one report. The explanation is that two tests were performed and are billable, and they had a single, combined outcome.

Tell the Donor the Outcome ■

The MRO should tell the donor the test's outcome, for example "The employer will be notified later today that the test is positive for marijuana." The MRO should invite the donor to call back if he or she has additional information about medication use or has any questions about the result. The MRO should take additional calls from the donor within reason. The MRO should try to answer,

Table 10-6. Reporting of Paired DOT Tests ■

Result Received First	Result Received Second	MRO Reports	Other Result?
Negative	Negative	Result received second	Do not report
Negative	Non-negative	Result received second	Do not report
Non-negative	Negative	Result received first, immediately	Do not report
Non-negative	Non-negative	Both results	N/A

within reason, technical questions raised by the donor. A donor who feels he or she was treated with disrespect may seek satisfaction by means of a lawsuit.

Inform the Donor of the Right to a Split Test or Retest ■

In some programs, such as those mandated by DOT, the specimen is split into two portions (Bottles A and B) at the time of collection and Bottle B is set aside while Bottle A is analyzed. If Bottle A is verified by the MRO as positive, adulterated, or substituted, the donor can challenge the laboratory result by having Bottle B analyzed at a different laboratory. In some other programs, employers allow donors to challenge laboratory results by having their specimens retested. If the donor has the right to a split test or a retest, he or she must ask for this within a defined time limit. The MRO notifies the donor of any right to a split test or retest and the time limit for requesting it. Under DOT regulations, the time limit is 72 hours during which the MRO is reachable, including by answering machine or voice mail. Certain state laws and employer policies give donors longer to decide. Under DOT regulations, the MRO tells the donor that prepayment for the test is not required and the employer may seek reimbursement from the donor for the cost of the test. It is important to remember that the MRO reports the verified result of the primary specimen (Bottle A) to the DER immediately after his/her determination that the test is positive, adulterated, or substituted. Reporting of the result is *not* delayed pending the donor's decision about the split specimen or pending the reconfirmation result from the laboratory.

Any right the donor has to a split test or retest remains even if the donor admits to the MRO having taken the illicit drug or having caused the adulteration or substitution finding. That right also remains even if the MRO suspects a required split was not collected. Many donors, when presented with the option for a split test or retest, are too upset about failing the drug test to make a reasoned decision or they think (or hope) they are being given the option of returning to the collection site to give a new specimen. The donor may ask the MRO, "What do you think I should do?" The MRO should respond that this is the donor's decision. DOT prohibits the MRO from demanding prepayment from the donor for a DOT split test, but requires the MRO to tell the donor that the employer may seek reimbursement for the cost of the test. The MRO should tell the donor that split testing is expensive (e.g., can cost $150–$200). Donors are less likely to ask for split tests and retests if they think they will have to pay for them. Applicants are less likely to ask for split tests and retests than are current employees, perhaps because the stakes are higher for current employees who fail their drug tests.

Only the donor can authorize a split test or retest. (By exception, courts can also order these when results have been challenged.) The donor authorizes the split test or retest by asking the MRO. Under DOT, the MRO must honor a verbal request. In non-DOT testing, some MROs insist on a written request in case the donor is later charged for the split and claims he/she never asked for it. The MRO records the date and time of the donor's request for analysis of the split specimen. If the donor makes a timely request, the MRO arranges for the split analysis. Under DOT rules, the MRO is not obliged to authorize analysis of the split specimen analysis if 72 hours have elapsed and the donor has no good reason or extenuating circumstances to explain the delay. If 72 hours elapse and the donor later presents the MRO with information documenting a serious illness, injury, or another reason that prevented a timely request, the MRO can still order the split analysis. If an MRO accepts a delayed request for a split test or retest, the MRO is obliged to cancel the original result if the additional test fails to reconfirm it. In DOT-mandated testing, the MRO must first consult with ODAPC before cancelling any test if more than 60 days has elapsed. (See "Changing the Report" at the end of this chapter.)

Usually the MRO or C/TPA selects the laboratory. Sometimes the employer selects the laboratory. Donors rarely express a preference for which laboratory handles their split test or retest, but any preferences they *do* express should be seriously considered because split tests and retests are performed on behalf of the donor. There is no regulatory requirement for the MRO to notify the employer that the donor has asked for the split test. In practice, many MROs do so, anyway.

Chapter 11 further describes the process for split specimen tests and retests.

"Can I Take Another Test, Doc?" ■

Almost every donor with a non-negative result would like a "do-over." During the interview, the donor may ask to take the test again. If the program allows for split tests or retests, the MRO offers that option. Otherwise, the MRO can respond that he or she is only calling about the test that was already performed and does not decide if this donor will be retested.

Reporting MRO Results ■

WHEN

DOT directs MROs to report positives, refusals to test, and cancelled tests requiring immediate recollection under direct observation so that employers receive them within 1 day of verification. DOT directs MROs to report all other tests so that employers receive them within 2 days of verification.

MROs report positive results and adulterated/substituted refusals to test promptly even when donors ask for split specimen tests. Results of split specimen tests are reported separately and typically a week or so after the primary results have been reported. The MRO has a responsibility to assure that the employer receives verified test results in a timely manner.

TO WHOM

The Employer/TPA
The MRO reports results directly to the employer or, at the employer's discretion, the employer's TPA. Under FMCSA, owner-operators must participate in testing programs administered by TPAs. Therefore, the MRO should report an owner-operator truck driver's results to that driver's TPA. If a self-employed donor does not belong to a TPA, the MRO reports the result directly to that self-employed donor. If a donor has paid for his/her own federally regulated drug test, the MRO reports the result to the employer (if known) because the federal rules require this. If a donor has paid for his/her own non-DOT drug test, the MRO reports the result to the donor unless the donor has provided written authorization to send the report elsewhere.

FAA
If the test is FAA regulated, the donor holds an airman medical certificate (i.e., is a pilot), and the verified result is positive or a refusal (i.e., adulterated, substituted, or shy bladder without medical explanation), the MRO notifies FAA. The MRO submits the person's name along with identifying information and supporting documentation within 2 working days after verifying a refusal or positive drug test result. Figure 10-4 is a form based on that designed by FAA for MROs to report positive drug tests and refusals to test to the federal air surgeon. (The employer informs FAA of refusals to test determinations made by the employer, e.g., employees who do not go for DOT tests as ordered.)

USCG
If the test is regulated by U.S. Coast Guard (USCG), and the verified result is positive or a refusal, the MRO reports the test in writing to the officer in charge of marine investigations at the area or the nearest marine safety office for any person holding a captain's license, merchant mariner's document, or certificate of registry. The donor's employer, prospective employer, or sponsoring organization is responsible for this reporting, but the MRO can do it on behalf of the employer or sponsoring organization. If the donor is self-employed or otherwise identifies no employer or sponsoring organization, the MRO provides the report directly to the USCG.

State Licensing Agency
There is no federal database of DOT drug test results. There is no nationwide system for removing a driver from CMV operation if he or she has a drug or alcohol test violation. Several states have enacted state registries that employers and state licensing agencies can query to help prevent continued CMV operation by drivers who have failed their drug and/or alcohol tests without completing the return-to-duty process. These laws, as of 2009, are summarized in Table 10-7. Some state laws ask MROs to report positive, adulterated, and substituted results. The DOT rule authorizes reporting of drug and alcohol test results to state regulatory agencies [49 *CFR* §40.331(g)].

Figure 10-4. Report Form for FAA Positive and Refusal to Test Results ■

Report of Verified Positive Drug Test
14 CFR Part 67 Airman Medical Certificate Holder

As the Medical Review Officer (MRO) for the company listed herein, in compliance with the provisions of 14 *CFR* Part 121, Appendix I, I am notifying you of a verified positive test result on the following individual who holds an airman medical certificate issued pursuant to 14 *CFR* Part 67.

Company name: _____

Airman's name: _____

Position or position applied for_____

Airman's social security number: _____ Date of birth: _____

Type of Test ✓   ☐ Pre-employment   ☐ Periodic   ☐ Random
                  ☐ Post Accident   ☐ Reasonable Cause   ☐ Follow-up

Date of Drug Test Collection: _____

Test received by MRO from: _____ on _____
                              laboratory name and city   date

Date verified as a positive drug test result by MRO: _____

Verified positive result(s) for ✓   ☐ Amphetamines ☐ Cannabinoids (THC) ☐ Cocaine Metabolites

OR   ☐ Opiates   ☐ Phencyclidine

Refusal to test ✓   ☐ Adulterated   ☐ Substituted

Date company management notified of verified positive test result by MRO: _____
✓☐ Testing of split specimen NOT requested, *OR* ☐ Date split specimen testing requested: _____.

Split specimen forwarded for testing to _____
                                          laboratory name and city

Date split specimen test result received_____ ✓ ☐ Reconfirmed the presence of the drug or drug metabolite(s),

OR

☐ I have not yet received the split specimen test result. I will forward it to the Federal Air Surgeon upon receipt.

I have enclosed the custody and control form ✓ ☐ copy 1 (or the laboratory report of the positive results); ☐ copy 2 of the custody and control form; the ☐ split specimen test result (if split testing requested); ☐ any other supporting documentation.

_____   _____
Medical Review Officer Signature   Date

_____   _____
Printed Name   Phone Number

Mail to: FAA/Drug Abatement Division, AAM-800, Room 806, 800 Independence Avenue, SW, Washington, DC 20591. *OR*, fax to: (202) 267-5200 *(secure fax)*

Donors

Several state laws require employers to notify donors in writing of their positive, adulterated, or substituted drug test results. Most of these laws require notification within a certain time, for example, within 5 working days after receipt of the positive test result.

These situations are the only federal or state laws that authorize release of drug test results to parties other than the employer. In the event of a safety risk or medical disqualification issue, the MRO may need to report relevant information to a third party, as described in the "Medical Qualification and Safety Concerns" section of this chapter. Employers and service agents need no written authorization from employees to release information to requesting federal, state, or local safety agencies with regulatory authority over them or employees.

Table 10-7. State Reporting of DOT/FMCSA Test Violations ■

State	Statute	What Is Reported	Who Reports?
Arkansas	Ark. Code Ann. §27-23-205	positive or refusal FMCSA-authorized alcohol tests; positive, refusal, substituted, or adulterated FMCSA-authorized drug tests	Both employers and consortia/third-party administrators
California	California V.C. Section 34520(c)	positive FMCSA-authorized drug and alcohol test "summaries"—notification (e.g., test date, reason for test, drug detected) without identifying the driver or motor carrier	consortium
	California V.C. Section 13376(b)(3)	positive or refusal FMCSA-authorized drug tests conducted on those holding special driver certificate for school buses, vehicles to transport developmentally disabled people, etc.	employers
New Mexico	N.M. Stat. Ann §65-3-14	positive drug test results	consortium or MRO
North Carolina	N.C. Gen. Stat. §20-37.19(c)	positive and refusal FMCSA-authorized drug and alcohol tests	employer
Oregon	Or. Rev. Stat. §825.410	positive FMCSA-authorized drug test, including identification of the drug that was detected	MRO
South Carolina	S.C. Code §56-1-2220	positive and refusal DOT drug and alcohol tests.	employers
Texas	Tex. Transp. Code Ann. §643.064	positive FMCSA-authorized drug tests	Form MCS-20 started by MRO; reported by employer or, if owner-operator, by MRO
Washington	Wash. Rev. Code §46.25.123	positive and refusal DOT drug or alcohol tests	employers report refusals; MROs and BATs report positives

WHAT TO REPORT

The MRO reports:

1. The verification outcome(s), i.e., negative, positive, refusal to test, or cancelled.
2. That the urine specimen is dilute, if this is the case.
3. That the donor should be retested, if this is the case.
4. Safety risk or medical disqualification concerns, if identified.

If the specimen is not urine (which is typically the presumed specimen), it is helpful for the MRO to identify the type of specimen on the report, e.g., "Hair Drug Test Report."

To Whom?	How?	Use of the Data
Office of Driver Services, Arkansas Dept. of Finance & Administration; Little Rock, AR	online, www.ark.org/drugtest, within 3 days of test	Employers must check the online database before putting drivers on the road.
California Highway Patrol, Commercial Vehicle Section; Sacramento, CA	mail	California originally planned to maintain a database of positive test results. However, no such database was developed. For compliance with the law, consortia must report positive tests, but without names.
Driver Safety Actions Unit, Sacramento, CA, with a copy to local California Highway Patrol Area Office	mail, using Positive Controlled Substance Test Result Report, within 5 days of receiving the test result	Driver's special certificate (not CDL) revoked for 3 years or until driver completes return-to-duty process.
Motor Vehicle Division; Santa Fe, NM		New Mexico plans on developing a database of positive drug test results.
Department of Motor Vehicles; Raleigh, NC	Form CDL-8 and copy of test result, by mail or fax (but originals must still be mailed), within 5 days of receiving the result	North Carolina revokes the driver's CDL until the driver successfully completes the DOT return-to-duty process.
Driver and Motor Vehicle Services Division; Salem, OR	CCF 2 and Form 735-7200, by mail or fax	Employers may not query the database because the program has not been well publicized and querying is not required.
South Carolina Department of Motor Vehicles	Form CDL-18 within 3 business days	Driver's CDL revoked until SAP process is complete.
Department of Public Safety, Motor Carrier Bureau; Austin, TX	Form MCS-20 and test report, within 10 days of receiving test result	With the driver's authorization, an employer can ask the motor carrier bureau about past positive results.
Department of Licensing; Olympia, WA	Form DR-500-013 by fax or mail, within 3 days of the test	Driver's CDL revoked until SAP verifies driver has begun treatment.

The following sections discuss the four components of the MRO's report in greater detail.

1. The Verification Outcome

Negative
The MRO reports the negative result.

Positive
The MRO reports that the result is positive and identifies the drug(s)/metabolite(s). The MRO's report does not include the concentration(s) of those drug(s)/metabolite(s), but the MRO can report those data later if the test is challenged in a legal or administrative process. The DOT rule directs MROs to *not* routinely report concentrations, lest employers inappropriately tailor their actions based on concentrations.

Refusal to Test
The MRO reports the result as a "refusal to test" and reports the reason. The reason may be that the specimen was "substituted" or "adulterated with <adulterant/acid/base>" and the donor had no medical explanation for this result—or the reason may be a refusal to undergo a required evaluation or other behavior as described in the "Refusal to Test" section of Chapter 6 of this book.

Cancelled
The MRO reports that the test is cancelled and the reason for cancellation.

2. Dilute
If the urine is dilute, the MRO indicates this on the report, e.g., "negative-dilute," "positive-dilute." When reporting a dilute result, DOT directs the MRO to explain what the employer should do as per 49 *CFR* §40.197. If the result is positive and dilute, the employer simply treats it as a verified positive result. If the result is negative and dilute, the employer's actions depend on the creatinine value as follows:

- Creatinine 2–5 mg/dL. The MRO tells the DER to retest the donor under direct observation immediately and with minimal advance notice. The retest is conducted just once and the second result is final, even if it is also dilute.
- Creatinine > 5 mg/dL. The MRO tells the employer that it has the option of retesting the donor once, not under direct observation (unless there is some other reason for doing so). Under the DOT rule, an employer may establish a policy of immediately retesting anyone with a dilute result or anyone with a certain type of dilute result, e.g., a random dilute, or a pre-employment dilute. (Retesting after a dilute-negative reasonable suspicion or post-accident test serves particularly little purpose, since the retest would take place at least several days after the incidents that prompted testing.)

Figure 10-5 presents a brief description to help explain dilute specimens to employers.

Consecutive Dilutes

If two consecutive urine tests are negative-dilute and the second was supposed to be a collection under direct observation, the MRO reviews the second test's CCF to ensure that a directly observed collection was documented. If "yes," then the MRO merely reports the negative-dilute result. If "no," the MRO does not report the result and instead directs the DER to immediately send the donor for another test, this time collected under direct observation.

3. Retest, if Needed

The donor may need to return to the collection site for another test, e.g., because of failure to properly collect a urine specimen under direct observation. The MRO would indicate this on the report to the employer.

4. Safety Risk or Medical Disqualification

If the MRO has identified a safety risk or medical disqualification concern, he or she can write "safety risk" or some other general comment on the drug test report or can inform the employer through some means separate from the drug test report. The MRO should reserve the medical details for the employer's occupational physician or other professional who is making the actual determination of fitness for duty.

The NRC rule directs the MRO to make additional interpretation of return-to-duty tests to determine if a positive is from new use or residual excretion.

HOW TO REPORT

The DOT rule allows MROs three different ways to report results:

1. Copy 2 of the CCF. The MRO enters the result in Step 6 and enters the date of the MRO's receipt of Copy 2. The date of receipt may have been auto-

---

Figure 10-5. Dilute Specimens ■

A dilute report on a urine drug test suggests that the donor drank a lot of fluids or added something to the specimen. Many people, even those who don't use drugs, drink a lot of fluids before their drug tests and produce dilute urine. Those who use diuretics and certain other medications can produce dilute urine, too. Very lean people are more likely to produce dilute urine.

Dilution of the urine makes it harder to detect drugs. The most effective measure to prevent dilute specimens is to minimize, where possible, the interval between an employee's notification for testing and the time at which he or she is tested, e.g., to no more than 3 hours.

Under U.S. Department of Transportation rules, most dilute, negative drug test results are cause for the employer to conduct one (and only one) retest, not under direct observation. If the specimen is extremely dilute (with creatinine of 2–5 mg/dL), the employer must retest the donor immediately and under direct observation. Employers should not take disciplinary action based on dilute test results. The dilute finding may have nothing to do with drug misuse.

---

stamped on the form if it was faxed to the MRO. Otherwise, the MRO writes the date on the form. The MRO can send a copy of Copy 2 to the employer and keep the original as hard copy. In regulated testing, if the result is non-negative, the MRO must sign and date the MRO block of Copy 2. In regulated testing, if the result is negative, the MRO can sign or initial Copy 2 or the MRO's assistant can stamp the MRO's signature in the MRO block. The DOT rule does not accept electronic signatures as replacements for original or stamped signatures. (An electronic signature means an electronic sound, symbol, or process attached to, or associated with, a document and executed with the intent to sign that document. An electronic signature is not an image reproduction of the MRO's signature.) Because Copy 1 has the laboratory report, the MRO must not send it to the employer, lest the employer be able to identify laboratory-positive/adulterated/substituted results that the MRO has changed to negative or cancelled.

2. A custom-designed form that includes the following information:
   a. Donor's full name.
   b. Specimen ID and donor ID numbers.
   c. Reason for the test, if known.
   d. Collection date.
   e. Date the MRO received Copy 2 of the CCF.
   f. Test result and date the MRO verified the result.
   g. For positive results, the name(s) of the drug(s)/metabolite(s).
   h. For cancelled tests, the reason for cancellation.
   i. For refusals to test, the reason for the refusal determination (e.g., in the case of an adulterated result, the name of the adulterant).

   Figure 10-6 presents an example of a form that can be used to report drug test results. MROs who use software to manager their drug test data typically produce reports from that software. Only one test is reported per form. A form, in comparison to Copy 2 of the CCF, is more legible and offers the flexibility with regard to format and additional information.

3. Electronic data transmission of negative results. For example, the MRO could securely transmit a data file with negative results or could post negative results to a secure website to which the DER has access. DOT prohibits reporting of non-negative results in this manner.

MROs who report results using custom-designed forms or electronic data files must also complete and retain Copy 2 of each CCF.

Positive results, refusals to test, and cancelled tests requiring immediate recollections should be immediately phoned to the DER if the report is not otherwise immediately delivered. Negative results can be phoned in, too, but these are usually less urgent. Phoned-in reports do not replace the need for hard-copy or electronic reports in the formats just listed. iMROs should not leave drug test results on DER voice mails or answering machines because there is no assurance that the DER will receive the message in a timely fashion. When transmitting result by phone, there should be some mechanism to mutually verify the identify of the MRO or MRO's staff, and the identity of the DER. A password would be good, but identities are often assured through familiarity between the MRO's staff and the DERs.

MROs can use any transmission device—for example, fax or mail—for transmitting hard-copy reports and must ensure that reports are transmitted

Figure 10-6. Urine Drug Test Report ■

Employee's Name: _____ SSN or Emp. ID: _____

Employer's Name: _____ Specimen ID: _____

Reason for Test: ❑ Pre-employment ❑ Random ❑ Post-accident
❑ Return-to-duty ❑ Periodic ❑ Reasonable suspicion ❑ Unspecified

Test Type: ❑ DOT (five-drug) test ❑ Non-DOT five-drug test ❑ Other: _____

Collection: Date: _____

Time: _____

❑ Check if donor did not appear at collection site

Date of MRO's receipt of CCF Copy 2: ___/___/___

Verification decision:
❑ Negative
If dilute-negative, check ❑ *and* check one of the following:
❑ employer must immediately retest under direct observation
❑ employer may retest once, direct observation not required

❑ Positive for:
❑ amphetamines
❑ cocaine
❑ marijuana
❑ opiates
❑ phencyclidine
❑ other: _____

❑ Refusal to test:
❑ specimen substituted
❑ specimen adulterated with: _____
❑ shy bladder with no medical explanation
❑ other:_____

❑ Cancelled: ❑ fatal or uncorrected flaw (describe: _____)
or ❑ invalid result with explanation (nonobserved retest if a negative result is needed)
or ❑ invalid result without explanation (need immediate, directly observed retest)
or ❑ shy bladder with medical explanation

MRO's name (print): _____

MRO's signature: _____

MRO's address: _____

Report date: _____

To: _____
Secure fax no.: _____
Initials: _____ Date: ___/___/___

Report positives on same or next day as verification

If this transmission is incomplete or illegible, please call us at 800-676-3784. This communication is of a confidential nature. If it has been misdirected to you, or if your fax machine is not in a secure access area, please contact us immediately.

Distribution: (1) Fax or mail original to employer, (2) Keep copy w/drug test record confidentially and received only by the appropriate designee(s). Most e-mails are not secure, although use of e-mail with encrypted attachments may be acceptable. The MRO should keep records of the transmissions; that is, what, when, how, and to whom each transmission was sent. The documentation can be simple. Small-volume MROs can just print a note on the upper corner of a copy of the employee report indicating how and to whom the report was sent. If reports are faxed, the fax machine can be programmed to automatically print a confirmation that the pages have been sent. E-mailed results can be programmed so that receipts are obtained when the e-mail has been received. Hard-copy mail can be sent with return-receipt provisions, but this is uncommon.

Data Management Software ■

Many employers, C/TPAs, and MROs manage almost all of their drug test data in electronic format. Some laboratories offer software for clients that allow computer-to-computer transfer of, or web-based access to, laboratory data. The largest, national MROs create and maintain their own software. Software can be purchased from third-party vendors. MROs and C/TPAs who are shopping for software should look for software that allows changes to data downloaded from laboratories and includes reporting and, perhaps, invoicing capabilities. Software without such capabilities is best suited for in-house administrators who manage company testing programs. Drug testing software typically include modules for managing the employee database, random selections and scheduling, result tracking, and summary reports.

The software programs that are designed for MROs and C/TPAs include one or more methods for reporting results to clients. Reporting options may include:

- *Automated fax reporting.* The software can be set up to automatically produce and fax reports of laboratory-negative results, upon receipt, and hold positive, adulterated, substituted, and invalid results in a file pending review by the MRO and his/her staff. (*Note:* DOT requires an administrative review of the MRO copy of the custody and control form at the MRO's office before negative results are reported.) The software is designed to match each test record to a designated employer representative and fax number. The software sends reports by way of fax modem to these reporting designates. Automated fax reporting presents two particular challenges: (1) The user must maintain a complete and current list of reporting designates and fax numbers, and (2) the recipients need secure (confidential) fax machines.
- *Automated voice reporting.* Some systems allow clients to call and receive automated voice reports of drug test data. These systems include processes for verification of client identification, e.g., through use of a password. After receiving the voice message, the client can request an automated fax report. Automated voice reporting has the advantage of confidentiality. Among its drawbacks, the client must access the system to determine if test results are available.
- *Web-based reporting.* The client logs into a password-protected website to access test results. Clients can view or download their data from these sites. Some systems send clients e-mail alerts when new results are posted. Clients

log into the computers' servers on which these data reside. These systems potentially offer clients more control over their data, since they can view complete data sets and generate certain reports from them. However, the systems do not automatically send the result to the client but instead require the client to retrieve the result from the system. Very large employers may prefer web-based reporting, since they may get results every day and will not mind logging in to check for result, and they can make good use of the reporting options. Other employers may find cumbersome the extra step of logging in and retrieving results.

- *Electronic reporting.* The MRO or TPA can send test results to a client's printer or computer, can send the data to a password-protected electronic mailbox for downloading by the client, or can post the data on an Internet site for password-protected access by the client. Electronic signatures (that is, use of a sound, process, or symbol that the sender affixes to the electronic report file) combined with encryption can help ensure confidentiality and reliable delivery of messages to the appropriate recipients. If the sender is transmitting the file to the recipient, the sender needs a process that ensures a reliable, updated set of addresses. Because electronic data can be altered without a trace, the sender and recipient should use a system that has auditing capabilities. Electronic reporting offers the advantages of immediacy and direct transfer of data into the recipient's database system.

MRO Recordkeeping ■

In regulated testing, the MRO keeps Copy 2 of the CCF. The MRO does not need the original Copy 2; a faxed copy or photocopy is sufficient. However, once Copy 2 is signature stamped (if negative) or signed (if non-negative) with the final outcome, the MRO must keep that stamped or signed piece of paper, at least in DOT-regulated testing. DOT considers the MRO's signature on that form as one of several signatures required to establish a forensically intact record. The other signatures (donor, collector, and, if positive, laboratory certifying scientist) are on the CCF form kept by the laboratory. DOT does not authorize use of electronic signatures in lieu of handwritten signatures. Thus, the requirement to maintain the paper Copy 2 with the handwritten signature is an obstacle to a completely paperless MRO recordkeeping system.

If the MRO uses a different form for reporting results, the MRO keeps a hard copy of that form, too. If the MRO uses an electronic data file to report negatives, the MRO must keep a copy of that file and, if audited, must be able to readily produce printed documents from it so that auditors can review the printouts rather than the electronic file. The MRO's drug test records also include information such as documentation to support an alternative medical explanation for a positive, adulterated, or substituted result, including any letters or notes received from a donor or donor's health care provider; documentation of MRO actions regarding the test, e.g., attempts to contact the donor; documentation of the donor interview; and any corrective statements obtained. Prudent MROs will keep these notes with the corresponding results.

The HHS *Guidelines* direct MROs to keep records for 2 years. DOT operating administrations have held that MROs, as agents of employers, must keep records for the same time frames as employers, i.e., at least 1 year for negative results and at least 5 years for non-negative results. This is partly in case inspectors auditing an employer suspect that a result has been changed from positive to negative—the only way to determine this is to ask the MRO for a copy of the results. MROs will also want to keep negative records for a year or two in case clients question bills—copies of the negatives can be resent to the client. MROs will want to keep positive, adulterated, and substituted records for several years in case donors sue or otherwise formally challenge their tests.

Workplace drug and alcohol test records should be kept separate from patients' medical records. Medical records are about evaluation and treatment of patients. Workplace drug and alcohol test records are about hiring and safety and are not medical records of patient evaluation and treatment. It is more practical to maintain the drug and alcohol test records in files separate from the medical records. If they are included with medical records, one or the other is likely to be inappropriately accessed by someone who has permission to see only the medical record or only the drug/alcohol test results. If there is a separate medical records department, and if the records are merged, that department's personnel may send a copy of the entire file, including both medical records and drug/alcohol tests, to an insurer who submits a medical release form asking for copies of the medical records. Storing the drug/alcohol test records separately also makes it easier to assemble them for copying, delivering, and statistical reporting of test data. While drug and alcohol test records are not medical records, they should be protected with similar security and confidentiality safeguards. There are no federal laws or other laws that directly address whether drug and alcohol test records must be maintained in, or outside of, patient medical records.

Collection sites and MROs with small numbers of tests may find it easiest to store drug and alcohol test records chronologically, for example, in folders (by month), hanging files, or boxes. Some MROs with large numbers of tests use microfilm or electronic imaging techniques to reduce space requirements.

Access to MRO Records ■

BY THE DONOR

Under the DOT rule, the MRO or service agent must provide to the donor a copy of his or her drug test result within 10 business days of receiving a written request from the donor [49 *CFR* §40.329]. The MRO should provide all records that are available related to that employee's test, to include written notes, checklists, or comments. The MRO may first redact sensitive medical, psychiatric, or mental health records that would be inappropriate to give to the donor [38]. The MRO may charge the donor for the cost of reproducing, handling, and sending a copy of the record.

If the donor wants his or her result sent elsewhere—for example, to an attorney or union representative—the MRO should first obtain the employee's written, signed authorization. This authorization should identify specifically what is to be released and who receives the result.

Some employers and service agents may see a risk in giving donors copies of the records. In practice, allowing donors to see the records often settles any questions they may have about the validity of the results.

BY THE EMPLOYER

The MRO should not routinely give the employer the individual laboratory reports or the interview notes. Disclosure of this information would allow employers to identify lab-positive results that the MRO has changed to negative. The interview notes often contain confidential medical information unrelated to the laboratory results. The MRO provides the interview notes to the employer only if the donor has provided a written consent for this release or if a legal challenge exists.

IN LEGAL PROCEEDINGS

The DOT rule allows MROs and other service agents to provide complete drug testing records to employers in certain legal proceedings [49 *CFR* §40.323(c)]. The term *legal proceedings* includes wrongful discharge lawsuits, arbitrations, unemployment compensation hearings, and criminal and civil lawsuits related to safety-sensitive duties, typically involving accidents. This is consistent with rules governing lawsuits, which provide for an exchange of information and documents as part of *discovery*. The MRO or C/TPA releases information directly to a court only if a valid court order (subpoena) has been received or if the donor provides written authorization for this release.

BY THE SAP

The MRO is authorized to provide, without the donor's consent, drug test-related information to the SAP evaluating that donor. This includes providing concentrations on individual results, as requested. The MRO should provide concentrations to SAPs only upon request.

BY PARENTS

MROs should not provide parents with results of drug tests performed on their children on behalf of employers. Parents may become interested in getting the results after an MRO has called their home to contact their children or after their children suddenly lose a job or job offer. The one exception to this advice is in Tennessee, where under state law any employer who has a drug-free workplace program approved by the state must notify the parents and guardians of a minor's drug test results [Tenn. Code Ann. § 50-9-109(1)(e)].

Programs include a policy of mandatory notification of parents.

BY DOT AND NTSB

MROs and other service agents must make test records and data available to relevant federal agency representatives (e.g., DOT, NTSB) upon request. If the records are in electronic format, the MRO may be required to produce them in printed documentation in a manner that is rapid and allows them to be audited.

TO OTHER THIRD PARTIES

The DOT rule prohibits the MRO from releasing information to other third parties without the donor's consent, with exceptions allowed for information affecting medical qualification or the performance of safety-sensitive duties, as described in the "Safety Risks and Medical Disqualification" section of this chapter [49 *CFR* 331(c)]. If a service agent gets a court order for release of DOT test information for which DOT does not authorize release, the service agent must seek legal relief. If the service agent is asked by an outside party for information about a drug test, the service agent should refer the outside party to the employer who ordered that test.

The MRO is authorized to inform an employer other than the one who ordered the test, about a positive result only if the donor provides consent. DOT requires an employer to ask new hires for releases to get past test results (as described in Chapter 4).

The Occupational Safety and Health Administration (OSHA) Access to Employee Exposure and Medical Records standard [29 *CFR* §1910.1020] allows employees and OSHA compliance personnel access to occupational health medical records. If drug test results are kept with other occupational health records, they will thereby be accessible to employees and OSHA compliance personnel.

Changing the Report ■

Only the same MRO who initially declared the test "positive" or "refusal to test" can change that verification decision. Under the DOT rule, the MRO may do so only in limited circumstances, as follows:

- If the MRO receives new evidence of a laboratory error.
- If the MRO has made an administrative error and reported an incorrect result.
- If the MRO receives additional information (that was not reasonably available at the time of verification) of a legitimate medical explanation for the test result. This includes information pertaining to non-contact verified results where the donor has now shown good reason for having been unavailable.

In the last situation listed, if the information is received more than 60 days after the original verification decision for a DOT-regulated test, the MRO must consult with ODAPC before making any changes.

Judges and arbitrators sometimes overturn tests for reasons other than those just listed. Those legal decisions do not change the test's outcome or return-to-duty requirements under the DOT rule. On occasion, this has created the perverse situation where a judge or arbitrator has ordered a worker reinstated to a DOT-regulated job while the DOT rule precludes that person from working in that job.

A negative drug test result from a second specimen is not cause for changing the positive result from the first specimen. The first and second test may differ in time frame and a variety of characteristics, including the rigor of the collection procedure, the specimen's dilution, and the analytes, cutoffs, and techniques used by the laboratory. To paraphrase an old saying, one cannot step in the same river twice. Likewise, one cannot collect the same drug test specimen at two different times.

Drug Tests and DOT Physicals ■

Some bus and truck drivers who are subject to DOT physicals are also subject to DOT drug and alcohol tests. The FMCSA requires a DOT physical exam of any

CMV driver in interstate commerce if his/her vehicle (1) weighs at least 10,001 lb, (2) transports more than eight people (including the driver) for compensation or more than 15 people (including the driver) not for compensation, or (3) is placarded for hazardous materials [49 *CFR* 390.5]. The FMCSA requires drug tests of CDL holders (and those holding a similar license issued by Mexico or Canada) if they drive a vehicle that (1) weighs 26,001 lbs or more, (2) carries 16 or more people (including the driver), or (3) is placarded for hazardous materials [49 *CFR* 382.107]. Some drivers must have DOT physicals but not DOT drug and alcohol tests. Some state regulatory agencies require DOT physicals for school van operators and other non-CMV workers.

The physical exam for CMV drivers includes a medical history, hands-on exam, vital signs (e.g., blood pressure), and basic, dipstick urinalysis (e.g., protein, sugar). If the patient is qualified, the examiner completes a medical examiner's certificate. The certificate is usually valid for 2 years but may be shorter if the examiner determines there is a need for closer monitoring. A current medical examiner's certificate is among several items necessary to obtain one's CDL from the state licensing agency. Any health care provider whose license permits him or her to perform physical examinations can be a medical examiner and perform a DOT physical. This varies by state and can include physicians, physician assistants, nurse practitioners, doctors of osteopathy, and chiropractors. The exams are recorded on the federal forms, which can be downloaded and/or printed from the federal websites or purchased in hard-copy from distributors of workplace health and safety publications. The medical examiner keeps the multi-page, double-sided medical examination report (*long form*) and gives the medical examiner's certificate (*the card*) to the driver. The CMV driver must have the card in his or her possession while operating a CMV. Some state rules require that the driver also have a copy of the long form. The CMV driver is not required to have copies of drug and alcohol test results in his or her possession.

The employer (*motor carrier*) keeps a copy of the card. The employer is not required or prohibited by federal law from getting the long form, which contains the history and physical findings. Confidentiality guidelines for occupational medicine physicians state that employers should not receive diagnoses or specific details—i.e., should not receive long forms—except where required by law or overriding public health considerations [39], but many employers want long forms. Some employers threaten to withhold payment or send their drivers elsewhere for exams if they do not get the long forms. Most health care providers routinely send long forms to employers. Some state licensing agents, particularly those for school bus drivers, require that drivers present long forms at the time of licensing or require that employers maintain copies if long forms. The health care provider that performs the exam should obtain the patient's authorization, using a HIPAA-compliant release form, before sending the long form to the employer or a state agency. Another approach is to give a copy of the long form to the patient, who can then give it to others as he/she sees fit. A facsimile should be considered as acceptable as an original signed form, but some employers want the original forms.

Drug tests and DOT physicals are separate events, even if both occur at the same visit. An examinee can pass one and fail the other. The medical examiner need not delay issuing a medical examiner's certificate while waiting for the DOT drug test result. While the medical examiner may think that the drug or alcohol test is important in assessing the patient's fitness, the single test is likely inadequate for this purpose. DOT has encouraged medical examiners to determine fitness based on the exams and consider the drug tests as separate, nonmedical, and unnecessary for determination of fitness. If a medical examiner is concerned about drug or alcohol use based on the standard DOT physical, he or she should evaluate the patient's history more closely, confer with the patient's personal physician, or conduct a hair test to check for repeated use over the preceding few months. Any drug test performed as part of a DOT physical is a non-DOT test, because DOT drug tests are not authorized in this context. Even if the medical examiner wants the DOT drug or alcohol test results, the examiner may not have ready access to them, particularly if another physician is the MRO.

The motor carrier is responsible for ensuring the potential driver does not operate its CMV(s) until the carrier receives both a copy of the medical examiner's certificate and a negative drug test report. If the driver has a positive drug test, the employer is responsible for removing the driver from service. Neither the medical examiner nor employer are obliged to retrieve, cancel, or otherwise nullify a DOT medical examiner's certificate on the basis of a positive drug test result.

DNA Testing ■

Genetic marker analyses can determine, in some cases to a high level of probability, whether the original specimen and a reference specimen were produced by the same person. These tests target proteins, blood-group antigens, and deoxyribonucleic acid (DNA). Genetic marker analyses work best with urine and oral fluid specimens that are fresh. DNA markers are obtained from cells in these specimens; from bladder cells that are sloughed off into the urine or from mucosal cells that appear in oral fluid. Cellular material is more plentiful in urine from women than urine from men. Cellular material is also more plentiful in urine and oral fluid specimens that are concentrated and are fresh. When urine and oral fluid specimens are stored and go through freeze/thaw cycles, the cellular material is degraded. Hair specimens can also be tested for DNA, but the hair shaft contains only mitochondrial DNA, and this test is expensive, has lower discriminatory power, and can only verify that the specimen came from a particular donor or any maternal relative of that donor. Specimens that are too small or might otherwise be inadequate for standard testing can often provide sufficient information through the use of polymerase chain reaction (PCR) procedures that amplify (replicate) portions of the DNA. If the laboratory can isolate protein or DNA markers in urine, it will also analyze a reference specimen (blood or saliva) from the donor for the same markers. The tests take approximately 6–8 weeks. (Without PCR, the cost is several hundred dollars; with PCR, the cost is approximately $1,000.) When it receives results, the laboratory reports *one* of two outcomes:

1. The person cannot be excluded as a donor of the challenged specimen test result. (The report also states the likelihood that the match is coincidental.)
2. The person is not the donor of the challenged specimen.

If the DNA test establishes that the original specimen and the reference specimen came from different people, this may mean one of four things:

1. An error occurred during the collection, shipment, or laboratory handling of the specimen.
2. The donor provided a substituted specimen at the original collection and provided his or her own specimen for the reference specimen.
3. The donor provided his or her own specimen at the original collection and provided a substituted specimen for the reference specimen.
4. The donor provided substituted specimens both for the original collection and for the reference specimen.

If proper collection procedures including chain of custody were performed, possibilities 2, 3, and 4 are more likely than 1. In general, MROs should not encourage use of DNA tests to establish ownership of the urine; the chain of custody serves this purpose instead. In DOT testing, DNA and serologic tests may be ordered only pursuant to a court order and DOT prohibits MROs from cancelling or otherwise negating test results based on these test results.

In a workplace setting, DNA and serologic tests in workplace are almost always performed on specimens that test positive, adulterated, or substituted. Negative test results are almost never challenged, and specimens that test negative are discarded promptly after testing.

References ∎

1. Department of Health and Human Services. *Medical Review Officer Manual for Federal Workplace Drug Testing Programs.* Rockville, MD: 2004.
2. Department of Health and Human Services. *MRO Manual.* Rockville, MD: 2004.
3. Peterson E, Rasmussen S, Daniel K, et al. Prescription medication borrowing and sharing among women of reproductive age. *J Women's Health* 2008;17(7):1–6.
4. Goldsworthy R, Schwartz N, Mayhorn C. Beyond abuse and exposure: Framing the impact of prescription-medication sharing. *Amer J Public Health* 2008;98(6):1115–21.
5. Daniel K, Honein M, Moore C. Sharing prescription medication among teenage girls: Potential danger to unplanned/undiagnosed pregnancies. *Pediatrics* 2003;111(5):1167–70.
6. Cohen P. American roulette—contaminated dietary supplements. *New England J Med* 2009;361: 1523–25. October 8, 2009.
7. Selavka C. Poppy seed ingestion as a contributing factor to opiate-positive urinalysis results: The Pacific Perspective. *J Forensic Sciences* 1991;36:685.
8. ElSohly M, Jones A. Morphine and codeine in biological fluids: Approaches to source differentiation. *Forensic Sci Rev.* 1989;1:13–22.
9. Rohrig T, Moore C. The determination of morphine in urine and oral fluid following ingestion of poppy seeds. *J Anal Toxicol* 2003;27:449–52.
10. Hill V, Cairns T, Chen-Chih C, Schaffer M. Multiple aspects of hair analysis for opiates: Methodology, clinical and workplace populations, codeine, and poppy seed ingestion. *J Anal Toxicol* 2005;29:696–703.
11. Department of Transportation. §40.159 Medical review officer—pH issue [Q&A]. Washington, DC: July 2008.
12. Clark WH, Sees KL. Drug testing and the toilet bowl blues. *JAMA* 1992;17:2377.
13. Lora-Tamayo C, Tena T, Rodriguez A. High concentration of ciprofloxacin in urine invalidates EMIT results. *J Anal Toxicol* 1996;20:334.
14. Inloes R, Clark D, Drobnies A. Interference of fluorescein, used in retinal angiography, with certain clinical laboratory tests. *Clin Chem* 1987;33:2126–27.
15. Crane T, Badminton MN, Dawson CM, et al. Mefenamic acid prevents assessment of drug abuse with EMIT assays. *Clin Chem* 1993;39:549.
16. Lora-Tamayo C, Tena T. High concentration of metronidazole in urine invalidates EMIT results. *J Anal Toxicol* 1991;15:159.
17. Price G, Doken W. Tolectin (Tolmetin) is a potent interfering substance for the Syva EMIT urine drug screen assays. *Clin Chem* 1990;36:1118.
18. American Medical Association. *Impaired Drivers and Their Physicians.* Chicago, IL: 1999. Policy E-2.24.

19. Malinowski M, Petrucelli E. Update of medical review practices and procedures in U.S. and Canadian driver licensing programs. Washington, DC: Federal Highway Administration, June 1997. DT FH61-95-P-01200.
20. *Roe v. Cheyenne Mountain Conference Resort.* 920 F Supp 1153. U.S. District Court–D Colo. 1996.
21. Federal Aviation Administration. *Guide for Medical Examiners,* 2009 Revision. Washington, DC: U.S. Department of Transportation, October 1999.
22. Committee on Fire Safety Occupational Medical and Health. Standard on Medical Requirements for Fire Fighters and Information for Fire Department Physicians. Quincy, MA: 2000 National Fire Protection Association (NFPA 1582).
23. Federal Motor Carrier Safety Administration. *Medical Advisory Criteria for Evaluation Under 49* CFR *Part 391.41.* Washington, DC: U.S. Department of Transportation. Updated April 8, 1998.
24. Coda B, Hill H, Hunt E, et al. Cognitive and motor function impairments during continuous opioid analgesic infusions. *Hum Psychopharmacol* 1993;9:383–400.
25. Kerr B, Hill H, Coda B, et al. Concentration-related effects of morphine on cognition and motor control in human subjects. *Neuropsychopharmacology* 1991;5:157–66.
26. Ghoneim M, Medwaldt S, Thatcher J. The effect of diazepam and fentanyl on mental, psychomotor, and electroencephalographic functions and their rate of recovery. *Psychopharmacology* 1975;44:61–66.
27. Linnoila M, Hakkinen S. Effects of diazepam and codeine, alone and in combination with alcohol, on simulated driving. *Clin Pharmacol Ther* 1974;15:368–73.
28. Saarialho-Kere U, Mattila M, Seppala T. Pentazocine and codeine: Effects on human performance and mood and interactions with diazepam. *Med Biol* 1986;64:293–99.
29. Redpath J, Pleuvry B. Double-blind comparison of the respiratory and sedative effects of codeine phosphate and (+/−)-glaucine phosphate in human volunteers. *Br J Clin Pharmacol* 1982;14:555–58.
30. Byas-Smith M, Chapman S, Reed B, Cotsonis G. The effects of opioids on driving and psychomotor performance in patients with chronic pain. *Clin J Pain* 2005;21:345–52.
31. Sabatowski R, Schwalen S, Rettig K, et al. Driving ability under long-term treatment with transdermal fentanyl. *J Pain Symptom Manage* 2003;25:38–47.
32. Sjogren P, Olsen A, Thomsen A, Dalberg J. Neuropsychological performance in cancer patients: The role of oral opioids, pain and performance status. *Pain* 2000;86:237–45.
33. Buvanendran A, Moric M, Kroin J, et al. Do chronic oral opioids impair driving skills? A randomised controlled trial. (Abstract) American Society of Anesthesiologists Annual Meeting, San Francisco, California, October 2007.
34. Jerome L, Habinski L, Segal A. Attention-deficit/hyperactivity disorder (ADHD) and driving risk: A review of the literature and a methodological critique. *Curr Psychiatry Rep* 2006;8(5):416–26.
35. American Society for Clinical Pharmacology and Therapeutics. Scientific Consensus Conference: Clinical Pharmacologic Implications of Urine Screening for Illicit Substances of Abuse. San Diego, California, March 7–8, 1988.
36. Moore KA, Levine B, Fowler DR. Prediction of impairment from urine bezoylecgonine concentrations. *J Anal Toxicol* 2003;383–34.
37. American Society of Addiction Medicine. Public Policy Statement on Drug Testing in Workplace Settings. *J Addict Dis* 2003;22:119–22.
38. Office of Drug and Alcohol Policy and Compliance. *Part 40 Questions and Answers.* Washington, DC: U.S. Department of Transportation. January 2002.
39. Confidentiality of Medical Information in the Workplace. Position Statement. American College of Occupational and Environmental Medicine. Elk Grove Village, IL. January 14, 2008.

Split Specimen
Tests and
Retests ■

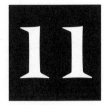

A *split specimen* is a specimen divided into two portions, or bottles, at the collection site. The two bottles are "A" or "primary" and "B" or "split." Bottles A and B are shipped together to a laboratory ("Laboratory A"). The laboratory tests Bottle A and keeps Bottle B sealed (or if there is a problem with Bottle A, the laboratory can test B instead). If the test result is verified positive, substituted, or adulterated, the donor can ask the MRO to have the second bottle sent to another laboratory ("Laboratory B") to reconfirm the result from the first bottle.

Split specimens are intended to help prevent false positive laboratory results. In practice, split specimen tests virtually never identify false positive laboratory results. Split specimen tests do sometimes lead to cancellation of positive results, but this usually occurs when a collection site fails to submit an adequate (or any) split specimen, thus precluding a split test. Other reasons for failure to reconfirm include leakage of the split specimen, the narrow specific gravity range criteria for "substituted specimen," a slow-acting adulterant in the specimen, and/or the degradation of unstable metabolites, such as 6-AM. Part 40, the HHS *Guidelines*, and certain state laws and employer policies require split specimen tests. Most nonregulated programs do not include split specimens.

A *retest*, as used in this chapter, refers to sending an aliquot from a single specimen to a different laboratory to doublecheck the first laboratory's positive, adulterated, or substituted finding. Under the NRC rule, the employer does not offer split specimens if the donor can authorize a retest of an aliquot from his or her original, single specimen. The great majority of programs without split specimens do not allow donors the opportunity to have aliquots from their specimens tested at second laboratories. If these programs were intended for such tests, they would probably have incorporated split specimen collections. Nevertheless, some programs without split specimen collections offer retests of the single specimens. Sometimes a judge, arbitrator, or other decision maker orders a retest of a single specimen in response to a challenged result.

Split tests and retests almost always involve urine. Enough urine is typically collected to allow for both the initial and confirmation assays and for a split test or retest. In tests of non-urine specimens, most or all of the specimen is consumed in the initial and confirmation assays, leaving too little specimen for a split test or retest. Because of the aforementioned specimen volume concerns and because there are no laws that require split tests or retests of nonurine specimens, split tests and retests are unusual for programs that test non-urine specimens. In hair testing, the next best thing is a promptly collected, second specimen. A second hair specimen collected within 1 to 2 weeks of the first hair specimen represents approximately the same window of detection and is sometimes used as an alternative to retesting the initial specimen. In oral fluid tests, some programs use two swabs to collect paired specimens, one of which is tested and the other used as the "split."

Reconfirmation Tests ■

Split tests and retests are performed to reconfirm the primary test results. Reconfirmation tests are different than the primary tests, as follows:

- A reconfirmation test should be—*must be* in regulated testing—performed at a different laboratory than the primary test. This offers a more independent validation of the primary result. While both laboratories may be owned by the same corporation, there is a greater perception of independence if they are not.
- The reconfirmation test looks only for the drug(s), adulterant, or substitution criteria that was identified in the primary result.
- The reconfirmation test for a drug or metabolite is a *confirmation* assay. A laboratory may first perform an immunoassay to determine a dilution factor in preparation for a confirmation assay, but would not use the immunoassay result to exclude the specimen from the confirmation assay.
- A reconfirmation test for a drug or metabolite identifies if the target analyte is present at or above the limit of detection (LOD). A LOD is the lowest concentration at which an analyte can be reliably shown to be present under defined conditions. Each laboratory sets its own LODs for each assay. LODs are much lower than cutoff values. LODs are used instead of cutoff values for several reasons, including:
  1. There is some variability in any assay's results. For example, the primary result may be positive just above the cutoff and the reconfirmation result may be negative just below the cutoff because of normal, acceptable variability.
  2. Concentrations of some drugs and metabolites drop over time, even in urine that is stored in a freezer. For example, the delta-9 tetrahydrocannabinol metabolite can be adsorbed onto the surface of the bottle and into precipitate matter in the urine. The heroin metabolite 6-AM is unstable and its concentration decreases over time.
  3. A slow-acting adulterant in the specimen can cause continued deterioration of the drug or metabolite, causing a reduction in concentration between the primary test and reconfirmation test.
- For reconfirmation of an adulterant, the laboratory only needs to perform one test for that adulterant. The reconfirmation test for an adulterated or sub-

stituted result needs to satisfy the same criteria that established the primary result as adulterated or substituted. The quantitative values in bottles A and B do not have to match. For example, if Bottle A's pH is 2.0 and Bottle B's pH is 2.1, the Bottle B result has reconfirmed the Bottle A result as each is outside the physiologic limit.

Processing Split Specimen Tests and Retests ■

If the result is verified positive, adulterated, or substituted and applicable policy gives the donor a right to a split specimen test or retest, the MRO informs the donor of this right, as described in Chapter 10. If within the allotted time frame the donor makes a request, the MRO sends a form or letter (e.g., Figure 11-1) to Lab A directing analysis of the split specimen or retest of the single specimen at Laboratory B. If an allowed request has been made and the MRO suspects the specimen may be insufficient or unavailable, the MRO should try to quickly ascertain this to allow for prompt cancellation and collection of a second specimen for testing. Otherwise, the MRO should report the initial result and order the split test or retest. If it later becomes clear that the split test or retest cannot be performed, the MRO cancels both tests. In DOT testing, a retest of urine from the

---

Figure 11-1. Example of MRO Request for Split Specimen Test ■

(Use the MRO letterhead, including MRO name and address)

By fax: (xxx) xxx–xxxx

Attn: Certifying Scientist
<laboratory name and address>

RE: Split specimen request
     Specimen ID # _____
     Collection Date: MM/DD/YY
     SSN 123-45-6789

Please arrange for testing of Bottle B from the above-referenced specimen for <drug/metabolite>. Please send Bottle B to <Laboratory B name, city, and state>. Lab B should send the result to my office at my secure fax number, <fax number>. Lab B should send the bill for the split specimen analysis to the account holder listed on the Custody and Control Form.

                              Sincerely yours,

                              <MRO's name>
                              Medical Review Officer

---

same bottle tested by Laboratory A cannot be used to satisfy a donor's request for a split specimen test.

Figure 11-2 illustrates the process for split urine specimen tests under the DOT Part 40 rule. A similar process applies to retests of single specimens.

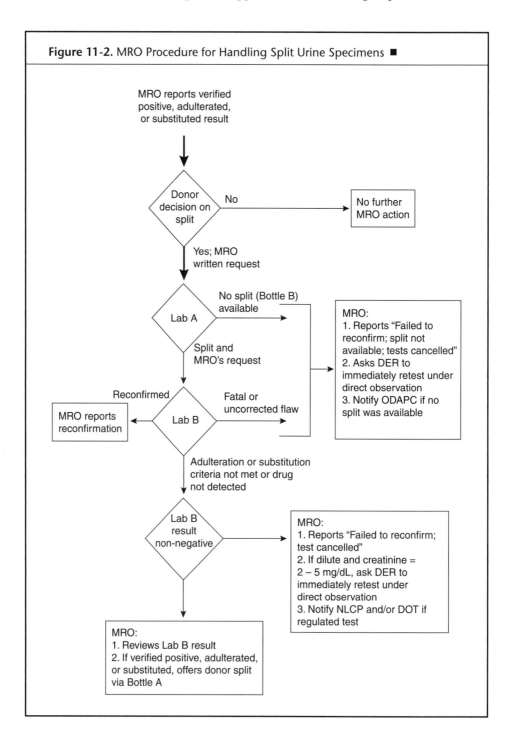

Figure 11-2. MRO Procedure for Handling Split Urine Specimens ∎

MRO reports verified
positive, adulterated,
or substituted result

Donor decision on split — No → No further MRO action

Yes; MRO written request

Lab A — No split (Bottle B) available →

Split and MRO's request

Reconfirmed — MRO reports reconfirmation ← Lab B — Fatal or uncorrected flaw →

MRO:
1. Reports "Failed to reconfirm; split not available; tests cancelled"
2. Asks DER to immediately retest under direct observation
3. Notify ODAPC if no split was available

Adulteration or substitution criteria not met or drug not detected

Lab B result non-negative →

MRO:
1. Reports "Failed to reconfirm; test cancelled"
2. If dilute and creatinine = 2 – 5 mg/dL, ask DER to immediately retest under direct observation
3. Notify NLCP and/or DOT if regulated test

MRO:
1. Reviews Lab B result
2. If verified positive, adulterated, or substituted, offers donor split via Bottle A

Upon receipt of the MRO's written request for analysis of Bottle B or a retest of Bottle A at a different laboratory, Lab A sends the following items to Lab B:

- A copy of the MRO's written request for a split test or retest
- Bottle B (for splits) or a resealed aliquot from Bottle A (for retests)
- A photocopy of the CCF

Lab B accessions the specimen, starts an internal chain of custody, performs re-confirmation testing, and sends a laboratory report for the result to the MRO. If the test has failed to reconfirm, Lab B reports why. The MRO reports the final outcome—reconfirmed or failed to reconfirm—to the designated employer representative (DER) in writing. In federally regulated testing, the MRO sends the employer an amended CCF with the split result entered at the bottom. The MRO also tries to notify the donor, typically by phone, of the split specimen result. The MRO files the Lab B result with the test record.

Failed to Reconfirm ■

The MRO, upon receipt of a failed to reconfirm laboratory report, checks the corresponding box in Step 7 of the Copy 2 of the CCF, prints the reason given by Lab B, and reports to the employer and the donor that the test is cancelled. Not only is the Bottle A result cancelled, but any personnel action the employer may have taken on the basis of the Bottle A result must also be reversed. The employer sends the donor for another test in the following circumstances:

- If the test was DOT and pre-employment, return-to-duty, or follow-up. In these situations, a negative result is required for performance of covered activities.
- The failure to reconfirm is due to a missing, invalid, adulterated, or substituted split specimen. DOT requires that the retest occur immediately using a collection under direct observation.

The MRO notifies the Office of Drug and Alcohol Policy and Compliance (ODAPC) of any failure to reconfirm of a DOT test. ODAPC reviews these and notifies HHS if no explanation for the discrepancy is identified. Figure 11-3 is a form developed by ODAPC for reporting of split-specimen cancellations. MROs can use similar forms with the same information or can report this information via ODAPC's website. The MRO should, as a courtesy, also notify Lab A of the failure to reconfirm.

Failures to reconfirm fall into four categories:

1. Failed to reconfirm primary result(s) *and* not adulterated or substituted

If the Lab A result is positive for a drug/metabolite and the Lab B result fails to reconfirm that drug/metabolite, Lab B will test the Bottle B specimen for adulterants and substitution. If Lab B does not identify the specimen as adulterated or substituted, it will report the failure to reconfirm to the MRO, who then notifies the employer and donor that the test is cancelled and (if

Figure 11-3. Split Specimen Cancellation Report to DOT ■

Note: Information is required only for those tests where donor requested test of split

1. Medical Review Officer Information

   Name:_____   Tel. No.: _____
   Address: _____   Fax No.: _____
   City: _____   State: _____   Zip: _____

2. Collection Site Information

   Name:_____   Tel. No.: _____
   Address: _____   Fax No.: _____
   City: _____   State: _____   Zip: _____

3. Date of Collection _____

4. Specimen I.D. _____

5. Laboratory A Accession _____

6. Primary Specimen Laboratory

   Name:_____   Tel. No.: _____
   Address: _____   Fax No.: _____
   City: _____   State: _____   Zip: _____

7. Date Primary Laboratory Reported or Certified Result _____

8. Split Specimen Laboratory (□ check here if not applicable)

   Name:_____   Tel. No.: _____
   Address: _____   Fax No.: _____
   City: _____   State: _____   Zip: _____

9. Date Split Laboratory Reported or Certified Split Specimen Result _____
   (□ check here if not applicable)

10. Primary Specimen Results in the Primary Specimen _____
    (e.g., name of drug, adulterant, etc.)

11. Reason for Split Specimen Failure-to-Reconfirm Result
    (drug/metabolite)

    □ split specimen failed to reconfirm for
    □ adulteration or substitution criteria not met
    □ split specimen reported as invalid
       □ split specimen not available for testing
       □ split specimen not collected
       □ split specimen leaked in transit to Lab B
       □ split specimen lost in transit to Lab B
       □ insufficient volume (no leakage)
    □ split failed to reconfirm: split specimen adulterated
    □ other (explain in comments)

Figure 11-3. continued ■

12. Action Taken by MRO
(e.g., notified employer of failure to reconfirm and requirement for recollection)

_____

_____

13. Additional Information Explaining Reason for Cancellation (Comments)

_____

_____

_____

14. Name of Individual Submitting the Report (if not the MRO)_____

Fax or mail to: Department of Transportation
                        Office of Drug and Alcohol Policy and Compliance
                                 1200 New Jersey Ave., SE
                                 Washington, DC 20590
                                  FAX: 202-366-3897

DOT) sends a report to ODAPC. This type of failure to reconfirm is typically caused by one of the following situations:

a. A collection error whereby Bottle A and Bottle B specimens come from different voids. The MRO can compare specific gravity and creatinine values from Bottle A and Bottle B. If the values are dissimilar, then the urine specimens probably came from different voids, maybe even different donors. In this situation, the collector should undergo error-correction training that focuses on the requirement to collect one void at a time and how to correctly split and seal it.

b. Lab B uses different GC/MS analytic procedures or instruments than Lab A. Lab B then has the option of performing a different GC/MS procedure on the split specimen or sending the specimen to another lab (Lab C) for the confirmatory test.

c. An undetected adulterant in Bottle B. For example, if Lab B finds that it can identify neither the drug/metabolite nor the internal standard that it added to the specimen, then Bottle B probably contained or still contains an undetected adulterant. Some adulterants act slowly and will degrade the real drug or metabolite during several days of contact without significantly affecting the internal standard that Lab B adds just prior to analysis.

2. **Failed to reconfirm primary result(s) _and_ invalid, adulterated, or substituted**

If Lab B fails to reconfirm the drug/metabolite and identifies Bottle B as adulterated or substituted, the MRO sets the Bottle A result aside and proceeds with review of Lab B's invalid, adulterated, or substituted result. If the B result is invalid, the MRO notifies the donor and the employer that the test is cancelled and directs the employer to immediately retest the donor with a directly observed collection. If the B result is adulterated or substituted and the donor provides a legitimate explanation for that result, the MRO reports the failure to reconfirm the positive result(s) and cancels both tests. However, if there is *no* legitimate explanation for the adulterated or substituted B result, the MRO reports this as a refusal to test and gives the donor 72 hours to ask that Lab A retest the specimen for the adulterant or for the substituted criteria.

3. Failed to reconfirm one or more, but not all, primary results and *not* invalid, adulterated, or substituted

If Lab B reconfirms one or more, but not all, drug(s)/metabolite(s), and does not identify Bottle B as adulterated or substituted, the MRO notifies the employer of which results reconfirmed and which results are cancelled (i.e., did not reconfirm). The employer takes action based on the reconfirmed results.

If codeine or morphine reconfirm but 6-AM does not, the MRO re-reviews the opiate positive result as if 6-AM was never detected. Thus, if the opiate concentrations in Bottle A are less than 15,000 ng/mL, the MRO now needs clinical evidence of opiate abuse to verify the result as positive. If opiate concentrations in Bottle A are ≥15,000 ng/mL, the MRO needs to interview the donor for legitimate medical explanations.

4. Failed to reconfirm one or more, but not all, primary results *and* invalid, adulterated, or substituted

The MRO notifies the donor and the employer of the reconfirmed result(s), the failed to reconfirm result(s), and the invalid, adulterated, or substituted Lab B result. The MRO need not review the invalid, adulterated, or substituted results from Lab B. Instead, the MRO tells the employer to take action based on the reconfirmed result(s).

5. Specimen not available for testing, or no split laboratory available

If the MRO orders a split specimen test and Lab A determines the split specimen is unavailable, Lab A reports to the MRO that the specimen was unavailable for testing. If Lab A sends the split specimen to Lab B, but Lab B finds its CCF or condition unacceptable (e.g., bottle leaked in transit), Lab B reports to the MRO that the specimen was unavailable for testing. The laboratory is supposed to indicate the reason for the unavailability.

The most common cause of failure to reconfirm is lack of a suitable split specimen. When this happens, the MRO follows these steps:

- Reports to the employer and the donor that the test must be cancelled and why.
- Direct the DER to immediately retest the donor under direct observation, with minimal advance notice given to the employee of this requirement.
- Notify ODAPC of the failure to reconfirm.

The result of the "collection under direct observation" retest will be the test of record for this testing event.

If an unusual adulterant was identified, there may be no split laboratory available to test for that adulterant. This would be handled in the same manner as a missing split specimen.

Payment for Split Specimen Tests and Retests ■

In regulated testing, MROs are responsible for assuring that each donor's request for a split specimen analysis or reanalysis is relayed to the laboratory promptly. The split analysis or reanalysis cannot be delayed or made conditional upon the donor's payment for this testing. Some employers have policies and procedures to help them get reimbursed by donors for costs of split specimens. The MRO can help employers start the "collection process" by informing them when donors have asked for split tests. For example, the MRO may add the remark, "Donor asked for split," on the report.

Many MROs and third-party administrators (TPAs) pay drug testing laboratories and pass along laboratory costs in their bills to clients. If the MRO orders a split analysis, A will charge the account holder for sending the split to Laboratory B, and Laboratory B will charge the account holder for analysis and handling of the split specimen. Split specimens also add to the workload of the MRO or TPA. MROs and TPAs are at financial risk for these expenses if their clients refuse to reimburse them. DOT takes no position on who pays for the split tests, except for generally stating that employers are responsible for costs associated with testing and cannot delay split tests because of payment issues. MROs and TPAs should expect and demand reimbursement from employers for their expenses associated with split tests and should include language to this effect in any contracts they have with their employer clients.

Urine and Other Specimens ■

Urine is the most commonly used specimen for workplace drug testing but has certain practical problems, most notably its vulnerability to dilution, adulteration, and substitution, and its relatively short detection period. Some employers test non-urine specimens for drugs because of their perceived advantages over urine specimens. Hair has been the second most commonly used specimen for drug testing. Oral fluid has been third. Both hair and oral fluid specimens are collected under direct observation, thereby reducing opportunities for tampering with the specimen. Different specimens have different windows of detection and sensitivity at detecting various drugs. Each specimen is good in its own way, and some are better than others for certain purposes. MROs are subject matter experts who can help their employer clients select appropriately should they choose to drug test using non-urine specimens.

Regulations ■

The HHS and DOT drug testing rules only authorize urine drug tests. During the 2000s, HHS looked closely at expanding its procedures to include tests of oral fluid, sweat, and hair, and even went so far as to issue a proposed set of laboratory accreditation procedures for non-urine specimen testing in 2004 (71 *FR* 19673). In 2008, HHS announced that there were significant issues that still precluded it from finalizing these procedures (73 *FR* 71858).

The DOT rule authorizes saliva and breath tests for alcohol. The DOT and NRC rules authorize clinical examinations of donors in certain situations (e.g., donors who cannot provide urine) to determine if there is clinical evidence of drug abuse, and those examinations can include alternative specimen tests, e.g., blood. In these clinical examinations, the drug test would be part of the evaluation. The examiner would issue an opinion about clinical evidence of drug abuse but would not report the drug test result to the employer. Some state laws allow certain specimens or prohibit certain specimens from use in workplace drug testing. State laws that require use of federally certified drug testing laboratories implicitly limit drug tests to urine, because the federal government only certifies *urine* drug testing laboratories.

Detection Times ■

Different types of specimens offer information about use over different periods of time, as illustrated in Figure 12-1. These differences make certain specimens better suited for certain types of testing, as shown in Table 12-1. For example, a hair test can identify repeated use over a long period of time and is thus well suited for pre-employment testing. However, because a hair test does not identify a single dose or recent use of drugs, hair tests are not well suited for post-accident or reasonable suspicion testing. Oral fluid provides a close correlation between use and time of collection, which makes it a good specimen for post-accident and rea-

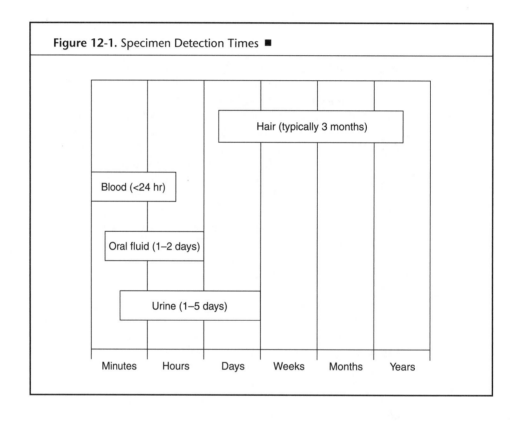

Figure 12-1. Specimen Detection Times ■

Table 12-1. Specimens and Reasons for Testing ■

Specimen	Pre-employment	Random	Post-accident	Reasonable Suspicion	Return-to-Duty	Follow Up
Hair	✓	✓			✓*	✓*
Oral fluid	✓	✓	✓	✓		
Urine	✓	✓	✓	✓	✓	✓

Adapted from: Mandatory Guidelines for Federal Workplace Drug Testing Programs. Notice of proposed revisions. *Federal Register* 2004;69(April 13):12,673–732.
*Should wait at least 3 months since last use when following common hair collection protocols

sonable suspicion testing. Urine drug tests are commonly used for post-accident and reasonable suspicion cases, although they are also limited because they do not differentiate "drugs on board today" from "brief recreational use of the drug a day or two before an accident or incident at work."

Non-Urine Specimens Compared with Urine Specimens ■

Table 12-2 lists the characteristics of specimens that are used for workplace drug tests. This table includes nails and blood even though they are used infrequently

Table 12-2. Comparisons Between Specimens ■

Specimen	Advantages	Disadvantages
Urine	Drugs and drug metabolites are concentrated	Limited window of detection
	Extensive scientific basis for testing methodology	Susceptible to adulteration, substitution, and dilution
	Extensive availability and experience by service agents	Biologic hazard for specimen handling and shipping to lab
	Broadest range of drugs/drug metabolites for which commercial testing is offered	Shy bladder problems may occur
	Laboratory certification program for federally mandated testing	Collections cannot be easily observed
	Performance testing is common	
	Results are frequently accepted in court	
	Uniform testing criteria (e.g., cutoffs) established	
	Easily tested by commercial screening methods	
	Least expensive	
Hair	Collection of head hair is less invasive or embarrassing than urine collection	If head hair is unavailable, some collectors take body or pubic hair, which seems invasive
	Long window of detection	May not detect recent drug use
	Detects parent drugs and metabolites (e.g., 6-acetylmorphine)	Insensitive for detection of occasional use, especially marijuana use
	It is hard to adulterate hair	Concern about possible hair-color bias
	Observed collection and thus minimal risk of tampering	Possible environmental contamination for some drug classes
	No need to refrigerate specimen	Cannot detect alcohol
	A second specimen collected within a week or two has about the same window of detection	Per-test cost is about twice that of urine
		Performance testing and specimen validity testing not well developed

continues

Table 12-2. Continued ■

Specimen	Advantages	Disadvantages
Oral fluid	Identifies recent drug use	Low drug/metabolite concentrations
	Noninvasive specimen collection	Short window of detection
	Observed collection and thus minimal risk of tampering	Less efficient than other testing methods in detecting marijuana use
	6-acetylmorphine and heroin are frequently present, i.e., can better identify heroin users	Collection volume is device-dependent
		Pad-type collection device does not lend itself to split specimen tests
	Can detect alcohol use, although with a procedure different from the drug test	Performance testing and specimen validity testing not well developed
		Variations in rate of saliva production
Blood	Most closely correlates with use	Shortest window of detection
	Can detect alcohol use	Invasive specimen collection
	Observed collection and thus minimal risk of tampering	Expensive
		Risk of infection from exposure
		Often collected in clinical settings that do not use chain-of-custody procedures
Nail	Long window of detection	Insufficient scientific data to support its use for routine workplace testing
	Observed collection and thus minimal risk of tampering	Possible environmental contamination for some drug classes
		Performance testing and specimen validity testing not well developed
		Cannot detect alcohol
		Limited number of labs that test nails for drugs

in comparison to urine, hair, and oral fluid. Non-urine specimens share certain advantages and disadvantages in comparison to urine, as follows:

Advantages of Non-Urine Specimens

- Collected under direct observation.
- Easier to ship and store.
- Fewer products and techniques available for adulteration and substitution.

Disadvantages of Non-Urine Specimens

- Not allowed in regulated testing and under certain state laws.
- Collection procedures and supplies are not standardized.
- Fewer collectors have experience with non-urine specimens.
- Fewer laboratories to choose from.
- Cost per test exceeds that for urine.
- Lower concentrations of drugs/metabolites requires the use of more sensitive and expensive analytic techniques.

- The specimen is used up in the analytic process by many laboratories (due in part to the lower concentrations and need for larger sample size), which may preclude any reanalysis or additional tests of the specimen.
- Less well understood, e.g., with regard to incorporation of drugs and issues of passive exposure, poppy seed ingestion, Vicks Inhaler, etc.
- No federal laboratory certification program.
- No formal industry standard cutoffs or analytic procedures.
- Scant (or no) reference materials are available for non-urine specimens, which hinders development of performance testing programs.
- Fewer illicit drugs to choose from for testing beyond the HHS five-panel. This is partly because fewer immunoassays have been formally designed, validated, and made available for testing of most non-urine specimens, with blood being a possible exception.
- More limited controlled drug administration studies available to guide interpretation.

Because of these disadvantages and because of comparatively limited use and limited case law, results from nonurine specimens can be harder to defend in front of an arbitrator, judge, or jury.

Conducting Multiple Tests at the Same Visit ■

Some employers collect two specimens (e.g., hair and urine) at the same testing event to get more information than one specimen provides. For example, an employer may conduct pre-employment tests with hair and urine to get hair's long detection window and urine's sensitivity for detecting recent use. If one specimen is positive and the other is negative, the donor may claim the inconsistency proves that the positive result is false. In fact, each test stands on its own merits; a negative result from one specimen does not invalidate a positive result from the other. The results may differ because of:

- Windows of detection.
- Stability of the drug(s) within the different matrices.
- Analytical sensitivity for the drug(s).
- Specificity for the drug(s).
- Panels of drugs for which the laboratory is testing and cutoff values for those assays.
- Adulteration or substitution of one specimen and not the other.

Medical Review of Non-Urine Test Results ■

The approach to reviewing non-urine drug test results is similar to that for urine drug test results. The knowledge base for interpretation of drug tests is well developed for urine, but not so much for non-urine specimens. The HHS and DOT procedures are a paradigm for workplace urine testing programs. There is no similar consensus about procedures for workplace non-urine specimen testing. Those who sell non-urine testing services offer information that supports the proper use of their products. Each MRO should keep in mind that *he or she* is responsible for the test interpretation and it is the *MRO's* signature that attests to the final outcome.

Problems with urine tests commonly involve specimen integrity issues (i.e., dilute, substituted, invalid, and adulterated specimens). Problems with non-urine specimens usually involve other issues, such as:

- Insufficient specimen volume for additional tests, such as *d*- and *l*-isomer tests for amphetamines, tests for specific adulterants, or reconfirmation analyses. (When the MRO believes an additional test should be performed but the specimen volume is insufficient, the MRO must cancel the test.)
- Uncertainty about distinguishing poppy seed use from heroin use. For urine, there are dozens of published scientific studies and there are federal procedures that have established a consensus on how to distinguish poppy seed use from opiate drug use. There is less information about this for hair tests and even less information about oral fluid tests.
- Uncertainty about distinguishing ethanol ingestion from passive exposure when testing for ethyl glucuronide in hair or oral fluid.
- Passive exposure to drugs. Urine tests at federal cutoff values will not be positive by passive exposure to drugs with rare exceptions for artificially intense exposure scenarios. The same cannot be said for hair and oral fluid tests, especially at low cutoffs used by some commercial laboratories.
- Non-beverage exposure to alcohol. Studies describe the detection of the metabolite ethyl glucuronide in urine and oral fluid after use of mouthwash, ethanol-containing hand sanitizers, and other non-beverage forms of ethanol (alcohol). There are more data about this phenomenon for urine than for oral fluid and scant information about this for hair.

Urine ■

INCORPORATION OF DRUGS INTO URINE

Urination is a major route for elimination of drugs/metabolites from the body. The kidney excretes drugs/metabolites into the urine by the same mechanism the kidney uses to remove end products of metabolism from the body. The urine concentrations of drugs/metabolites usually peak in the first 24 hours after use. Concentrations then decrease after last use over several days or weeks depending on the characteristics of the drug/metabolite. Over the elimination period, urinary drug/metabolite concentrations vary depending on factors such as urinary flow rates and urine pH. Increases (or decreases) in urine volume cause decreases (or increases) in drug/metabolite concentrations. Drugs/metabolites that are bases are excreted to a greater extent if the urine is acidic, whereas acidic drugs/metabolites are excreted to a greater extent if the urine is alkaline.

SPECIMEN COLLECTION CONCERNS

With urine, the collection step is the most problematic part of testing. Donors urinate in privacy in workplace testing. This allows an opportunity to adulterate or substitute their specimen. Donors can also drink a great deal of fluids and dilute their specimens, possibly reducing drug/metabolite concentrations below cutoffs. There is a wealth of publically available information and products to help cheat on urine drug tests. There is much less information and products to cheat on non-urine tests, in part because these tests are newer and less prevalent than urine in workplace settings.

WHEN TO CONDUCT URINE TESTS

The great majority of workplace drug tests are conducted with urine. Table 12-2 lists some of the advantages to urine tests in comparison to other specimens. Urine is used for all types of workplace tests, i.e., pre-employment, post-accident, etc. If an employer wants to test for an uncommon analyte—for example, certain prescription opiates—the employer may have to conduct a urine test because commercial hair and oral fluid testing laboratories offer tests for comparatively fewer analytes.

If a test is performed to measure impairment or use associated with a very recent accident, blood or oral fluid are better choices than urine. If a test is performed to identify use beyond the past few days, hair is often a better choice than urine.

Hair ■

INCORPORATION OF DRUGS INTO HAIR

Drugs can be incorporated into hair by at least three routes:

1. **Transfer from blood into the follicle.** Drugs and metabolites diffuse from blood through the dermal papilla and into the hair follicle and are thereby incorporated into newly forming hair cells in the hair shaft.
2. **Transfer from sweat and oil into the shaft.** Drugs and metabolites are secreted by the apocrine sweat glands and sebaceous glands. These secretions can be adsorbed into the hair shaft.
3. **External contamination of the shaft.** Drugs from the environment can settle on, and be absorbed into, hair. Pubic hair and body hair are more porous and thus may be more susceptible to external contamination than scalp hair.

Hair growth alternates between periods of growth (*anagen* phase) and rest (*catagen* and *telagen* phases). At any moment, approximately 85 to 90% of the hair is growing and 10 to 15% is resting. Hair growth varies among people and by body region. Scalp hair grows at a rate of about 0.4 mm per day (or 1.2 cm per month). Hair from other body regions grows more slowly. In workplace testing, the specimen typically consists of about 3 cm of length cut from the scalp and kept in orderly bundles of strands, which corresponds to about 3 months of growth.

Once incorporated into hair, drugs and metabolites for the most part remain in place and unchanged, but there can be changes over time. For example, there is some evidence that cocaine may be hydrolyzed to benzoylecognine [1]. Perming, straightening, and coloring hair may decrease certain drug/metabolite concentrations. Washing hair can at least partly remove ethyl glucuronide.

Each strand of hair consists of a follicle (bulb) below the skin surface and a shaft above the skin surface. Direct incorporation occurs into developing hair cells during the time drugs and metabolites are in the bloodstream. Drugs/metabolites incorporated into the follicle below the scalp appear above the scalp after about a week. Thus, drugs/metabolites that are incorporated by follicle-based cell formation remain below the scalp for about a week, and during this time are inaccessible for testing because hair specimens are cut from above the scalp. Some refer to hair testing as *hair follicle* testing, a term that exaggerates its abilities. The hair follicle is below the scalp surface and is neither collected nor tested. As the hair grows, the shaft—and, with it, any sequestered bands of drug/metabolite—are pushed outward. While hair grows a discrete length each day, the concentration of drug or metabolite, when plotted out along the hair shaft, looks like more of a bell curve than a discrete, 1-day band (see Step 1 in Figure 12-2). If the person uses drugs repeatedly, the drugs/metabolites will be present along the hair shaft in multiple bands (see Step 2 in Figure 12-2). Hair tests are conducted on lengths of hair that are cut and digested. Hair tests measure the average use over time and, at typical cutoffs, identify repeated use rather than single use.

SEGMENTAL ANALYSIS

Segmental analysis refers to cutting and analyzing hair in sections (see Step 3 in Figure 12-2) and comparing the concentration changes between sections to estimate when the person used the drug (see Step 4). If segmental analysis is ordered from the laboratory, the laboratory will subdivide the specimen into segments

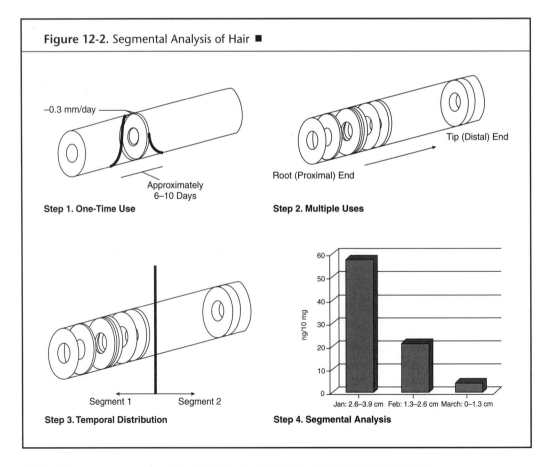

Figure 12-2. Segmental Analysis of Hair ■

Step 1. One-Time Use

Step 2. Multiple Uses

Step 3. Temporal Distribution

Step 4. Segmental Analysis

and test each segment using both screening analyses for presumptive determinations of relative drug use levels and confirmatory methods to get concentrations. Typically, hair is aligned and cut in 1 cm segments, each approximating 1 month's growth. The precision of segmental analysis can be reduced by absorption of drugs and metabolites onto distal segments from sweat and oil secretions from the scalp. The laboratory's washing of specimens prior to analysis can reduce such issues, but they must nevertheless be considered. The precision is also reduced by the variation in growth rates between strands of hair. If a person used drugs a few months ago but not recently, the drug/metabolite concentration in his or her hair should be lower in segments close to the scalp than in segments further away from the scalp. Segmental analyses performed on positive hair specimens may identify drug/metabolite in all segments, but at different concentrations. The reviewer is then left wondering how much of a change is required to definitively determine if someone used, or stopped using, drugs between segments. There are no definitive criteria for this. The test offers information about patterns of use over time, but is too imprecise for distinguishing use from non-use over periods of time in workplace drug testing programs. Because of the liability risk associated with assigning time frames for specific segments being tested, some hair testing laboratories will not perform segmental analysis or will not perform it for workplace testing programs. Segmental analysis may be useful for monitoring a person's compliance with drug therapy and investigating suspected drug-facilitated sexual assaults or in other criminal cases.

COLOR/ETHNIC BIAS

The potential "color" bias in hair testing arises from the affinity of some drugs to bind with the pigment melanin. There are two types of melanin in hair: eumelanin, which is present at much greater quantities in most hair, and pheomelanin. Eumelanin gives hair its darker color and is present in higher concentrations in people of Asian and African descent. After ingesting or being exposed to the same amount of a drug, individuals who have darker hair will have a greater amount of drug incorporated into their hair than individuals who have lighter hair.

The "ethnic bias" in hair testing refers to the likelihood that, for any given exposure, a positive test is more likely among people with dark, thick hair (e.g., African Americans) than among people with light, thin hair (e.g., northern Europeans). This may be from drug binding with eumelanin. It may also be from differences in drug use behaviors, potencies, hair treatments, and even environmental exposure.

Some laboratories have tried to remedy concerns about hair color by extracting melanin from the hair during specimen preparation. Whether this eliminates any effect of hair color remains unclear.

PASSIVE EXPOSURE

Laboratories wash hair samples to remove surface contaminants and reduce the possibility of positive results caused by environmental contamination. Whether this is effective remains unclear. Some laboratories apply reporting criteria whereby drug-positive results are reported only if one or more metabolites are also present at or above certain threshold concentrations or if the metabolite-to-parent ratio exceeds some threshold. The assumption is that significant concentrations of metabolites establish use of the drug as opposed to external contamination of the hair. However, some of these "metabolite" analytes are present in environmental residues that are deposited onto hair, and some arise from cocaine deposited on hair that is transformed by non-metabolic processes. This remains an area of debate. However, it appears that extensive external exposure to at least some drugs can cause positive results [2,3,4].

WHEN TO CONDUCT HAIR TESTS

Based on the long detection window, hair is best suited for pre-employment and random testing. Unless at least 3 months have elapsed since last use, testing of scalp hair is a poor choice for return-to-duty and follow-up drug testing. This is because a donor may test positive for drugs for at least 3 months even if he or she has stopped using, due to the presence of "telogen" hair that can remain present after they have stopped growing and incorporating drugs. Hair is a poor choice for reasonable suspicion/cause and post-accident testing because it takes at least 7 days for drug or drug metabolites to appear in hair, and thus the specimen collected just after the event will not identify use just before the event.

Hair offers an average measure of use over a relatively long period of time. In comparison to urine, a positive hair test is a better indicator of chronic use. Hair testing is best suited for tests where a long window of detection is desirable. Hair testing can also be useful in evaluating a person's fitness to perform safety-sensitive duty because it can help identify if the person has repeatedly used a drug over recent months. Hair tests have been observed to have higher positive rates than urine tests in workplace settings, by about two-thirds, with particularly higher rates for detection of cocaine and methamphetamine [5].

Hair tests are not designed—using commonly applied cutoffs and hair lengths tested—to detect a single use and probably not even a few uses. A well-timed urine test is relatively more sensitive at identifying one or several uses of a drug.

Hair tests do not directly identify ethanol due to its volatility and its potential absorption from external sources. Hair tests to monitor for alcohol use should instead target the ethanol metabolites ethyl glucuronide or fatty acid ethyl esters [6]. Availability of hair testing for synthetic opioids and other drugs beyond the HHS five-panel is limited.

Because of the possibility of positive hair test results from heavy external contamination with cocaine, hair tests for cocaine should be avoided on those who have occupational exposure to cocaine [3].

Oral Fluid ■

INCORPORATION OF DRUGS INTO ORAL FLUID

The terms *oral fluid* and *saliva* are often used interchangeably. Oral fluid is the technically correct, albeit awkward, term. Oral fluid contains saliva, cellular material, and other components that, in combination, are more properly called *oral fluid*. More than 14 glands in the head and mouth excrete saliva. Saliva flow varies from 0.5 L/day to 1.5 L/day and can be stimulated to a peak flow of approximately 10 mL/min.

Most drugs passively diffuse from plasma into saliva, but some (e.g., steroids) are actively secreted from plasma into saliva. Cannabinoids and benzodiazepines are strongly bound to proteins in plasma and thus diffuse into saliva at low rates, which accounts for their low concentrations in oral fluid. The marijuana metabolite THCA, which is commonly targeted in tests of other specimens, does not diffuse in significant concentrations from plasma into saliva. Oral fluid tests for marijuana instead target the parent drug, THC, which can get into oral fluid both by transfer from plasma to plasma and by residues that absorb in the mouth from inhaled marijuana smoke, even second-hand smoke.

Most drugs/metabolites are detectable in oral fluid within minutes after use. Their concentrations drop rapidly and, depending on the cutoffs, may become undetectable within 24 hours after last use. This roughly parallels the rise and fall of plasma concentrations, and thereby provides some degree of correlation with pharmacodynamic effects. The presence of the parent drug in oral fluid may also provide a better correlation with ongoing pharmacodynamic effects than with urine testing.

Drugs can be directly deposited onto the mucosal surface of the mouth and upper airways. This is particularly true of drugs that are smoked, snorted, or dissolved under the tongue but does not appear to occur by ingestion of capsules or coated pills. Drug/metabolite deposits on the oral mucosa can become incorporated into oral fluid.

Drug/metabolite concentrations in oral fluid are at least tenfold lower than in urine and are especially low for benzodiazepines and cannabinoids. Their measurement therefore requires highly sensitive assays, including tandem mass spectrometry as part of confirmation methods.

PASSIVE EXPOSURE

Oral fluid tests can be positive due to recent passive exposure to cannabis smoke. Cannabis residues deposited while smoking are cleared from the oral cavity within 30–60 minutes [7]. Cannabis residues from passive inhalation are cleared more quickly, e.g., usually within 30 minutes [8]. Experiments using intense environmental exposure and low cutoffs have measured THC-positive oral fluid results for up to 60 minutes after passive exposure [9]. The consensus appears to be that passive inhalation must be intense and recent to cause positive oral fluid results. The risk of positive results from passive exposure appears to be limited to 30 minutes after such exposure. Passive exposure does not appear to be a problem for cocaine and heroin, because tests for those drugs target metabolites of these drugs that are not present in significant concentrations in environmental smoke.

SPECIMEN COLLECTION CONCERNS

Most oral fluid collection devices consist of a pad on a stick that is placed in the mouth. Saliva flow can be stimulated by chewing gum, cough drops, and merely putting the oral fluid collection device in the mouth. Concentrations of drugs in stimulated oral fluid specimens tend to be lower than in non-stimulated specimens. Drug/metabolite concentrations are also dependent on the fluid pH.

The pad is removed from the mouth and placed in a buffer solution, which dilutes the specimen. One can estimate but not precisely measure the volume of oral fluid collected on a pad-on-stick device. Likewise, the drug/metabolite concentration in the oral fluid is estimated based on the measured value in the oral fluid/buffer mix and the expected ratio of that mix. Recovery and stability of drugs and ethanol varies among collection devices. Certain drugs—e.g., THC and benzodiazepines—are adsorbed to some devices rather than going into solution, which can lead to false-negative results [10]. Many devices collect less than 1 mL of oral fluid, limiting available samples for multiple drug confirmations. There is variability in the oral fluid volume obtained within and between devices and imprecision in the calculated concentrations. At least one collection device that is commercially available is designed to collect a known volume of neat oral fluid. Concentration calculations from neat oral fluid are relatively straightforward.

POINT-OF-COLLECTION ORAL FLUID TESTS

Performance of point-of-collection test (POCT, or on-site) test devices for oral fluid varies widely and is generally below that of laboratory-based oral fluid tests [11]. They are particularly insensitive at identifying marijuana use. This is because many use the same types of immunoassays as are used for urine tests, i.e., immunoassays targeted at the metabolite THCA. However, THC is the predominant analyte in oral fluid; this is what laboratories target. THCA concentrations in oral fluid are low, but THC concentrations are much lower, limiting diagnostic sensitivity of most POCT oral fluid tests.

WHEN TO CONDUCT ORAL FLUID TESTS

Oral fluid offers information about very recent use. Drugs that are smoked or snorted can be detected in oral fluid immediately after use. Drugs that are swallowed can be detected in oral fluid within 1–2 hours. By comparison, drugs are first detectable in urine 2–6 hours after use.

In comparison to other specimens, the window of drug detection in oral fluid more closely parallels that in plasma. Some have therefore looked at oral fluid as a surrogate for blood testing, even accepting it as an indicator of impairment. While there are no data that correlate positive oral fluid tests with impairment, the assumption is that a positive oral fluid test result at least represents very recent use and may be more closely related to impairment.

Oral fluid can detect drug use within the past hour or so, which urine can miss. This makes it well suited for reasonable suspicion/cause and post-accident testing. The short window of detection of oral fluid testing makes it less useful for return-to-duty and follow-up drug testing. The short window of detection may also reduce detection and the deterrence value of oral fluid in comparison to other specimens. Oral fluid tests have been used for workplace testing, roadside testing of impaired drivers, and in treatment monitoring and emergency room testing. DOT allows use of an oral fluid (saliva) test for alcohol screens in its workplace testing programs. In some foreign countries, for example, Australia—oral fluid is the most commonly used specimen in workplace testing programs [12].

Nail ■

Nails grow slowly. Drug tests of nails provide little information about recent use and instead measure use from several months ago. The collection procedure—clipping nails—seems easy and non-invasive. As with other directly observed collections, the donor has little opportunity for adulteration or substitution.

INCORPORATION OF DRUGS INTO NAILS

The nail is a hard, translucent material composed of interlocking, dead keratinous cells. The nail is approximately 0.5 mm thick, is usually thicker in men than women, and thickens with age. Fingernails grow at an average rate of 3 mm per month (range 1.9–4.4 mm per month). The lifespan from formation of new nail to growth long enough to clip is about 6 months for fingernails. Toenails grow at about one-third the rate of fingernails. The growth rate varies among people and even between digits.

Most of the nail is formed at the germinal matrix below the skin just before where the nail exits. About 20% of the nail is also formed as the nail grows out over the nail bed, causing the distal end to grow thicker. The mechanism of drug entry and incorporation into the nail matrix probably involves drug deposition both during formation in the germinal matrix and during formation along the nail bed. Drugs/metabolites can also be incorporated into the top surface of the nail to a limited extent from environmental exposure and from sweat and other secretions from the body. The distal segment of a nail that is clipped off for a workplace drug test can be used to identify use during much of the nail's approximately six-month lifespan.

NAILS, ALCOHOL, AND DRUGS

A wide variety of drugs, including each of the drugs/metabolites in the federal test panel, can be detected in nails. Detection of marijuana use requires highly sensitive methods similar to those used for oral fluid and hair. Nail testing cannot be used to identify use of ethanol, but alcohol biomarkers have been detected in nails, as has cocaethylene, which is formed by combined use of ethanol and cocaine.

WHEN TO CONDUCT NAIL TESTS

Some hair testing laboratories offer nail tests as an alternative for donors who have no hair. There are no independent laboratory proficiency testing programs to help ensure the reliability of nail tests. Neither the government nor any professional organization has issued guidelines or standards for the use of nails for workplace testing. The published literature on nail testing for drugs is scant in comparison to other matrices. Nail testing for drugs may have value for certain forensic applications, such as postmortem examinations for heavy metals and some other exposures, but there are too many unknowns to establish its reliability for use in workplace testing programs. Several national MRO services have made it their policy to avoid involvement with nail drug testing programs.

Blood ■

Under ideal circumstances, the concentration of drug/metabolite in blood correlated with the concentration at the brain and therefore should be related to the degree of cognitive impairment. However, there is very little data available correlating blood concentrations with impairment. One exception is for alcohol for which there are many years of data correlating impairment and blood concentration. Blood testing is rarely used in workplace settings because it is considered too invasive and because the federal regulations do not authorize it, with limited exceptions, as described later in this chapter.

INCORPORATION OF DRUGS INTO BLOOD

Because most drugs are rapidly metabolized and eliminated, blood tests offer a brief detection window. Drugs in blood are typically detectable from minutes to hours after use depending on the drug and the dose. Blood levels of certain prescription drugs can be correlated with dosage, clinical effects, or both. Fewer data are available for correlation of blood concentrations of illicit drugs and impairment.

BLOOD ANALYSIS

Most drugs and their metabolites are eliminated from the body in urine. Their concentrations in urine are typically about 10 to 100 times greater than in blood. Because of the low concentrations, blood drug testing requires the laboratory to use sophisticated screening and confirmation analysis techniques. This can be time consuming and expensive.

BLOOD, ALCOHOL, AND DRUGS

Alcohol

This section presents brief summaries about blood tests for certain drugs. Readers should consult pharmacology and toxicology texts for more detail.

Blood alcohol concentrations (BACs) can be correlated with intoxication. State "driving under the influence" laws define intoxication at 0.08 BAC or higher. DOT defines impairment as 0.04 BAC (as measured in breath) or higher, because 0.04 is the threshold for being able to consistently measure impairment of functions associated with the safe operation of complex equipment.

Most studies relating alcohol concentration to impairment are based on either whole blood specimens or whole blood concentrations as reflected in breath specimens. Clinical laboratories usually test plasma or serum (which, for purposes of this discussion, are equivalent) instead of whole blood. The ratio of plasma (or serum) to blood alcohol is between 1.15 and 1.2. When interpreting the degree of intoxication associated with a plasma or serum alcohol concentration, the first step is to divide the value by 1.15–1.2, to calculate the whole blood alcohol concentration.

Amphetamines

A prescription-strength oral dose of amphetamine typically results in a peak plasma concentration of 110 ng/mL. The plasma half-life for the *d*-isomer is about 12 hours. The plasma half-life of the *l*-isomer is about one-third longer. Doses of 5 to 10 mg amphetamine typically result in blood concentrations between 20 to 60 ng/mL.

Cocaine

After a typical dose of cocaine (e.g., 50 mg), blood concentrations peak at around several hundred ng/mL. After repeated or high doses, blood concentrations can peak as high as several thousand ng/mL. Cocaine can be identified in blood for at least 8 hours after a typical dose and for up to 24 hours or more after a high dose. The detection period is longer for the cocaine metabolites benzoylecgonine and ecgonine methyl ester.

Marijuana
Peak plasma THC concentrations of 100–200 ng/mL can occur after smoking potent marijuana. Plasma THC and THCA concentrations drop below 1 ng/mL within a few hours after a single use. Concentrations may remain above 1 ng/mL for more than 24–48 hours after repeated use. Whole blood THC and THCA concentrations are lower than plasma concentrations, with a blood-to-plasma ratio of approximately 0.5.

Opiates
Heroin has an elimination half-life of about 3–6 minutes and is rarely detected in blood or other body fluid samples. The heroin metabolite, 6-acetylmorphine (6-AM), also has a short plasma half-life, about 15 minutes, and is rarely detected in blood. The plasma half-life of morphine is about 2–3 hours. The plasma elimination half-life of codeine is about 3.3 hours.

Phencyclidine
The plasma half-life of PCP is usually less than 24 hours, but has been reported as long as 3 days in cases of PCP overdose.

WHEN TO CONDUCT BLOOD TESTS

The DOT rule authorizes blood testing in limited circumstances:

- The U.S. Coast Guard (USCG) allows blood alcohol tests in reasonable suspicion and post-accident circumstances.
- The Federal Railroad Administration (FRA) requires blood specimen analyses for drugs and alcohol in investigation of railroad accidents. The blood samples are analyzed at an FRA-designated laboratory, using limits of detection rather than standard federal cutoff levels and including tests for an expanded panel of psychoactive substances.
- The Federal Motor Carrier Safety Administration (FMCSA) and Federal Transit Administration (FTA) allow employers to use, for purposes of compliance with DOT post-accident regulations, the results of blood alcohol testing conducted by a law enforcement agency under that agency's independent authority.

As noted in the "Regulations" section of this chapter, the DOT rule also authorizes clinical examinations to assess drug abuse, and these exams may include tests of nonurine specimens, such as blood.

References ■

1. Ropero-Miller J, Stout P. Analysis of cocaine analytes in human hair: Evaluation of concentration ratios in different hair types, cocaine sources, drug-user populations, and surface-contaminated specimens. Grant report to the U.S. Department of Justice Office of Justice Programs National Institute of Justice. Document number 225531, received January 2009.

2. Stout P, Ropero-Miller J, Baylor M, Mitchell J. External contamination of hair with cocaine: Evaluation of external cocaine contamination and development of performance-testing materials. *J Anal Toxicol* 2006;30:490–500.
3. LeBeau M, Montgomery M. Considerations on the utility of hair analysis for cocaine. *J Anal Toxicol* 2009;33:343–44.
4. Romano G, Nunziata B, Spadaro G, et al. Determination of drugs of abuse in hair: Evaluation of external heroin contamination and risk of false positives. *Forensic Sci Int* 2003;131:98–102.
5. Quest Diagnostics. New hair data validate sharp downward trend in cocaine and methamphetamine positivity in general U.S. workforce, according to Quest Diagnostics Drug Testing Index. Madison, NJ: Quest Diagnostics, Inc. Nov. 20, 2009.
6. Society of Hair Testing. Consensus of the Society of Hair Testing on hair testing for chronic excessive alcohol consumption. Roma, Italy. June 16, 2009.
7. Heustis M, Cone E. Relationship of delta 9-tetrahydrocannabinol concentrations in oral fluid and plasma after controlled administration of smoked cannabis. *J Anal Toxicol* 2004;28:394–9.
8. Niedbala S, Kardos K, Salamone S, et al. Passive cannabis smoke exposure and oral fluid testing. *J Anal Toxicol* 2004;28:546–52.
9. Niedbala S, Kardos K, Fritch D, et al. Passive cannabis smoke exposure and oral fluid testing, II: Two studies of extreme cannabis smoke exposure in a motor vehicle. *J Anal Toxicol* 2005;29:607–15.
10. Langel K, Engblom C, Pehrsson A, et al. Drug testing in oral fluid—evaluation of sample collection devices. *J Anal Toxicol.* 2008;32:393–401.
11. Bosker W, Huestis M. Oral fluid testing for drugs of abuse. *Clin Chem* 2009;55:1910–31.
12. Dyer K, Dyer K, Wilkinson C, et al. The detection of illicit drugs in oral fluid: another potential strategy to reduce illicit drug-related harm. *Drug and Alcohol Review* 2008;27:99–107.

Alcohol and Specific Drugs ■

Alcohol ■

Alcohol is a sedative drug. Figure 13-1 presents its chemical structure. While the term *alcohol* also refers to a class of chemicals that includes methanol and iso-propanol, in the context of workplace testing, *alcohol* means *ethanol.*

USE

Alcohol use by adults is legal in the United States. Alcohol is the most widely used intoxicant in the world.

ALCOHOL ABUSE AND DEPENDENCE

Alcohol abuse and alcohol dependence are characterized by a compulsion to drink despite adverse consequences. During 2001–2002, the prevalence of alcohol abuse and dependence in the U.S. was 8.5%, according to the National Institutes of Health. Early indicators of heavy drinking include personality problems, family problems, legal and financial problems, increased use of sick leave, and increasing medical problems and somatization. In the early stages, clinical findings are few and subtle. As alcoholism progresses, the person's health and workplace performance deteriorate. Patients with longstanding alcohol problems may present with alcohol-related diseases such as cirrhosis or pancreatitis.

An accurate diagnosis of alcohol abuse or dependence requires a thorough history of the person's drinking behavior and its consequences. Several screening

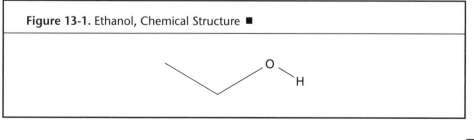

Figure 13-1. Ethanol, Chemical Structure ■

questionnaires are available to help identify alcohol problems. The four CAGE questions, for example, are quickly administered and easily remembered by the mnemonic: "C" for cut down, "A" for annoyed, "G" for guilty, and "E" for eye-opener [1] (see Figure 13-2). "Yes" responses to two or more CAGE questions are thought to be clinically significant and may indicate alcohol dependence.

METABOLISM AND EXCRETION

When a person consumes alcohol, the blood alcohol concentration (BAC) rises while alcohol is absorbed from the intestine, plateaus while alcohol is distributed to and equilibrates with tissues, and falls during metabolism and excretion. Alcohol is absorbed into the blood in 30–60 minutes. If a test is performed during the absorptive period, the measured value may be less than the person's subsequent peak BAC. Alcohol is soluble in water and barely soluble in fat. Once absorbed, alcohol distributes to the blood and throughout the body, predominantly in aqueous fluids (like blood) and tissues. As a general rule, the heavier a person, or the greater proportion of body weight that is water, the greater the volume of alcohol that must be consumed to reach a specific alcohol concentration in the body. The proportion of body weight that is water is 55–65% in men and 45–55% in women. The volume of distribution, V_d, is a term relating the dose and blood concentration of ethanol after absorption and equilibration with body tissues, as follows:

$$V_d = dose/BAC$$

This value is approximately 0.68 L/kg (range 0.51 to 0.85) in men and 0.55 L/kg (range 0.44 to 0.66 L/kg) in women. The apparent V_d for alcohol varies between people depending on stomach contents, sex, previous alcohol intake history, metabolic capacity, and amount of body fat. Consumption of food slows absorption, causes a decrease in peak BAC, and thereby causes an increase in the apparent V_d. Alcoholics have lower apparent V_d values than nonalcoholics of the same sex.

Approximately 90% to 95% of ingested alcohol is oxidized in the liver, first to acetaldehyde, then to carbon dioxide and water. About 1–2% of ingested alcohol is excreted unchanged in the urine. Alcohol is eliminated from the body at a rate of about 0.015–0.018 g/dL/hr, equivalent to about one drink per hour. Alcohol elimination rates are highly variable, ranging at least as broadly as 0.010–

Figure 13-2. CAGE Assessment ■

1. Have you ever felt you ought to cut down on your drinking?
2. Have people annoyed you by criticizing your drinking?
3. Have you ever felt bad or guilty about your drinking?
4. Have you ever had a drink first thing in the morning to steady your nerves or get rid of a hangover (eye-opener)?

0.024 g/dL/hr in the general population. Even within the same person, the rate of alcohol elimination can vary over time. Drinkers metabolize alcohol more quickly—e.g., 0.017 g/dL/hr for a moderate drinker and 0.020 g/dL/hr for a heavy drinker (60 or more drinks per month)—until cirrhosis develops, at which point the metabolic rate is reduced. Alcohol metabolism rates are also increased at very high BAC. Use of barbiturates can increase one's alcohol metabolism rate.

A number of software programs and interactive web pages are available for calculating BAC following alcohol consumption. These calculations require entry of the person's weight and gender, the volume of alcohol consumed, and the time period during which it was consumed. The volume of alcohol depends on the volume and type of alcoholic beverage. Table 13-1 lists the alcohol content of various beverages and products as a percentage by volume. *Proof* refers to the percentage by volume multiplied by two. For example, rum is 80–100 proof, and contains 40–50% alcohol by volume.

Because alcohol is eliminated from the body in a somewhat predictable manner, one can estimate the BAC at a time several hours earlier by assuming a straight-line decrease in BAC. This technique, called *back extrapolation,* can be used to estimate a person's BAC at the time of an accident or reasonable suspicious incident, based on the BAC measured several hours later. This is performed by multiplying the elapsed time by the elimination rate and adding this value to the measured BAC. Extrapolation uses certain assumptions and approximations that introduce potential inaccuracies. Ideally, extrapolation is conducted starting with a blood alcohol concentration because starting with a surrogate for blood (e.g., breath) introduces an additional variable and potential for error. Extrapolation results should be presented to account for low, high, and average metabolic rates, thereby accounting for the range of possible results. For example, Figure 13-3 presents a range of back-extrapolated BAC values based on low (0.010 g/dL/hr), average (0.015 g/dL/hr), and high (0.020 g/dL/hr) alcohol metabolism rates. The DOT Part 40 rule does not allow for extrapolation of alcohol test results. Thus, alcohol test results cannot be used to identify employees who may have violated the "pre-duty abstinence" periods required of certain DOT-covered safety-sensitive employees. By contrast, the NRC rule directs the MRO to take alcohol test results in the 0.02–0.04 range and back-extrapolate them to the time the worker was on duty.

Table 13-1. Alcohol Content of Some Common Products ■

Product	Ethanol, % by Volume
Beer	3.2–6
Cough medicine	5–17
Mouthwash	15–25 up to 75
Rum	40–50
Scotch	40–50
Vodka	40–50
Wine, fortified (e.g., sherry, vermouth)	14–20
Wine	5–13

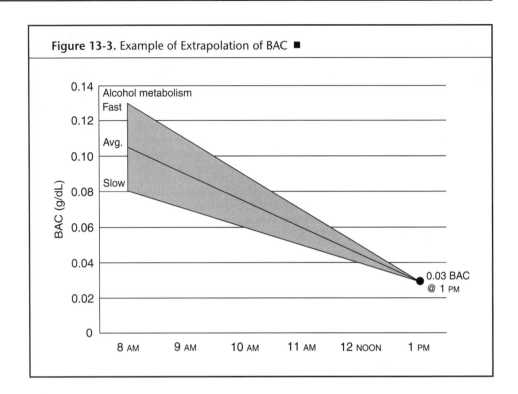

Figure 13-3. Example of Extrapolation of BAC ■

(Figure shows BAC (g/dL) on the vertical axis from 0 to 0.14 and time on the horizontal axis from 8 AM to 1 PM. Labels: Alcohol metabolism — Fast, Avg., Slow. Endpoint marked 0.03 BAC @ 1 PM.)

LABORATORY ANALYSIS

Breath and oral fluid alcohol tests are noninvasive, provide immediate results, and are required for use in workplace testing under the Department of Transportation (DOT) and Nuclear Regulatory Commission (NRC) rules. Tests of breath and oral fluid are used to approximate the person's BAC.

Blood

BAC is the most direct measure short of testing cerebrospinal fluid to assess the concentration, and thus the effect, of alcohol on the brain. The concentration of alcohol in blood is expressed as milligrams or grams of ethanol per 100 mL of blood, written as "mg/dL" or "g/dL." The popular methods for measuring ethanol in a clinical laboratory are the Conway microdiffusion assay, the alcohol dehydrogenase assay, immunoassays, and, especially in forensic laboratories, gas chromatography with or without mass spectrometry.

Urine

Urine alcohol testing is accepted by a few states for purposes of establishing driving while intoxicated, but it is not authorized by the federal drug testing rules. Most employers who test urine for alcohol do so because they already test urine for drugs and adding alcohol to the urine panel is convenient. Because of the poor correlation between random urine alcohol and BACs, employers who want to test for alcohol should instead test breath.

Urine alcohol concentration can be correlated with BAC with certain caveats. The urine alcohol concentration is related to the average BAC during the time the urine was produced, which can extend for several hours before collection. A random urine specimen's alcohol concentration is not necessarily related to the donor's BAC at the time of specimen collection. Therefore, it cannot be used to indicate unequivocally whether the person was impaired or intoxicated at the time of specimen collection. A two-step collection procedure can be used to obtain urine produced during a period more closely approximating the time of collection and thus more closely related to current BAC. The procedure for two-step urine collection is described in Chapter 6 of this book. If the urine alcohol concentration in the second step collection is divided by 1.3, it approximates the BAC during the time the urine was produced (i.e., at about the time of collection). However, there is tremendous variation in the urine-blood ratio, with studies suggesting a range at least as wide as 0.53 to 2.17. Also, residual urine may remain in the bladder after the first void, diluting the "freshness" of the second specimen.

It is possible to have production of alcohol in a specimen obtained from a person who did not consume alcohol. This phenomenon is uncommon, but it can happen if all three of the following conditions are present:

1. The urine contains glucose, i.e., the donor is a diabetic.
2. The urine is contaminated with certain microorganisms, such as *Candida albicans.*
3. The urine has been stored at room temperature without a preservative for 1 day or more prior to analysis. (This is usually the case for workplace urine specimens, which are rarely prepared with perservatives and are usually shipped to laboratories by nonrefrigerated courier services.)

When urine is tested for alcohol for workplace purposes, it should also be tested for glucose. If glucose is detected, the urine alcohol concentration may be elevated because of contamination with microorganisms.

Saliva
The analysis of alcohol in saliva is performed on-site using a point-of-collection test device, rather than sending the specimen to an off-site laboratory. The Q.E.D. Saliva Alcohol Test device (Orasure Technologies, Inc., Bethlehem, Pennsylvania) is among the most widely used devices for saliva alcohol testing in workplace settings. It is a cotton pad on a stick (like a Q-Tip) that, when in contact with alcohol, displays a color change through a reaction with alcohol dehydrogenase. If the saliva alcohol concentration correlates with a BAC above a cutoff value, this is evidenced by a color change on the device after several minutes. Alcohol concentration in saliva is about the same as alcohol concentration in blood at a steady state, although there is much variability in this ratio. Each device also has a built-in quality control mechanism to help ensure the validity of results. The Q.E.D. Saliva Alcohol Test device has been granted waived status under the Clinical Laboratory Improvements Amendments.

Hair
The direct determination of ethanol itself in hair is not possible due to its volatility and its potential absorption from external surfaces. Instead, tests for chronic alcohol use should target the ethanol metabolites ethyl glucuronide (EtG) or fatty acid ethyl esters. A negative result does not prove abstinence, but a positive result indicates use or exposure. The extent to which incidental exposure to ethanol

can lead to EtG in hair is unclear. The Society for Hair Testing has proposed using a 30 pg/mg scalp hair cutoff for EtG to identify chronic excessive alcohol consumption [2].

Breath

Breath is the specimen usually used in workplace testing. Chapter 14 discusses workplace breath alcohol testing.

INTERPRETING RESULTS

Alcohol tests are not reviewed to determine if the donors have legitimate medical explanations. The donor should not have an unacceptable alcohol level just before, during, or just after performing safety-sensitive duties, without regard to the source of alcohol. An occasional employee may claim that consumption of cough medicine, mouthwash, or another ethanol-containing product caused his or her positive result. These products contain low concentrations of ethanol (see Table 13-1) and their proper use will not cause a detectable level of alcohol in workplace testing.

BACs can be correlated with intoxication, as illustrated in Table 13-2. Most studies relating alcohol concentration to impairment are based on either whole blood specimens or whole blood concentrations as reflected in breath specimens. Clinical laboratories usually test plasma or serum—which, for purposes of this discussion, are equivalent—instead of whole blood. The ratio of plasma (or serum) to blood alcohol is between 1.15 and 1.2 [3]. When interpreting the degree of intoxication associated with a plasma or serum test result, the first step is to divide the value by 1.15–1.2 to arrive at the corresponding value for whole blood.

The DOT program has set 0.02 BAC in breath as an action level for temporary removal from safety-sensitive job tasks. An employee with a BAC of 0.02–0.039 is *temporarily* removed from safety-sensitive job tasks and does not have to complete the return-to-duty process. The length of time the employee is removed is set by each DOT agency rule and ranges from 8–24 hours (see Table 2-1). The DOT based its program on zero tolerance and selected 0.02 as the cutoff value because some breath test devices are unreliable below 0.02, because some people may experience some degree of impairment in this range, and because this concentration may represent a rising or increasing alcohol concentration.

The DOT program has set 0.04 BAC in breath as a rule violation which, like a positive drug test, requires removal from safety-sensitive job tasks. Return to safety-sensitive duties can occur only after successful completion of the return-to-duty process. The 0.04 concentration is considered the minimal threshold for being able to consistently measure impairment of functions associated with the safe operation of complex equipment. The probability of an auto crash begins to rise when the driver's blood alcohol concentration exceeds 0.04 and rises dramatically when it reaches 0.10.

Employers with non-DOT alcohol testing programs often use the DOT thresholds, although some use 0.08, which is the per se threshold for driving under the influence in the United States. The consensus opinion is that everyone is too intoxicated to drive at 0.08 BAC. In some states, drivers with concentrations at or

Table 13-2. Stages of Acute Alcoholic Influence/Intoxication ∎

Blood Alcohol Concentration (g/100 mL)	Stage of Alcohol Influence/ Intoxication	Clinical Signs/Symptoms
0.01–0.05	Subclinical	Behavior nearly normal by ordinary observation. Slight changes detectable by special tests. Computation speed diminished. Mental acuity decreases.
0.03–0.12	Euphoria	Mild euphoria, sociability, talkativeness. Increased self-confidence; decreased inhibition. Diminution of attention, judgment, and control. Mild sensory-motor impairment. Slowed information processing. Loss of efficiency in fine-motor performance tests.
0.09–0.25	Excitement	Emotional instability; loss of critical judgment. Impairment of perception, memory, and comprehension. Decreased sensory response; increased reaction time. Reduced visual acuity, peripheral vision, and glare recovery. Sensory-motor incoordination; impaired balance. Drowsiness.
0.18–0.30	Confusion	Disorientation, mental confusion; dizziness. Exaggerated emotional states (e.g., fear, rage, sorrow). Disturbances of vision (e.g., diplopia) and of perception of color, form, motion, dimensions. Increased pain threshold. Increased muscular incoordination, staggering gait, slurred speech. Apathy, lethargy.
0.25–0.40	Stupor	General inertia; approaching loss of motor functions. Marked muscular incoordination; inability to stand or walk. Vomiting; incontinence of urine and feces. Impaired consciousness; sleep or stupor.
0.35–0.50	Coma	Complete unconsciousness; coma; anesthesia. Depressed or abolished reflexes. Subnormal temperature. Incontinence of urine and feces. Impairment of circulation and respiration. Possible death.
0.45+	Death	Death from respiratory arrest.

Source: Dubowski KM. Alcohol determination in the clinical laboratory. *Am J Clin Pathol* 1980;74:747–50.

above 0.05 are also considered "under the influence" if there is corroborating evidence, for example, a positive roadside sobriety test. For drivers under 21 years of age, the state thresholds are either zero tolerance or 0.02.

ALCOHOL BIOMARKER TESTS

Tests of alcohol biomarkers, predominantly in urine, are used to indirectly determine whether someone has consumed alcohol in the last 12–35 hours. Tests of alcohol biomarkers in hair can be used to identify alcohol consumption for even longer time periods, but with less sensitivity. Urine tests for alcohol biomarkers are used to monitor people for abstinence. For example, they are used to monitor physicians, airplane pilots, and others who had alcohol problems and have agreed to abstain and undergo monitoring as a condition of licensure or employment. Drinking alcohol off duty is otherwise allowed and a positive alcohol biomarker test result would be meaningless as far as fitness for work is concerned. Alcohol biomarker tests have little to do with detection of impairment at work.

Urine tests for alcohol biomarkers commonly target ethyl glucuronide (EtG) and ethyl sulfate (EtS). Ethanol is metabolized to both, as shown in Figure 13-4. After a single moderate intake of alcohol, EtG can be detected in blood for 10–14 hours, in urine for 25–35 hours, and in oral fluid for 14 hours [4, 5]. After heavy drinking, EtG and EtS can be detected longer, e.g., in urine for up to 5 days. EtS is somewhat more specific than EtG at detecting alcohol use. This is because certain bacteria that may contaminate urine can effect concentrations of EtG, but not EtS [6,7].

Hair tests for alcohol biomarkers target EtG and fatty acid ethyl esters (FAEE) can be entrapped in hair, where they can be detected long after use. Hair testing has not been used to monitor sobriety. The Society of Hair Testing has recommended an EtG cutoff of 30 pg/mg and a combined EtG+FAEE cutoff of 0.8 ng/mg to identify "excessive" but not "social" alcohol consumption [2]. This cutoff is high enough that passive exposure will not cause positives.

Urine testing for EtG and EtS became much more widespread in the 2000s, particularly for monitoring of impaired professionals. Laboratories were using low cutoffs, e.g., 100 ng/mL. Studies then demonstrated that use of ethanol-based mouthwash could cause urine EtG levels as high as 345 ng/mL [8,9] and skin exposure to ethanol-containing hand sanitizers could cause urine EtG levels above 100 ng/mL [9,10]. In 2006, SAMHSA issued a warning about use of alcohol biomarker tests because, given the cutoffs, they were not distinguishing between inadvertent exposure and deliberate consumption [11]. There is as yet no consensus on a urine EtG cutoff level that offers adequate analytical sensitivity and eliminates positives due to non-beverage alcohol. That cutoff may well be in the 1,000–2,000 ng/mL range for EtG in forensic testing programs. This cutoff

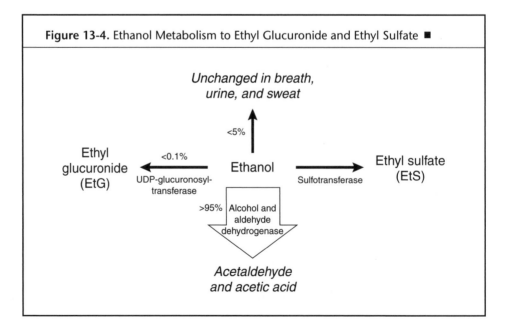

Figure 13-4. Ethanol Metabolism to Ethyl Glucuronide and Ethyl Sulfate ■

would avoid positives from skin exposure and mouthwash, but not necessarily from consumption of ethanol-containing cough syrups and other medications. Consumption of beverage ethanol can cause urine EtG results as high as the tens of thousands of ng/mL.

Amphetamines ■

The term *amphetamines* refers to a group of stimulants that includes amphetamine, methamphetamine, methylene-dioxymethamphetamine (MDMA), methylenedioxyamphetamine (MDA), and methylenedioxyethylamphetamine (MDEA). The federal five-drug panel originally targeted amphetamine and methamphetamine, primarily to identify illicit methamphetamine use. SAMHSA planned on adding tests for MDMA, MDA, and MDEA in 2010. Figure 13-5 presents the chemical structures of amphetamine, methamphetamine, and MDMA.

THERAPEUTIC USES

d-Amphetamine and *d*-methamphetamine are Schedule II controlled substances. (The "*d*" corresponds to the *dextro* isomer—or, more specifically, enantiomer—which has greater stimulant properties than the "*l*" or *levo* isomer.) *d*-Amphetamine and *d*-methamphetamine are used for the treatment of attention-deficit disorder (ADD) and attention-deficit hyperactivity disorder (ADHD), narcolepsy, and learning disorders associated with fetal alcohol syndrome.

Figure 13-5. Amphetamine, Methamphetamine, and MDMA, Chemical Structures ■

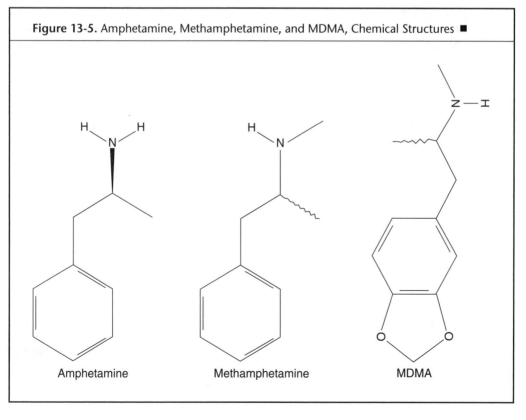

Amphetamine　　　　Methamphetamine　　　　MDMA

Vicks VapoInhaler and some similar generic products contain *l*-methamphetamine, also called levmetamfetamine or *l*-desoxyephedrine. Use of these products can cause positive test results for amphetamine or methamphetamine. This has been reported for urine, but is uncommon. This has not been reported, or well studied, for non-urine specimens. Vicks VapoInhaler is sold over the counter and is a plastic lipstick-size tube with one or more holes at one end and, inside the tube, a solid core that releases *l*-methamphetamine. Other products that carry the Vicks brand name do not contain *l*-methamphetamine.

Table 10-2 lists medications prescribed in the United States that contain or are metabolized to amphetamine or methamphetamine.

ILLICIT USES

Methamphetamine can be easily synthesized in clandestine laboratories. This type of synthesis originally used 2-phenylpropanone (P2P) as the precursor, producing a mix of *d*- and *l*-methamphetamine. When P2P availability was restricted, pseudoephedrine became the primary precursor with the side "benefit" of producing pure *d*-methamphetamine. When sales of large amounts of pseudoephedrine were restricted, illicit producers reverted to other precursors, including synthesized P2P, thus once again producing a mix of *d*- and *l*-methamphetamine. Illicit methamphetamine is used by smoking, intranasal inhalation, injection, and oral ingestion.

Some people take *d*-amphetamine medications to stay alert or remain awake for long periods of time. Groups at particular risk for nonmedical use of amphetamines include truck drivers, athletes, and students. A single dose enhances attention and performance for about 2–4 hours. A worker who has recently taken amphetamine may appear nervous, suspicious, and hyperactive. Stimulation fades and is replaced by exhaustion. Prolonged abuse of amphetamines can result in paranoia, delusions, and hallucinations (*amphetamine psychosis*).

MDMA, MDA, and MDEA have become popular drugs of abuse for youth at "rave" parties where they are used as short-term stimulants. They are Schedule I drugs under the Controlled Substances Act; that is, they have no legitimate medical use. Ecstasy is the street name for both MDMA and MDA. Eve is the street name for MDEA. Some products that users mistakenly refer to as Ecstasy actually contain caffeine, *d*-methamphetamine, cocaine, or PCP.

METABOLISM AND EXCRETION

A small proportion of methamphetamine is metabolized to amphetamine, just 4–7% for the *d*-form and 2% for the *l*-form. The isomeric structure is preserved during metabolism; *d*-goes to *d*, *l* goes to *l*. After methamphetamine use, both methamphetamine and amphetamine may be present in the urine but the amphetamine concentration is usually lower and may be below the cutoff. Metabolism of methamphetamine to amphetamine has long been considered one way, but at least one study raises the possibility of amphetamine being metabolized to methamphetamine (or the presence of methamphetamine as a contaminant of amphetamine) [12]. In that study, amphetamine concentrations exceeded methamphetamine concentrations by more than 200 times.

The elimination half-life of *d*-methamphetamine is about 12 hours and ranges from 8 to 17 hours. The elimination half-life of *l*-methamphetamine is slightly longer.

Several prescription drugs are metabolized to amphetamine or methamphetamine, as listed in Table 10-2. Methylphenidate (Ritalin) does not contain, and is not metabolized to, amphetamine or methamphetamine. MDMA, MDA, and MDEA also are not metabolized to amphetamine or methamphetamine. Both MDMA and MDEA are metabolized to MDA. Following MDMA administration, MDMA is excreted in the range of 8–45% of the administered dose; and MDA is excreted in the range of 0.3–1.0%. Following MDEA administration, MDEA is excreted in a range of 16.4–21.5% and MDA is excreted in a range of 2.0–3.8%.

Urine

A single therapeutic dose (e.g., 10 mg) of amphetamine or methamphetamine can cause a positive urine test result for about 24 hours depending on urinary pH and individual metabolic differences. Multiple high doses can cause positive urine test results for 2–4 days after last use.

Oral Fluid

Detection periods for amphetamine and methamphetamine for oral fluid are shorter than those for urine. Studies suggest that workplace oral fluid tests can detect use of amphetamine and methamphetamine for no more than 48 hours after last use, although high and repeated dosing might extend this period.

LABORATORY ANALYSIS

Urine

Immunoassays used to test for amphetamine and methamphetamine are targeted toward methamphetamine. These immunoassays are more selective now than in the past, but many still have cross-reactivity to a variety of drugs including ephedrine, pseudoephedrine, phentermine, mebeverine, and promethazine. They also have some cross-reactivity to MDMA. However, for appropriate sensitivity, laboratories that test for MDMA, MDA, and MDEA use immunoassays targeted for MDMA.

In regulated testing, the laboratory can report a result as methamphetamine-positive only if amphetamine is also present at or above 100 ng/mL. HHS introduced this reporting rule because of an analytic problem identified in the early 1990s in which a few specimens with large concentrations of ephedrine or pseudoephedrine tested false-positive for methamphetamine but amphetamine was inexplicably absent. After use of methamphetamine, amphetamine should be present as a metabolite of methamphetamine. The reporting rule in regulated testing was one of several measures instituted to avoid the pure-methamphetamine positive results that occurred through the aforementioned analytic problem. This reporting rule is used in regulated tests but not necessarily in nonregulated tests.

Another approach for eliminating the potential for false positive results from ephedrine and pseudoephedrine is to incorporate a pre-oxidation step into the extraction. In this protocol, oxidation with periodate destroys ephedrine and pseudoephedrine, thereby preventing their conversion to methamphetamine later during the analysis.

Immunoassay tests are mostly selective for the *d*-methamphetamine isomer. Routine confirmation tests are not selective for the *d*-isomer. An additional GC/MS procedure known as chiral analysis can be performed to determine the relative proportions of *d*- and *l*- for amphetamine or methamphetamine. This is helpful in determining if the result was caused by use of certain medications that are metabolized to the *d*- or *l-isomer* (see Table 10-2). Hair testing laboratories typically perform *d*- and *l*-isomer proportions only on request, not routinely. If the laboratory has too little hair left over to perform requested *d* and *l* isomers analysis, the MRO should cancel the test.

Hair
Some hair testing laboratories require the presence of amphetamine at or above LOD to report a methamphetamine-positive result because this reduces the possibility of positive results caused by external contamination with methamphetamine.

Oral Fluid
The immunoassay targets methamphetamine and has cross-reactivity to amphetamine, MDMA, and MDEA. The laboratory will report a methamphetamine-positive result without regard to whether amphetamine is also present.

INTERPRETING RESULTS

Amphetamine
Most amphetamine-positive, methamphetamine-negative results are due to use of prescription medication. If a donor with an amphetamine-positive result claims use of Ritalin, the MRO should ask the donor to double check that the medication truly is Ritalin because a donor may mistakenly claim use of Ritalin when he or she actually took Adderall. Ritalin use cannot cause an amphetamine-positive drug test, but Adderall use can. Fenproporex produces amphetamine as a metabolite and is prescribed as a diet pill in some countries other than the United States, mainly in Brazil.

Methamphetamine
Most methamphetamine-positive results are due to use of illicit methamphetamine. Certain prescription medications are metabolized to *d*-methamphetamine (see Table 10-2). Methamphetamine-positive results could also be due to the use of over-the-counter *l*-methamphetamine.

Vicks VapoInhaler
Chiral analysis can help determine the methamphetamine's source. The mnemonic "*d*" is for "drug" and "*l*" is for "legal," which helps MROs remember that the "*d*" isomer corresponds to illicit methamphetamine or a prescription drug, whereas the "*l*" isomer corresponds to Vicks VapoInhaler or other over-the-counter nasal inhalers that contain *l*-methamphetamine. Chiral analysis usually finds mostly *d*-methamphetamine, thus ruling out use of the over-the-counter

nasal inhaler. Positive test results from *l*-methamphetamine are uncommon, in part because the immunoassays are selective for the *d*-isomer. Given the costs and delays involved in ordering chiral analysis, MROs should (a) work with a laboratory that routinely performs this test, (b) establish a standing order for chiral analyses of all methamphetamine-positive results, or (c) order chiral analyses only when the interview findings suggest that Vicks Inhaler may have caused the result. Findings that suggest use of Vicks VapoInhaler include (1) specimen that is methamphetamine- and amphetamine-positive and the donor gives a history of using Vicks VapoInhaler or its equivalent within several days before the test, and, (2) a specimen that is methamphetamine- or amphetamine-positive and the donor says he or she used selegiline or another medication that is metabolized to *l*-amphetamine and *l*-methamphetamine.

If the MRO thinks *d*- and *l*-chiral testing is necessary, the MRO should order it. Payment for chiral analysis, like payment for other parts of drug testing, is ultimately the employer's responsibility, even when the MRO has to pay the laboratory fee up front.

When asking the donor about the use of Vicks VapoInhaler, the MRO should not first ask, "Did you use Vicks VapoInhaler," but should instead explore this indirectly: "Did you use any cough, cold, or allergy medicines?" If the donor says "Yes," the MRO can ask, "What type? Syrup? Pills? Mouth spray? Nasal spray or inhaler?" The problem is, some donors when confronted with positive results are liable to say "yes" in response to every drug the MRO asks them about, hoping that this will excuse their result. The experience of most MROs is that chiral analyses always, or almost always, confirm the use of the *d*-isomer.

Chiral separation assays of *d*- and *l*-isomers do not provide results that are 100% *d* or 100% *l* for two reasons: (1) impurities in the chiral derivatizing agent cause about 5% imprecision in the result, and (2) illegally manufactured amphetamine and methamphetamine often contain mixtures of *d*- and *l*-isomers. Tests conducted after use of pure *l*-methamphetamine generally detect 97–98% *l*-methamphetamine. HHS has advised MROs to use an 80/20 guideline for urine testing: If more than 80% of the methamphetamine is the *l*-isomer, this can be attributed to use of Vicks VapoInhaler and is not evidence of illicit drug use, regardless of the total concentration. If 20% or more of the methamphetamine is the *d*-isomer, the MRO can safely conclude that the employee used a prescription or illicit drug.

It is unknown if use of *l*-methamphetamine-containing nasal inhalers can cause methamphetamine-positive results in nonurine specimens. Until scientific studies have been conducted that rule this out, it seems prudent to assume they can.

MDMA, MDA, and MDEA
MDMA, MDA, and MDEA are illegal drugs for which there is no legitimate medical explanation.

PASSIVE EXPOSURE

Some reports have been published of young children who had methamphetamine in their urine shortly after they were taken from homes where adults used or manufactured methamphetamine. These children had urine methamphetamine concentrations below the federal workplace cutoffs. Their exposure was most likely from ingestion, for example, by putting their fingers in the mouth after they touched contaminated surfaces. Law enforcement and clean-up workers may be exposed to methamphetamine as part of their jobs, but if they use proper personal protective equipment, the extent of exposure can be minimized. A study published in 2006 describes drug tests conducted on workers who handled large quantities of methamphetamine as part of their jobs while wearing personal protective equipment. Some tested positive for methamphetamine, but the mean urine methamphetamine concentration was just 18 ng/mL and the maximum was 262 ng/mL [13]. The current confirmatory cutoff for methamphetamine is 250 ng/mL.

Barbiturates ■

THERAPEUTIC USE

Barbiturates are used as sedative-hypnotics and anticonvulsants. At therapeutic doses, barbiturates do not noticeably affect simple motor performance but can impair complex psychomotor and cognitive performance. Butalbital is most often prescribed in combination with salicylates (Fiorinal) or acetaminophen (Fioricet) and is used for treatment of headaches and for sedation. Mephobarbital and phenobarbital are anticonvulsants. Several phenobarbital-containing medications are used for treatment of gastrointestinal disorders.

ILLICIT USE

Decades ago, barbiturate abuse was of greater concern. Today, they are rarely taken for recreational abuse. Some positive results occur because of borrowed barbiturate products, e.g., taking someone else's Fiorinal for a headache.

METABOLISM AND EXCRETION

Barbiturates are rapidly absorbed when taken orally, have a 10- to 60-minute onset of action, and, depending on the agent, cause effects that last 5–8 hours. Short-acting barbiturates such as butalbital typically can be detected in urine for a day or less after use. Long-acting barbiturates, such as phenobarbital, can be detected for more than a week after use. Long-acting barbiturates can accumulate in the body, and after chronic use, detection periods can lengthen.

LABORATORY ANALYSIS

The federal test panels do not include tests for barbiturates. Employers who test for barbiturates do so in nonregulated programs. Immunoassays for barbiturates are usually targeted at secobarbital and have varying cross-reactivity to other barbiturates. GC/MS analyses are generally targeted at a panel of barbiturates consisting of amobarbital, butalbital, pentobarbital, phenobarbital, secobarbital, and, less often, butabarbital. The screening cutoff value is generally higher than the confirmatory cutoff—for example, 300 ng/mL for screening and 200 ng/mL for confirmation.

INTERPRETING RESULTS

The two most frequently detected barbiturates are phenobarbital and butalbital. Butalbital is commonly prescribed, sometimes borrowed, and rarely taken for recreational abuse. Because most MROs reject borrowed medication as an explanation, a large proportion of the positives verified by MROs represent borrowed medication.

Benzodiazepines ■

More than a dozen benzodiazepines are commercially available in the United States. Table 13-3 lists the more commonly prescribed benzodiazepines. Some are now available as generic medications.

THERAPEUTIC USE

Physicians prescribe benzodiazepines for the treatment of anxiety, insomnia, muscle spasms, alcohol withdrawal, and seizures. The widely prescribed sleeping pills zolpidem (Ambien) and eszopiclone (Lunesta) have effects similar to benzodiazepines, but they are <u>not</u> benzodiazepines.

ILLICIT USE

The benzodiazepines with the shortest half-life and highest potency (e.g., alprazolam, triazolam) and greatest lipophilia (e.g., diazepam) have the most abuse potential. People who abuse benzodiazepines frequently abuse other drugs as

Table 13-3. Benzodiazepine Half-Lives ■

Benzodiazepine (Brand Name)	Half-life (hr)
1. alprazolam (Xanax)	10–15
2. chlordiazepoxide (Limibitrol)	5–30
3. clonazepam (Klonopin)	18–50
4. clorazepate (Tranxene)	2
5. diazepam (Valium)	30–60
6. estazolam (ProSom)	10–24
7. flurazepam (Dalmane)	50–100
8. lorazepam (Ativan)	10–25
9. midazolam (Versed)	1.3–2.5
10. nordiazepam (active metabolite)	30–100
11. oxazepam (Serax)	5–20
12. prazepam (Centrax)	0.6–20
13. quazepam (Doral)	39–53
14. temazepam (Restoril)	3–13
15. triazolam (Halcion)	1.5–5.5

well. For example, addicts may use benzodiazepines to self-medicate for opiate drug withdrawal or to modulate the adverse effects of cocaine or methamphetamine. Benzodiazepine overdoses are rarely fatal except when combined with other drugs. Chronic use of benzodiazepines can cause physical tolerance. If its use is suddenly stopped, withdrawal symptoms such as vomiting, sweating, and convulsions may occur.

METABOLISM AND EXCRETION

Benzodiazepines are usually taken by mouth but can also be taken intravenously. The liver produces many metabolites (see Figure 13-6). A benzodiazepine's duration of effect depends on the half-life of the parent drug and the half lives of any active metabolites. For example, prazepam is long acting because its pharmacologically active metabolite, desmethyldiazepam, has a half-life of 30–100 hours. Short half-life benzodiazepines (e.g., alprazolam and triazolam) can be detected in urine for no more than a few days after last use. Long half-life benzodiazepines (e.g., diazepam and chlordiazepoxide) can be detected in urine for up to several weeks or months after chronic use.

LABORATORY ANALYSIS

The federal test panels do not include tests for benzodiazepines. Employers who test for benzodiazepines do so in nonregulated programs. The immunoassay

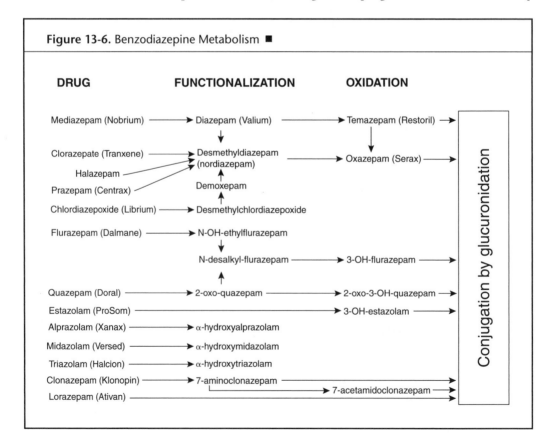

Figure 13-6. Benzodiazepine Metabolism ■

screens for benzodiazepines are directed at nordiazepam (also known as *desmethyldiazepam*), nitrazepam, and oxazepam. They have varying reactivity to other benzodiazepines. Typical cutoffs for benzodiazepine testing are 200–300 ng/mL for screening and 100 ng/mL for GC/MS. Confirmation is usually targeted at nordiazepam, oxazepam, temazepam, α-hydroxyalprazolam, and sometimes diazepam. Additional confirmation tests may include α-hydroxytriazolam, 7-aminoclonazepam (and clonazepam), lorazepam, and flurazepam. Benzodiazepine confirmation tests are challenging because of the numerous benzodiazepines prescribed, their low doses, and the low urinary concentrations of metabolites.

Oxaproxin (Daypro), a nonsteroidal anti-inflammatory drug, can cause false-positive results on some older benzodiazepine enzyme screening tests. Use of oxaproxin does not cause positive confirmatory results for benzodiazepines.

INTERPRETING RESULTS

MROs should be especially careful in interpretation of benzodiazepine-positive results. There is potential for misidentification due to complex and overlapping metabolic pathways.

Several nonprescription benzodiazepine-containing products are produced abroad. For example, Black Pearls (also known as Tung Shueh, Cows Head, and Chiufong Toukawan pills) are illegally imported from East Asia and sold in some health food stores in the United States. Although unstated on the labels, Black Pearls contain diazepam and their use can cause benzodiazepine-positive urine test results.

Cocaine ■

Cocaine is found in the leaves of the coca plant, grown principally in the northern South American Andes Mountains and to a lesser extent in India, Africa, and Java. Cocaine is a potent central nervous system stimulant that results in a state of increased alertness and euphoria. Figure 13-7 presents the chemical structure of cocaine.

THERAPEUTIC USE

No prescription products contain cocaine. Cocaine has a limited medical use in the United States as a topical anesthetic and vasoconstrictive agent. Plastic surgeons, otolaryngologists, and ophthalmologists are among the specialists who might apply a 1–4% solution of topical cocaine as a presurgical anesthetic. An emergency department physician may apply topical cocaine before packing an intractable nose bleed. Rarely, a physician may dispense a cocaine-containing solution for the patient with recurrent nose bleeds to use at home. An emergency department physician may apply TAC, a solution of tetracaine, adrenaline, and cocaine, to anesthetize skin before suturing lacerations, particularly in children. Positive drug test results have been reported from the use of cocaine-containing preparations for topical anesthesia and as a diagnostic test for Horner's syndrome. Some dentists administered cocaine as an anesthetic in the early twentieth century, but dental use of cocaine is now rare or nonexistent.

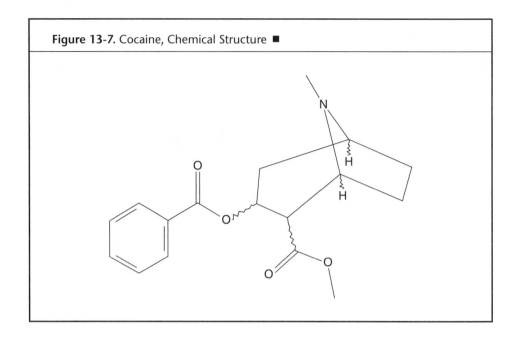

Figure 13-7. Cocaine, Chemical Structure ■

ILLICIT USE

Cocaine abuse has a long history and deep roots in the drug culture in the United States. It has a strong addictive potential. Cocaine is sold on the street in two forms: the hydrochloride salt (powder) and crack. The hydrochloride salt form of cocaine can be snorted or dissolved in water and injected. Crack is cocaine that has not been neutralized by an acid to make the hydrochloride salt. Crack cocaine comes in rock crystals that can be heated and the vapors smoked. The term crack refers to the crackling sound heard when it is heated.

METABOLISM AND EXCRETION

Cocaine has numerous metabolites, including benzoylecognine (BE) and ecgonine methyl ester (EME). Cocaine is pharmacologically active, but BE and EME are not. Cocaethylene (CE, also known as *ethylcocaine*) is formed in the liver when cocaine and alcohol are used together. While CE is considered a marker for combined use of cocaine and alcohol, traces of cocaethylene have also been identified in confiscated illicit cocaine samples, i.e., it is created during processing. CE crosses the blood-brain barrier and this may explain why so many cocaine users use alcohol—for a greater and longer high.

Urine

After cocaine use, urine contains little cocaine but more BE and EME. In a person who is not a regular cocaine user, the biologic urinary half-lives of cocaine, BE, and EME after a single dose of cocaine are 1.5 hours, 7.5 hours, and 3.6 hours, respectively, according to one study [14]. With repeated use, half-lives lengthen. BE can be detected in urine for up to 2–3 days after cocaine use by a person who is not a regular cocaine user and for up to 4–5 days after repeated use at a cutoff of 150 ng/mL.

Oral Fluid

After smoking or snorting cocaine, concentrations in oral fluid rise quickly due to mucosal contamination and fall within a few hours. Cocaine and BE are detectable in oral fluid for up to 1–2 days after the last use of cocaine and possibly longer after repeated, high-dose use [15].

LABORATORY ANALYSIS

Urine

Screening and confirmation tests of urine target BE because it is the predominant metabolite and because it has a longer half-life than cocaine. Screens respond also, but not as well, to EME. Confirmation procedures are specific for BE. In regulated urine testing, the screening cutoff concentration (150 ng/mL) is higher than the confirmation cutoff concentration (100 ng/mL) because specimens can degrade and benzoylecgonine concentrations can drop over time. However, in practice this is of little concern because confirmation assays are performed promptly after screening.

Hair

Hair tests target both cocaine and BE and may also target CE or norcocaine.

Oral Fluid

Laboratories target both cocaine and BE in oral fluid.

INTERPRETATION

The MRO should ask the donor who tests positive if he or she recently had a medical procedure or been treated at an emergency room. If "yes," the MRO should ask about procedures that might have included local anesthesia. If the history suggests medical use of cocaine within 2–3 days of the drug test, the donor should be asked to have a copy of the pertinent medical record sent to the MRO or should give the MRO authorization to communicate with the treating physician. Medical use of cocaine is rare, so MROs should be skeptical and demand firm, independent corroboration of any such claim. Anesthetics other than cocaine that have the suffix "-caine"—for example, procaine, lidocaine, and benzocaine—are structurally different than cocaine and do not cause cocaine-positive drug test results.

PASSIVE EXPOSURE

Passive inhalation of cocaine vapor may produce urine concentrations of benzoylecgonine just above the federal cutoff values under artificially intense experimental conditions. For example, in one study of passive cocaine exposure, several adults had peak urine benzoylecgonine concentrations of 22–123 ng/mL for up to 7 hours after intense exposure in an unventilated room, and none had concentrations at or above the federal cutoff of 150 ng/mL [16]. Published case reports of bezoylecgonine-positive urine from young children rescued from crack houses may reflect ingestion of cocaine residues deposited on surfaces rather than passive inhalation of cocaine smoke.

Experiments that have looked at whether handling cocaine can cause positive urine test results have found cocaine metabolite only under the most extreme of circumstances and even then at low (below cutoff) levels. Consider these three examples:

1. A person handled money that had been immersed in coca paste. His peak urine cocaine metabolite concentration was 72 ng/mL [17].
2. TAC applied on intact skin caused a peak urinary concentration of 55 ng/mL [18].
3. Laboratory workers who ground cocaine powder and prepared cocaine training aids for detection dogs underwent urine drug tests. Only two of 233 urine specimens tested positive for cocaine metabolite at or above 100 ng/mL [19]. Ventilation and work practice improvements were put into place. Follow-up urine tests then found much lower cocaine metabolite concentrations, all lower than the workplace cutoffs [20].

Trace amounts of cocaine are excreted in semen. However, exposure to semen from cocaine-using sexual partners does not cause positive urine drug test results when using the federal cutoffs [21].

Traces of BE can be identified in hair from environmental exposure. BE can get into hair by direct deposition from the environment [22] and by non-metabolic transformation of cocaine residues deposited on the surface of hair [23, 24]. Hair testing laboratories wash specimens prior to analysis in an attempt to remove surface residues. Many, but not all, hair testing laboratories have reporting rules whereby cocaine-positive results are reported only if a cocaine metabolite is present in significant concentration. The decontamination wash and use of metabolite-based reporting criteria reduces but does not necessarily eliminate the possibility of positive hair test results caused by environmental exposure to cocaine. MROs should be particularly alert to cocaine-positive hair test results where no metabolite has been reported. The absence of cocaine metabolite makes passive exposure more plausible.

Contamination of the oral cavity during and immediately after administration of cocaine (through smoking) has been reported [25, 26]. In these reports, the initial high cocaine concentrations observed in oral fluid rapidly dissipated within approximately 30 minutes after drug administration. Cocaine and benzoylecgonine also enter oral fluid through diffusion from the blood stream.

COCAINE IN FOOD AND BEVERAGES

The coca leaf is a narcotic under the Comprehensive Drug Abuse Prevention and Control Act of 1970. U.S. customs inspectors have been instructed to confiscate cocaine-containing tea products [27], but some tea nevertheless slips through. Coca tea (also called mate de coca) is sold abroad, over the Internet, and even by some restaurants and health food stores in the United States. Most of these products come from Peru or Bolivia. Their distributors claim they contain no or negligible amounts of cocaine. Studies of coca tea products available in the United States indicate around 5 mg of cocaine per tea bag [28,29]. For comparison, a "line" of cocaine hydrochloride contains an estimated 20–30 mg of cocaine. Studies of coca tea consumption have reported benzoylecgonine-positive urine test results as high as 5,000 ng/mL [28,30,31,32].

Lysergic Acid Diethylamide ■

ILLICIT USES

Lysergic acid diethylamide (LSD) is a Schedule I drug available in liquid, powder, tablet, and capsule form. Figure 13-8 presents the chemical structure of LSD. This drug is abused for its hallucinogenic effects. The adverse reactions associated with its use include "flashbacks," where the original psychedelic experience is repeated (which may occur for years), and sense-distorting effects including fear or paranoia. Various governments around the world outlawed LSD after a number of fatal accidents were reported. Such accidents involved, for example, people under the influence of LSD jumping off high buildings, thinking they could fly.

METABOLISM AND EXCRETION

LSD is generally taken in small doses, e.g., 20–140 µg. LSD is metabolized rapidly, has a short half-life, and is an unstable compound. Following absorption, only 1–3% of the parent molecule is excreted in urine. To increase the window of detection for LSD use, assays target the metabolites because they have longer half-lives and are present in higher concentrations than LSD. LSD has a half-life of about 5 hours. The half-life of *N*-demethyl-LSD (*nor*-LSD) is 10 hours. The metabolite 2-oxo-3-hydroxy-LSD has been reported in concentrations of up to 25 times higher than LSD in urine. LSD use can be detected in urine for 2–5 days after use. LSD is infrequently included in nonregulated testing programs, in

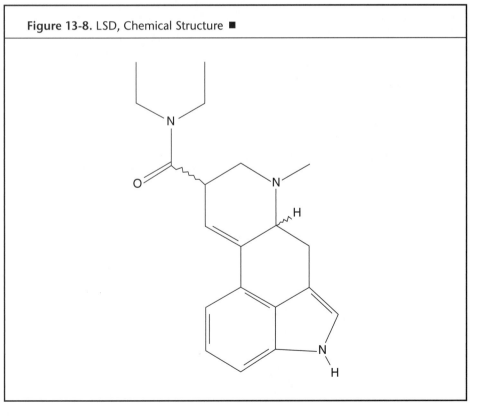

Figure 13-8. LSD, Chemical Structure ■

part because of the difficulty associated with confirming the presence of the metabolites.

Marijuana ■

Marijuana is a mixture of the dried flowering tops and leaves from the hemp plant, *Cannabis sativa*. The most active psychoactive ingredient in marijuana is tetrahydrocannabinol, or "THC." Figure 13-9 presents the chemical structure of THC.

THERAPEUTIC USE

Dronabinol contains synthetic THC, the principal psychoactive agent found naturally in marijuana. Dronabinol is FDA approved for treatment of chemotherapy-induced nausea and for appetite stimulation in the treatment of AIDS-related anorexia. Sativex is a cannabis extract that contains THC and other cannabinoids and is available as a mouth spray by prescription in certain foreign countries, including Canada, the United Kingdom, and Spain. Nabilone (Cesamet) is a synthetic cannabinoid that does not contain, and does not cause, positive results for THC.

As of 2010, 14 states—Alaska, Arizona, California, Colorado, Hawaii, Maine, Michigan, Montana, Nevada, New Jersey, New Mexico, Oregon, Vermont, and Washington—allow use of prescribed marijuana for certain medical reasons. Some of these reasons are nonspecific, e.g., chronic pain. There is some scientific evidence that marijuana helps patients with chronic and otherwise unmanageable pain and vomiting, and this is why THC is available in prescription form as dronabinol. Medical marijuana advocates claim that smoking marijuana has more immediate effects and allows the user to take just enough to ease symptoms. Marijuana remains a Schedule I drug and its use is thus illegal under federal law. In 2009, the U.S. Department of Justice announced that it would no longer prosecute marijuana users and distributors who abide by state medical marijuana laws.

Figure 13-9. THC, Chemical Structure ■

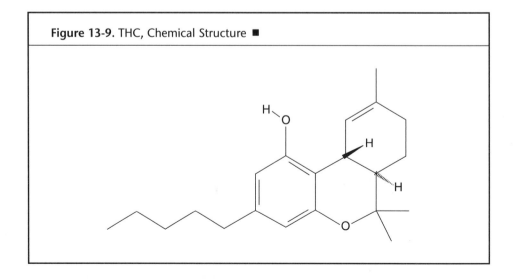

Federal court decisions have upheld an employer's right to fire workers who test positive for marijuana; that is, claims of medical marijuana use do not preclude an employer from firing someone who tests positive for THC.

ILLICIT USE

After tobacco, alcohol, and caffeine, marijuana is the most commonly used drug throughout the world. Marijuana and hashish (a concentrated cannabis extract) is smoked in cigarettes and sometimes ingested with baked items or tea. Marijuana is a hallucinogen that produces euphoria followed by drowsiness. The THC content of marijuana varies. In the mid-1970s, it averaged less than 1%. It has steadily increased through selective cultivation to reach, on average, about 8.5% in 2008 [33]. Recreational doses of marijuana vary. A single intake of smoke from a pipe or joint is called a *hit* (approximately 1/20th of a gram). The lower the potency, the more hits are needed to achieve the desired effects.

Hashish consists of the cannabinoid-rich resinous material of the cannabis plant, which is dried and compressed into a variety of forms (e.g., balls, cakes). The THC content of hashish is typically about two to three times higher than that of marijuana. Hash oil is a viscous brown or amber-colored liquid extract of cannabinoids from plant material.

Hemp usually refers to varieties of the cannabis plant that have low concentrations of the psychoactive cannabinoids or to the stalks and seeds of the plant, which also are low in psychoactive cannabinoids. In many countries, including the United States, hemp cultivation is prohibited by legislation because of the presence of the psychoactive cannabinoids.

METABOLISM AND EXCRETION

Inhaled cannabinoids are immediately absorbed and cause psychomotor effects within minutes. Plasma THC concentrations can peak at 100–200 ng/mL and typically drop below 1 ng/mL within a few hours. Ingested cannabinoids are more slowly absorbed and are metabolized by the liver before wider distribution throughout the body. Cannabinoids are highly lipophilic and are extensively stored in adipose tissue. While stored, they undergo some slow metabolism and gradually reenter the bloodstream at very low concentrations, primarily in conjugated forms that are not detected by standard drug testing. Despite the urban myth that says otherwise, weight loss is not known to increase cannabinoid concentrations.

Urine

THC is oxidized to 11-hydroxy-THC (11-OH-THC), which has equipotent psychoactivity. 11-OH-THC is rapidly oxidized to 11-nor-delta-9-tetrahydrocannabinol (THCA), which is not psychoactive. THCA is the metabolite that usually appears in the greatest concentration in urine and is the target for both screening and confirmation tests. A nonuser who takes one dose of THC can test positive in urine for approximately 3 days using a GC/MS cutoff of 15 ng/mL. After multiple high doses, and if low cutoffs are used, THCA can be detected in urine for up to several weeks and perhaps longer after last use. There are, however, extreme case reports of THCA detected in urine for 36–95 days after cessation of intake [34,35,36].

Hair
THCA is an acidic chemical and as such is not as readily incorporated into hair as more basic chemicals such as cocaine and methamphetamine. THCA is found in hair only at very low concentrations. THC is found in higher concentrations in hair, but the detection of THCA in hair is required to eliminate the potential for positive results due to environmental contamination.

Oral Fluid
Oral mucosal contamination from cannabis smoke is the main source of THC collected and measured in oral fluid analysis. THC and THCA diffuse from plasma into saliva only at very low concentrations.

After smoking marijuana, THC concentrations in oral fluid rise quickly and fall quickly, generally below 1 ng/mL within 12 hours. The apparent THC concentration is further reduced by THC that sticks to the pad used in most collection devices, and by dilution of fluid as it is extracted from the pad.

Passive exposure to marijuana smoke can cause THC concentrations in oral fluid at concentrations above cutoff (e.g., 4 ng/mL) for brief periods, as described in the "Oral Fluid—Passive Exposure" section of Chapter 12.

LABORATORY ANALYSIS

Urine
Most cannabinoid immunoassays are designed with a 50 ng/mL cutoff but some have cutoffs of 20 or 100 ng/mL. The 20 ng/mL cutoff is typically used by nuclear power plants and other settings in which higher sensitivity is desired. A 100 ng/mL cutoff appeared in the HHS *Guidelines* in 1988 and is still used by some nonregulated programs even though HHS reduced the screening cutoff to 50 ng/mL in 1994.

The immunoassays used by laboratories are targeted at THCA but detect multiple cannabinoids. Many immunoassays used on POCTs are less specific for THCA and have more crossreactivity to metabolites. The confirmatory result represents only THCA. The immunoassay cutoff is set higher than the confirmatory cutoff because the immunoassay measures multiple cannabinoids.

THCA-positive results after use of either marijuana or dronabinol are often less than 100 ng/mL and rarely more than several hundred ng/mL. Delta-9-tetrahydrocannabivarin (THCV) is a natural component of cannabis products and does not exist in dronabinol. The presence of THCV in a urine specimen indicates that the donor used marijuana or another natural cannabis product. A few laboratories offer THCV tests. The laboratory charge for a THCV test is about $150.00. In response to written requests, DOT has authorized THCV testing of specific THC-positive specimens.

False-positive immunoassay test results for marijuana metabolites have been reported after use of efavirenz (Sustiva, an antiviral drug used in the treatment of HIV infection), pantoprazole (Protonix, an anti-ulcerative drug), and quinacrine (Mepacrin, used to treat giardiasis, and no longer commercially distributed in the United States). The Syva EMIT immunoassay from the 1970s cross-reacted with ibuprofen, but this immunoassay product is long gone. GC/MS confirmatory analysis is specific for THCA and does not identify other drugs or metabolites.

Oral Fluid

THC is the primary analyte for marijuana in oral fluid. Any THCA present in oral fluid after use of marijuana is at concentrations in the pg/mL range. Laboratories have been trying to develop capability of testing for THCA, but this is technically challenging because of the low concentrations. THC is present in oral fluids at concentrations one or two orders of magnitude greater than THCA.

INTERPRETATION

Use of dronabinol and Sativex can cause THCA-positive drug test results. Chapter 10 discusses MRO interpretation of "medical marijuana" explanations.

The DOT drug testing rules do not authorize downgrading of a laboratory-positive test result based on the possibility that it represents old use. By contrast, the NRC rule does ask MROs to determine if positive return-to-duty test results represent new use or residual excretion. This question often arises in return-to-duty DOT testing, when an employee has been temporarily removed after a THC-positive test result. If the person's return-to-duty test result is positive, he or she cannot return to safety-sensitive work and must again be referred to the Substance Abuse Professional for an initial evaluation. In a situation in which the person has a history of chronic and high-dose marijuana use, he or she should wait until at least 4 weeks after his or her last use to avoid a positive return-to-duty test urine result caused by residual excretion.

The long excretion profile of THCA makes it difficult to determine if a positive result conducted long after last admitted use represents residual excretion or recent use. Although the rate of THCA excretion in urine is relatively constant, its concentration changes with changes in urine dilution. The variability in concentration due to dilution can be adjusted for by dividing each THCA concentration by the respective urine creatinine concentration. If one divides the later test's THCA/creatinine ratio by the earlier test's THCA/creatinine ratio and the result is 1.5 or more, this suggests marijuana use between the first and second test. The 1.5 threshold is not that sensitive; it misidentifies some new use as residual excretion, but its identification of new drug use is almost always correct. More sensitive but less-specific thresholds, such as 0.5, have also been studied [37,38]. Figure 13-10 illustrates a set of calculations using a 1.5 threshold.

Donors contacted by MROs about their THC-positive results usually have no legitimate explanation. On occasion, they call the MRO back later saying they forgot to mention they took dronabinol. They might go to great lengths to prove this, including forging medical records and persuading physicians to prescribe them dronabinol, with prescriptions dated after the tests were conducted. Marijuana use is common but prescriptions for dronabinol are not. MROs should therefore be especially careful to corroborate any donor's explanation that he or she used dronabinol.

THC has psychoactive effects, so use of THC-containing drugs such as marijuana and Marinol may be a disqualifier from performance of safety-sensitive

Figure 13-10. Example of Calculation Using Normalized THCA ■

Test	THCA, ng/mL	creatinine, mg/dL	THCA/Creatinine
1st	25	70	0.36
2nd	56	80	0.70
			0.70/0.36 = 1.94

The 1.94 ratio exceeds 1.5, thereby indicating use of marijuana between the first and second tests.

duties. As one might expect with a prevalence of use in the general population, marijuana use is often identified in people who have had accidents and other mishaps. Simulator studies have shown impaired performance after marijuana use, in some persisting longer than the euphoric effects. While illicit use of marijuana is a clear disqualifier from commercial motor vehicle operation under the FMCSA medical standards, use of dronabinol is permitted if prescribed by a licensed medical practitioner who is familiar with the driver's medical history and assigned duties and has advised the driver that the marijuana will not impair safety.

PASSIVE EXPOSURE

Urine

Experimental studies conducted in the 1980s showed that it was highly unlikely that a non-smoking person could unintentionally inhale enough marijuana smoke from other users to cause a positive drug test using the 15 ng/mL confirmatory cutoff concentration used in federally regulated testing [39, 40]. In one passive exposure study that reached concentrations above 15 ng/mL, exposure conditions were unrealistically severe [41]. Since the 1980s, marijuana has become two to three times more potent. On the other hand, immunoassays used to measure a broad range of cannabinoids are now more specific for THCA. The more potent marijuana and the use of immunoassays that are more specific for THCA have opposite effects on the likelihood of passive inhalation causing a positive drug test result. There are unfortunately no recent research studies that re-examine this issue. MROs should assume—and, in federally regulated testing, must assume—that passive exposure to marijuana does not cause positive drug tests. SAMHSA's 1997 *Medical Review Officer Manual* advises MROs that passive inhalation does not constitute an alternative medical explanation [42]. Part 40 also directs MROs not to change positive drug tests based on explanations of passive inhalation [49 *CFR* 40.151(d)].

Use of hemp-oil body lotions is not a plausible cause of a THC-positive urine test. There are no human experimental data that directly address this. The plausibility seems far-fetched when one calculates what might occur based on concentrations of THC in hemp-oil products, estimated transfer rates of THC through skin, and other variables [43].

Hair

An experiment on the effect of cannabis-containing commercial shampoo on hair drug test results found no THC-positive results from such use [44].

Oral Fluid

Laboratory-based oral fluid drug tests target the parent drug THC, which is present in smoke, rather than the metabolite THCA, which is not present in smoke. THC that is inhaled, whether by actively smoking or passively exposed, is incorporated into oral fluid and can cause a positive test result. Experiments indicate that passive exposure to marijuana smoke may cause THC-positive oral fluid test results for up to about 30–60 minutes following exposure [45, 46, 47]. While some studies suggest the interval is shorter (e.g., no more than 10 minutes), enough data have been published to warrant a longer, smoke-free interval to rule out any possibility of passive exposure causing a positive result.

CANNABIS IN FOOD AND BEVERAGES

Marijuana eaten in brownies or other foods can cause psychoactive effects and THC-positive urine drug test results [48]. Food containing marijuana has a fibrous texture and tastes bad. Someone who eats food containing significant amounts of marijuana usually knows something was added to the food.

Some recreational marijuana users and cancer and AIDS sufferers brew tea from marijuana leaves. Marijuana tea is more common in the West Indies where marijuana is culturally accepted. Between 8% and 22% of the THC is released by boiling the marijuana leaves. Consumption of such tea can cause a THC-positive drug test [49,50].

Food products containing hemp seeds or extracts are popular, perhaps as much for their novelty as for their nutritional value or taste. Hemp is comprised of the stalks and seeds of the cannabis plant and may contain trace amounts of THC. Hemp stalks and seeds contain little THC but can be contaminated with larger amounts of THC from the plant's leaves, flowers, and resins. Hemp oil is processed from the seeds and contains THC from this outside contamination of the seed hull with cannabinoids. In the mid-1990s, reports first surfaced that people who consumed hemp-seed products—hemp oil products, in particular—could test positive for THC. Hemp-containing products sold in the United States at that time had THC levels ranging from nondetectable to more than 100 µg/g. Hemp oils sold abroad had THC levels as high as several thousand µg/g. Manufacturers have since reduced THC levels in hemp oil sold in the United States by shelling the seeds and washing them before pressing. Consequently, THC content in hemp oil dropped to around 5 µg/g by 2000 [51]. In 2003, the Drug Enforcement Agency (DEA) modified the Controlled Substances Act to more clearly categorize THC-containing food products as Schedule I, i.e., illegal [21 *CFR* §1308.35(a)(2)]. THC content in hemp oil subsequently dropped even lower [52]. The probability of a THC-positive drug test due to ingestion of hemp products sold in the United States is now remote. Personal-care products (e.g., shampoos, lotions) are not regulated under the Controlled Substances Act because they are not intended for human consumption. Studies have shown that use of these products does not cause urine specimens to test positive for THC using the federal cutoffs. Dietary hemp oils with considerable THC concentrations, enough to cause positive drug test results, are still available in other countries.

Methaqualone ■

Methaqualone is a central nervous system depressant. It causes fatigue, dizziness, sluggishness, and paresthesias. High doses can cause delirium, convulsions, and coma. In the 1970s, methaqualone became a popular drug of abuse because it was considered an aphrodisiac. In 1983, methaqualone was removed from the market and reclassified as a Schedule I drug. It is rarely detected in workplace drug testing programs, and several large forensic drug testing laboratories stopped offering methaqualone tests in the late 1990s. Figure 13-11 presents the chemical structure of methaqualone.

METABOLISM AND EXCRETION

Methaqualone is taken orally. Its effect lasts for 4–8 hours. The elimination half-life of methaqualone is 10–42 hours. Methaqualone is extensively metabolized by the liver. The laboratory assays used in workplace drug testing are targeted at methaqualone and not its metabolites. Immunoassay and confirmation cutoff values are typically 300 ng/mL.

INTERPRETING RESULTS

The rare specimen that is methaqualone positive is usually a performance test sample rather than a real employee specimen. If a real donor specimen is methaqualone positive, the MRO should try to interview him or her and verify the result as positive.

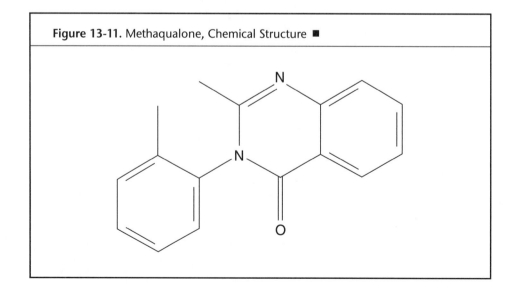

Figure 13-11. Methaqualone, Chemical Structure ■

Nicotine ■

Tests for cotinine are used to identify use of nicotine. Tests for cotinine do not distinguish between nicotine from cigarette smoking and nicotine from replacement therapy, e.g., nicotine gum. By contrast, anabasine is a tobacco metabolite present after smoking but not after use of nicotine replacement therapy.

Tests for breath carbon monoxide can help identify cigarette smokers, particularly if performed on an unannounced basis. Because carbon monoxide levels go back to normal within about a day of stopping smoking, tests for carbon monoxide are sensitive only at detecting recent use.

Most laboratories use an oral fluid cotinine cutoff of 200 ng/mL. Research indicates that a cutoff as low as 50 ng/mL can reliably distinguish nicotine users from nonusers [53]. Passive exposure to cigarette smoke can cause oral fluid cotinine, but at concentrations of only a few ng/mL, i.e., below the cutoffs [54].

Opioids: Introduction ■

The term "opioids" refers to drugs prepared from opium or synthesized drugs that have morphine-like activity. Opioids can be classified as follows:

1. Natural opiates, contained in the resin of the opium poppy, including morphine and codeine.
2. Semi-synthetic opiates are created from the natural opiates. Semi-synthetic opiates include diacetylmorphine (heroin), hydrocodone, hydromorphone, oxycodone, and oxymorphone.
3. Fully synthetic opioids, such as fentanyl methadone, oxycodone, propoxyphene, and tramadol.

Heroin is synthesized by reacting morphine with acetic acid. Because heroin has a brief half life and is hard to detect, urine tests to identify heroin abuse instead target the metabolites morphine and 6-acetylmorphine.

In 1997, two expert panels in the United States introduced clinical guidelines that encouraged expanded use of opioids for chronic pain. In the years since those guidelines were published, retail purchases of opioid pain relievers increased dramatically (Table 13-4). Prescription opioid abuse is now considered one of the greatest drug problems in the United States. For example, Americans are only 4% of the world's population, but consume 80% of the world's opioids [55].

Employers who can select their own test panels (i.e., are not limited to the test panels required by certain federal or state rules) may include tests for prescription opioids because they think it will improve safety. Some employers also select expanded panels because they cost little more than five-drug panels.

Figure 13-12 depicts opioid metabolic pathways of greatest interest in workplace testing programs. Table 13-5 lists certain pharmacologic data for opioids.

Ingestion of small to moderate amounts of opioids produces a short-lived euphoric feeling followed by several hours of relaxation. Opioids are physically and psychologically addictive. Dependence can develop after taking large doses for several weeks.

Table 13-4. Retail Sales of Opioid Medications (Grams) 1997–2006 ■

	1997	2006	% Change
Methadone	518,737	6,621,687	1,177
Oxycodone	4,449,562	37,034,220	732
Fentanyl base	74,086	428,668	479
Hydromorphone	241,078	901,663	274
Hydrocodone	8,669,311	29,856,368	244
Morphine	5,922,872	17,507,148	196
Meperidine	5,765,954	4,160,033	−28
Codeine	25,071,410	18,762,919	−25

Source: Office of Diversion Control. Retail Drug Summary. Springfield, VA: U.S. Dept. of Justice. 2002, 2008.

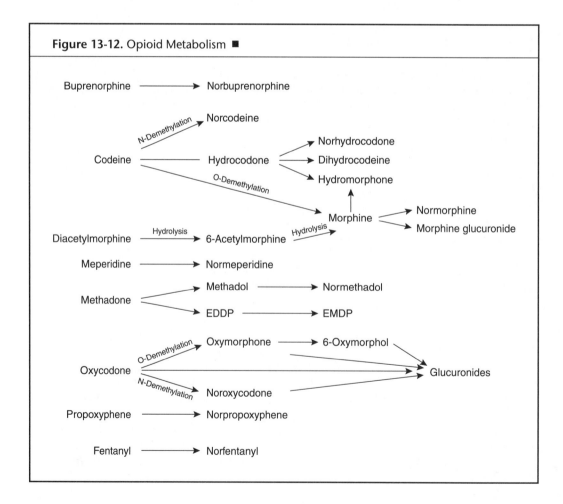

Figure 13-12. Opioid Metabolism ■

Table 13-5. Comparative Data on Some Prescription Opioids ■

Drug (Metabolite)	~$T_{1/2}$ (hr)	Detection Period in Urine	CSA Schedule
Buprenorphine	20–37	2–4 days	III
Codeine	2.5–4	1–3 days	III–V[1]
Fentanyl	4	1–3 days[2]	II
Heroin	very short	–	I
(6-Acetylmorphine)	0.5	8 hrs	
Hydrocodone	4	2–4 days	III
Hydromorphone	2.6–4	2–4 days	II
Meperidine	2.4–4	2–4 days	II
Methadone	15 single dose	2–4 days	II
	48–72 repeated dosing		
Morphine	2–3	1–3 days	II
Oxycodone	2–3	2–4 days	II
Oxymorphone	7–11	1–3 days	II
Propoxyphene	6–12	2–7 days casual up to 30 days chronic	IV
(Norpropoxyphene)	30–36	7 days	

[1]CSA Schedule III when just codeine. Schedule V when combined with acetaminophen or with NSAID.
[2]1–3 days for single dose. Slow, prolonged release while wearing fentanyl patch.

Codeine, Morphine, and Heroin ■

Figure 13-13 presents the chemical structures of codeine, morphine, and heroin.

THERAPEUTIC USE

Codeine is used as an analgesic and cough suppressant. Some states allow over-the-counter sales of small amounts of codeine or opium, for example, codeine in cough syrups and opium in anti-diarrhea preparations. Purchasers in those states sign receipts at pharmacies for these over-the-counter products. Even in these states, some pharmacies choose to not sell codeine- or opium-containing products. Codeine-containing pills are sold over the counter in Canada (e.g., 222, AC&C) and Mexico.

Morphine is used to treat moderate to severe pain. Morphine is administered intravenously in hospitals and other health care settings, and is contained in some prescription medications.

ILLICIT USE

Heroin can be injected, smoked, or sniffed/snorted. The availability of high-purity heroin, however, and the fear of infection by sharing needles has made snorting and smoking heroin more common. Street heroin can be cut with codeine, fentanyl, or other drugs.

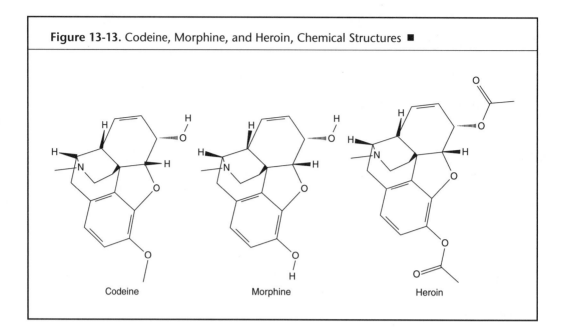

Figure 13-13. Codeine, Morphine, and Heroin, Chemical Structures ■

Codeine   Morphine   Heroin

METABOLISM AND EXCRETION

Heroin is rapidly metabolized to 6-acetylmorphine (6-AM), which is metabolized to morphine. The half-life of heroin is approximately 2–5 minutes. Because heroin's half-life is so short, it is hard to detect in biological specimens. Urine drug testing laboratories instead test for heroin metabolites (6-AM, morphine) instead of the parent drug. The presence of 6-AM is pathognomic for heroin use, but its absence does not rule out heroin use.

Codeine is metabolized to morphine, norcodeine, and (after large doses) hydrocodone. Morphine is metabolized (after large doses) to hydromorphone.

Urine
The metabolite 6-AM can be detected in the urine for up to 8 hours after heroin use. Urine tests for 6-AM are most likely to be positive when the specimen's morphine concentration is high (more than 5,000 ng/mL) and the codeine-to-morphine ratio is low (less than 0.125). 6-AM is stable for up to 10 days in refrigerated urine and up to 2 years in frozen urine.

After codeine use, codeine or morphine may be detected in urine. There is usually more codeine than morphine, but the codeine-morphine ratio is not a reliable measure by which to determine if someone took only codeine *or* took codeine and morphine.

High concentrations of morphine (> 50,000 ng/mL) are often observed in patients taking this drug. Morphine is not metabolized to codeine. The traces of codeine that may be found in commercial morphine are too small to account for codeine-positive workplace drug test results [56].

Hydrocodone is a minor metabolite of codeine. Limited data have been published in recent years that show low concentrations of hydrocodone in urine after substantial doses of codeine. A urine specimen with a codeine concentration that is quite high (> 5,000 ng/mL) and a hydrocodone concentration that is quite low (around 100 ng/mL) could be explained by use of only codeine.

Hydromorphone is a minor metabolite of morphine. Limited data have been published in recent years that show low concentrations of hydromorphone (e.g., no higher than 1,500 ng/mL) in urine when the morphine concentration is high (e.g., 10,000 ng/mL or higher).

Hair

The three primary opiate analytes reported for workplace drug testing are codeine, morphine, and 6-AM. In hair, morphine and 6-AM are normally found at highest concentrations.

Hydrocodone is a minor metabolite of codeine, a hydrocodone-positive hair test result can occur as a result of codeine use [57].

Oral Fluid

Following heroin use, 6-AM and morphine are detectable in oral fluid, with 6-AM concentrations peaking between 0.5 and 8 hours after smoking. Heroin as the parent (unchanged) drug can be detected in oral fluid for about an hour after use and for up to 24 hours after smoking or intranasal use.

Norcodeine, not morphine, is detected in oral fluid following use of codeine. Therefore, the detection of morphine in oral fluid can be interpreted as use of heroin or morphine.

LABORATORY ANALYSIS

Immunoassays for 6-AM are targeted at 6-AM. Immunoassays for codeine and morphine are targeted to either morphine (usually) or codeine (less often). Given the structural similarity of codeine and morphine, the immunoassay—whether targeted at one or the other—identifies both drugs well. The immunoassay also has crossreactivity to hydrocodone and hydromorphone, though less strong because the structures of these semi-synthetic opiates differ from those of codeine and morphine. Synthetic opioids, such as oxycodone, have structures that diverge further from morphine or codeine, and thus codeine/morphine immunoassays detect synthetic opioids less well. Effective detection of synthetic opioids such as oxycodone requires use of immunoassays that are specifically targeted at those drugs.

Confirmation tests for opiates at regulated urine testing laboratories and at oral fluid testing laboratories are limited to codeine, morphine, and 6-AM. Some hair testing laboratories also perform confirmation tests for heroin.

In regulated testing, the laboratory cutoffs for codeine and morphine screening and confirmation are 2,000 ng/mL and for 6-AM screening and confirmation are 10 ng/mL. Some nonregulated laboratories screen and confirm for morphine and codeine with 300 ng/mL cutoffs. This is the cutoff that was used in regulated testing until 1998, when HHS raised it to 2,000 ng/mL to make testing more specific for heroin.

Most commercial hair testing for workplace programs targets codeine, morphine, and heroin. 6-acetylmorphine, a metabolite that is specific to heroin, can be found at relatively high concentrations in hair, whereas morphine is the major metabolite in urine.

INTERPRETING RESULTS

The "Codeine/Morphine/6-AM Result Review" section of Chapter 10 describes the interpretation of codeine-, morphine-, and/or 6-AM-positive results.

Buprenorphine ■

Buprenorphine is a semi-synthetic opioid with partial agonist activity at mu receptors. In non-dependent subjects, it produces typical opioid effects but to a limited extent. In patients physically dependent on mu-receptor agonists such as heroin and oxycodone, use of buprenorphine can prevent symptoms of withdrawal.

THERAPEUTIC USE

Buprenorphine is relatively new in the United States and has been used in Europe for much longer. Buprenex is an injectable formulation used to treat pain. Two sublingual buprenorphine products, Subutex and Suboxone, are used for opiate replacement therapy in addicts. Subutex contains buprenorphine. Suboxone contains buprenorphine and naloxone, a drug used to reverse opioid effects. Naloxone is included in this sublingual product because it is absorbed poorly by mouth but is effective intravenously, thus discouraging intravenous abuse of the product. Suboxone is quite expensive, so its use in public treatment programs may be limited. Figure 13-14 presents the chemical structure of buprenorphine.

Subutex and Suboxone are prescribed by addiction medicine physicians who have been certified by attending a special training course and submitting their qualifications to the Substance Abuse and Mental Health Services Administration (SAMHSA). Physicians also must agree to refer patients for drug addiction counseling. After registering with SAMHSA, physicians receive a special identification number from DEA that appears on all buprenorphine prescriptions they administer. The DEA-issued identification numbers assigned to each certified physician aids law enforcement and antidiversion officials in tracking any diversion of the drugs.

ILLICIT USE

Buprenorphine use does not create a pleasant high. Nevertheless, clusters of buprenorphine abuse have emerged in areas where the drug has been extensively prescribed, for example, in some parts of Scandinavia. Drug abusers can crush and inject or snort Subutex. If they inject or snort crushed Suboxone, the naloxone component may cause withdrawal symptoms.

METABOLISM AND EXCRETION

The mean elimination half-life of buprenorphine is 37 hours. It is metabolized to norbuprenorphine, which is pharmacologically active and has a slightly longer elimination half-life. Buprenorphine doses can range widely among people treated with buprenorphine as a substitute for other opioids. Urine concentrations range widely, too, from the single digits to more than 1,000 ng/mL.

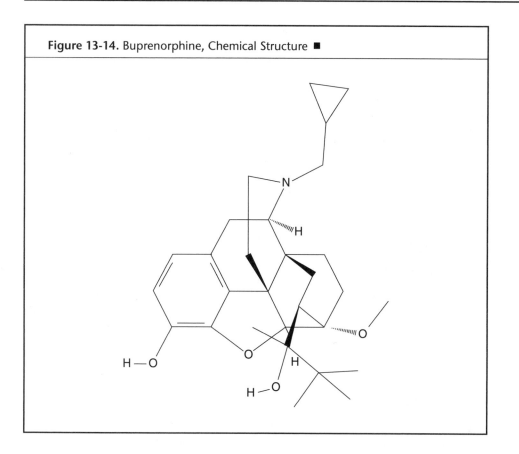

Figure 13-14. Buprenorphine, Chemical Structure ■

LABORATORY ANALYSIS

Availability of laboratory testing for buprenorphine is limited. This is true for urine and particularly true for hair. For many laboratories, this is a "send out"; i.e., the laboratory sends the specimen to a reference laboratory that can perform the test. Buprenorphine is not detected by usual opiate screening procedures. The laboratory may screen with an immunoassay targeted at buprenorphine or nor-buprenorphine, or it may go directly to confirmatory analysis for buprenorphine or norbuprenorphine. Analytic sensitivity and urine cutoff levels must be set low, e.g., 2 ng/mL for confirmation in urine. To achieve this, confirmation assays use particularly sensitive techniques, such as tandem MS.

INTERPRETING RESULTS

Tests for buprenorphine are typically conducted for monitoring compliance of patients who receive it as part of an opiate addiction treatment program. In this context, positive results are expected and negative results suggest the patient is diverting the drug instead of taking it. Workplace testing for buprenorphine may be conducted for reasonable suspicion in a nonregulated (non-DOT) setting, for example, in a health care institution where an employee is suspected of stealing it. If a donor has a buprenorphine-positive workplace test and says he or she received it for opiate addiction treatment, the MRO may need to contact the treating physician to corroborate the explanation (as opposed to contacting the pharmacy or asking for a copy of the label). This is because buprenorphine is sometimes, especially during early treatment, administered as observed dosing in the office instead of by prescription.

Use of prescribed buprenorphine by a commercial motor vehicle (CMV) operator may raise a safety concern. The MRO should tell the employer that the CMV operator should be further evaluated to determine fitness for duty because of use of a prescribed medication. Buprenorphine is a relatively new drug and its use has not yet been addressed under the Federal Motor Carrier Safety Administration (FMCSA) rules and guidance for medical qualification of commercial motor vehicle (CMV) operators.

Fentanyl ■

THERAPEUTIC USE

Fentanyl is potent and short-acting. It is a Schedule II drug, most widely used as a transdermal patch (Duragesic, Mylan) to treat chronic pain. It is also available as an oral lozenge (Actiq, Fentora) and as an injection (Sublimaze) used to assist with anesthesia, typically for outpatient surgery. Figure 13-15 presents the chemical structure of fentanyl.

ILLICIT USE

Outside the hospital setting, most illicit use of fentanyl comes from diverted pharmaceutical products that are intended for pain management. Drug abusers can remove fentanyl from some designs of transdermal patches and take the entire supply at once. Some illicit fentanyl is synthesized at clandestine laboratories. Fentanyl has been used in combination with heroin and cocaine in certain drug markets. Users may or may not be aware that they are purchasing and using fentanyl. In workplace settings, fentanyl tests are typically conducted in reasonable suspicion tests or monitoring of impaired health care professionals. Fentanyl is among the more commonly abused substances by medical personnel and is the drug most often abused by anesthesiologists.

METABOLISM AND EXCRETION

Fentanyl is almost completely metabolized, with less than 10% excreted in urine as an unchanged drug. Norfentanyl, the primary metabolite, has minimal pharmacologic activity. It is detectable in the urine longer and usually at greater concentrations than fentanyl and its inclusion in the laboratory analysis provides additional evidence of fentanyl use. Use of fentanyl can be detected in urine for no longer than 3–4 days after the last dose.

LABORATORY ANALYSIS

Because of its potency, fentanyl is administered in low therapeutic doses and very sensitive techniques are required to identify and quantify fentanyl and norfen-

Figure 13-15. Fentanyl, Chemical Structure ■

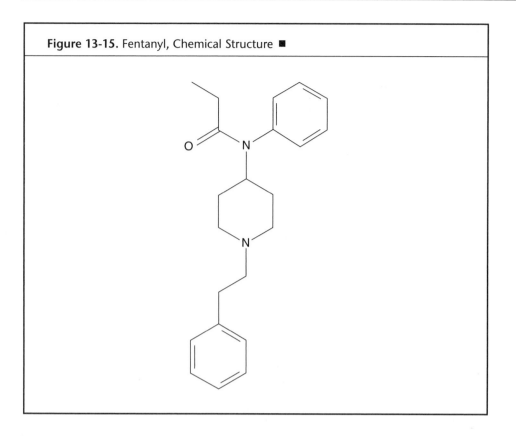

tanyl in biologic specimens. Fentanyl is not detected by usual opiate screening procedures and may be detected by specific confirmatory techniques. Because of the cost implications, laboratories charge more for this. Analytic sensitivity and urine cutoff levels must be set low, e.g., 0.3 ng/mL for confirmation in urine. To achieve this, confirmation assays use particularly sensitive techniques, such as tandem MS. Hair testing for fentanyl is uncommon but is commercially available at several laboratories.

INTERPRETATION

Workplace tests for fentanyl are typically reserved for situations involving reasonable suspicion or follow-up testing. Given the short half-life and low concentrations, it is important to remember that a negative result does not rule out use.

Hydrocodone ■

Hydrocodone is a semi-synthetic opioid derived from codeine and thebaine. In amounts less than or equal to 15 mg per dose, and when combined with acetaminophen or other non-controlled drugs it is Schedule III. The looser regulatory controls of Schedule III, in comparison to Schedule II, are partly accountable for its widespread use. Americans are only 4 percent of the world's population but consume 99% of the world's hydrocodone [55]. Figure 13-16 presents the chemical structure of hydrocodone.

THERAPEUTIC USE

Hydrocodone is prescribed for pain relief and as a cough suppressant.

ILLICIT USE

Hydrocodone's Schedule III status has helped make it easier to get it for illicit use than Schedule II drugs, such as oxycodone. Schedule III drugs can be ordered by phone and can be ordered with refills. Schedule II drugs, by contrast, can only be ordered by written prescription and not with refills. Hydrocodone abuse often occurs because of over-prescription, theft, "doctor shopping," and bogus call-in or written prescriptions.

METABOLISM AND EXCRETION

About one quarter of a single dose is eliminated in urine as unchanged drug. About 1–5% of a hydrocodone dose is metabolized to and excreted in urine as hydromorphone. Data suggest that after use of only hydrocodone, the hydrocodone concentration should exceed the hydromorphone concentration by a factor of at least four. About 3% of a hydrocodone dose is metabolized and ex-

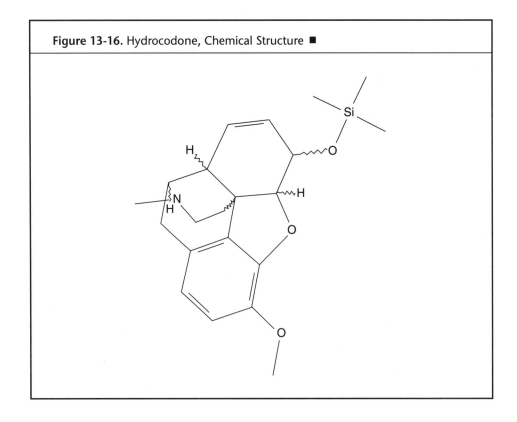

Figure 13-16. Hydrocodone, Chemical Structure ■

creted in urine as dihydrocodeine. Thus, a donor who has recently used hydrocodone may test positive for hydromorphone or dihydrocodeine.

LABORATORY ANALYSIS

Most commercial immunoassays for opiates cross-react with hydrocodone. Laboratories typically use 300 ng/mL as the confirmation cutoff for hydrocodone in urine. This is the same cutoff as was first used for morphine and codeine in the federal drug testing panel. Laboratories use lower cutoffs for confirmation testing of hydrocodone in hair (e.g., 0.3 ng/mg) and oral fluid (e.g., 10 ng/mL).

INTERPRETING RESULTS

MROs change nearly 90% of hydrocodone-positives they review to negative. Most prescription use involves pills prescribed for pain. Some involve hydrocodone-containing cough syrup.

As described in the "Codeine, Morphine, and Heroin" section of this chapter, use of high doses of codeine can result in low concentrations of hydrocodone. As just noted, use of hydrocodone can account for the presence of hydromorphone or hydrocodeine in urine in combination with high concentrations of hydrocodone.

Hydromorphone ■

THERAPEUTIC USE

Hydromorphone is sold in both tablet and injectable forms. It is shorter acting and more potent than morphine. It is primarily used in hospitals and other health care settings and is thus a target when testing health care workers suspected of stealing drugs. Figure 13-17 presents the chemical structure of hydromorphone.

ILLICIT USE

Hydromorphone tablets can be dissolved and injected as a substitute for heroin. Prior to the current popularity of hydrocodone and oxycodone among drug abusers, hydromorphone formulations were the leading opioid products for abuse and diversion.

METABOLISM AND EXCRETION

About 30% of a hydromorphone dose is eliminated in urine as conjugated hydromorphone and 6% as free hydromorphone. Hydromorphone is a metabolite of hydrocodone, as described in the "Hydrocodone" section of this chapter. It is also a minor metabolite of morphine, as described in the "Codeine, Morphine, and Heroin" section.

LABORATORY ANALYSIS

Hydromorphone will cross-react to a variable extent with most commercial opiate immunoassays. GC/MS confirmation can identify and quantify the presence of hydromorphone.

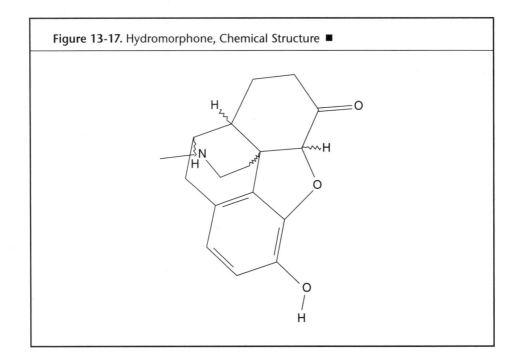

Figure 13-17. Hydromorphone, Chemical Structure ∎

INTERPRETING RESULTS

MROs change more than three-quarters of hydromorphone-positives they review to negative. Use of hydromorphone, hydrocodone, and high doses of morphine can account for the presence of hydromorphone in urine.

Meperidine ∎

Meperidine is a synthetic opioid that had been widely prescribed during much of the 20th century but has fallen out of favor relative to other opioid painkillers in recent years for all but a few, specific indications.

THERAPEUTIC USE

Meperidine is used for pre-anesthesia and pain relief, particularly in obstetrics and post-operative situations. Meperidine is available in tablets, syrups, and injectable forms under generic and brand name Schedule II preparations. Figure 13-18 presents the chemical structure of meperidine.

ILLICIT USE

Meperidine can be abused in a manner similar to other opioids. Demerol has been abused by crushing, chewing, snorting, or injecting the dissolved product. It is a drug primarily used in hospitals and other health care settings and is thus a target when testing health care workers suspected of stealing drugs.

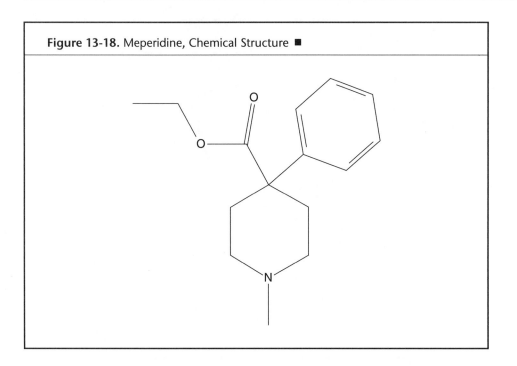

Figure 13-18. Meperidine, Chemical Structure ■

METABOLISM AND EXCRETION

About 7% of a meperidine dose is excreted unchanged in the urine with about 17% as normeperidine, a metabolite with about half the analgesic activity of meperidine. Normeperidine has an elimination half-life of 24–48 hours and can accumulate with frequent doses.

LABORATORY ANALYSIS

Laboratory tests for meperidine use typically target both meperidine and normeperidine. Urinary concentrations for meperidine and normeperidine of 1,000–10,000 ng/mL are typical following therapeutic use.

Methadone ■

Methadone is a synthetic opioid with a long duration of effect. Methadone produces many of the same effects of other opioids. High doses of methadone can block the euphoric effects of heroin, morphine, and similar drugs. Figure 13-19 presents the chemical structure of methadone.

THERAPEUTIC USE

Methadone has historically been used as a substitute for heroin and has been administered or prescribed in opiate addiction programs. Since the late 1990s, methadone has also been widely prescribed to help treat chronic pain. While a

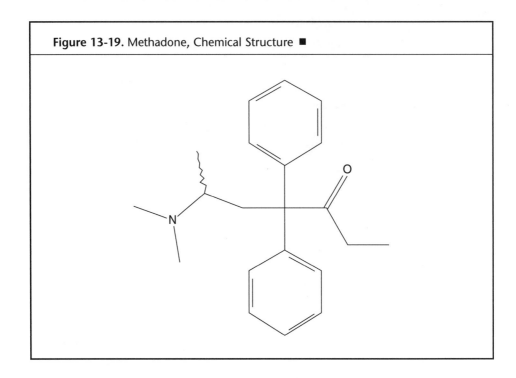

Figure 13-19. Methadone, Chemical Structure ■

physician must have a separate DEA registration to prescribe methadone to treat opiate addiction, no such registration is required to prescribe methadone for pain.

Methadone is administered orally, typically at daily doses of 30–100 mg, and as high as 180 mg/day. Some patients stay on methadone indefinitely, while others move from methadone to abstinence. An addict in a treatment program initially receives each methadone dose individually and directly from the program. Over time, as the patient's condition stabilizes, the patient may be given the next day's dose to bring home so that he or she need not return for methadone every day. He or she does not get prescriptions for methadone and does not buy methadone at pharmacies.

ILLICIT USE

Methadone is abused for its sedative and analgesic effects. Some patients in methadone maintenance programs continue the use of heroin and other drugs. Some sell their take-home methadone. The dramatic increase in sales of methadone in the United States (see Table 13-5) for pain treatment has helped fuel a corresponding increase in methadone abuse in recent years.

METABOLISM AND EXCRETION

Methadone is rapidly absorbed from the gastrointestinal tract and can be detected in the blood within 30 minutes, reaching a peak concentration at about 4 hours. It has a slow onset of action and therefore a lower potential for abuse than faster-acting opioids. Methadone has a slow metabolism and high-fat solubility, making it longer lasting than morphine-based drugs. Methadone has a typical elimination half-life of 15–60 hours with a mean of around 22. It is metabolized by the liver primarily into two inactive metabolites: 2-ethylidene-1,5-dimethyl-3, 3-diphenylpyrrolidine (EDDP) and 2-ethyl-5-methyl-3,3-diphenyl-1-pyrroline (EMDP). The percentage of a dose excreted in the urine as unchanged methadone and EDDP varies with the pH of the urine. Urinary excretion of unchanged parent drug is 5–50%, and excretion of EDDP, 3–25%. EDDP is detectable in the urine longer and usually at greater concentrations than methadone and its inclusion in the laboratory analysis provides additional evidence of methadone use.

LABORATORY ANALYSIS

Testing programs that wish to target methadone need to use screening tests specific for methadone or the metabolite EDDP. The opiate immunoassays used in regulated testing for codeine, morphine, and 6-AM have no significant cross-reactivity for methadone or EDDP. Confirmation tests for methadone are targeted at either methadone alone or methadone and EDDP. Urine concentrations of donors who use methadone therapeutically can be as high as 20,000–50,000 ng/mL.

Patients in methadone maintenance programs have on occasion not taken their methadone but spiked their urine specimens with small amounts to ensure positive results in tests conducted to monitor adherence. This practice results in a high concentration of methadone and no metabolites. This is among the reasons for including EDDP when testing for methadone.

Drugs that have been reported to cross-react with certain methadone immunoassays include disopyramide, diphenhydramine, meperidine, and doxylamine succinate.

INTERPRETING RESULTS

Tests for methadone are sometimes conducted for monitoring compliance of patients who receive it as part of an opiate addiction treatment program. In this context, positive results are expected and negative results raise questions about whether the patient is diverting the drug instead of taking it. If a donor has a methadone-positive workplace test and the donor says he receives it for opiate addiction treatment, the MRO may need to contact the treating physician to corroborate the explanation (as opposed to contacting the pharmacy or asking for a copy of the label). This is because methadone is sometimes, especially in early treatment of opiate addicts, administered as observed dosing in the office instead of by prescription.

Use of methadone is always a disqualifier from CMV operation, according to guidance from the Federal Motor Carrier Safety Administration (FMCSA) [58]. This guidance was developed when methadone was used almost exclusively to treat addiction to heroin and other opiates and was based in part on the belief that these people are untrustworthy. The prohibition remains and applies to any methadone use, even for pain control.

Oxycodone ∎

Oxycodone is a semi-synthetic opioid. Of all countries, the United States had the highest total consumption of oxycodone in 2007 (82% of the world total) [59].

THERAPEUTIC USE

Oxycodone is the most commonly prescribed opioid in the United States. Trade names include OxyContin, Percocet, Percodan, and Tylox. Oxycontin is a slow-release formulation that contains more oxycodone than Percocet or Percodan. Its name is a contraction of oxycodone and the word *continuous*. Figure 13-20 presents the chemical structure of oxycodone.

ILLICIT USE

Because of a shortage of heroin, social unacceptability of heroin, and an ample supply of oxycodone in the United States, misuse of oxycodone has surged. Some drug users crush OxyContin and thereby release all of the oxycodone at once and snort or inject the contents for an immediate and short-lasting rush similar to heroin.

METABOLISM AND EXCRETION

Only 10% of a dose of oxycodone is excreted unchanged in the urine. Oxycodone undergoes N-demethylation to yield noroxycodone, a major metabolite, which has only modest analgesic potency. Oxycodone also undergoes O-demethylation to yield oxymorphone, a minor metabolite that has high analgesic potency. Thus, after use, urine may be positive for oxycodone, oxymorphone, or noroxycodone.

Less than 15% of an oxycodone dose is metabolized to oxymorphone, however, oxymorphone has a longer half-life than oxycodone. Oxycodone/

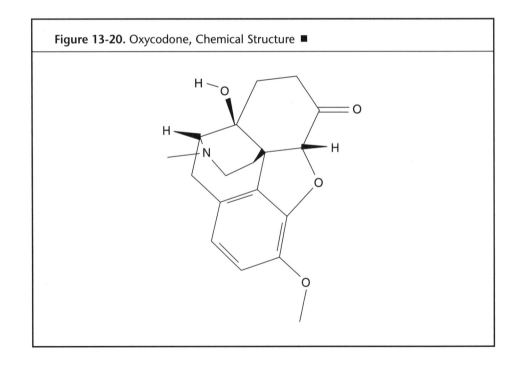

Figure 13-20. Oxycodone, Chemical Structure ■

oxymorphone ratios after oxydodone use vary widely and do not provide reliable information for discriminating between oxycodone use and oxymorphone use.

LABORATORY ANALYSIS

Oxycodone screening is effective only if the screening assay is specific for oxycodone. The standard opiate immunoassays used in most workplace testing programs have little cross-reactivity for oxycodone. Naloxone has been reported to have cross-reactivity with certain oxycodone immunoassays [60]. Confirmation tests identify oxycodone.

INTERPRETING RESULTS

MROs change about three-quarters of oxycodone-positive results they review to negative. Many oxycodone abusers have prescriptions, and this limits the effectiveness of workplace testing for oxycodone.

Oxymorphone ■

Oxymorphone is a semi-synthetic opioid. Figure 13-21 presents the chemical structure of oxymorphone.

THERAPEUTIC USE

Oxymorphone is sold in the United States as an injectable or suppository (Numorphan) and for oral use (Opana) in regular and extended-release tablet formulations.

ILLICIT USE

Oxymorphone was not widely abused before the advent of Opana in 2006 because the previous formulation, Numorphan, had limited availability and was not for oral use. As use of Opana the pill has increased, abuse of the drug has likewise increased.

METABOLISM AND EXCRETION

The elimination half-life of oral oxymorphone is 7–11 hours. Oxymorphone is extensively metabolized in the liver, forming two major metabolites, oxymorphone-3-glucuronide and 6-OH-oxymorphone, and resulting in less than 1% of the free parent drug being excreted in the urine.

LABORATORY ANALYSIS

Oxymorphone screening is conducted with immunoassays directed at oxycodone or at both oxycodone and oxymorphone. Confirmatory testing specifically identifies oxymorphone.

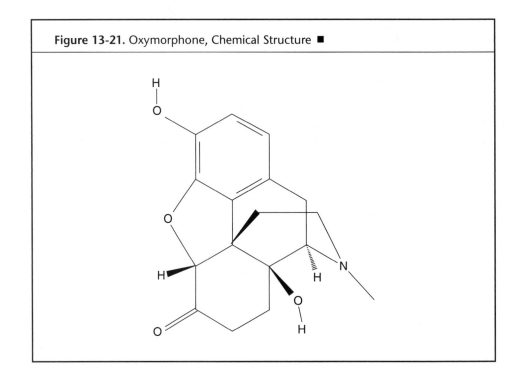

Figure 13-21. Oxymorphone, Chemical Structure ■

INTERPRETING RESULTS

The MRO reviewing an oxymorphone-positive result should consider use of either oxymorphone or oxycodone. As described in the "Oxycodone" section of this chapter, oxymorphone is a metabolite of oxycodone.

Propoxyphene ■

Propoxyphene is a synthetic opioid. Figure 13-22 presents the chemical structure of propoxyphene.

THERAPEUTIC USE

Propoxyphene is prescribed for treatment of mild to moderate pain. Some physicians prescribe it for opioid-demanding patients as a way of mollifying their demands for stronger narcotics that have higher abuse potential. Propoxyphene has a relatively weak analgesic effect. With repeated, frequent use, its cardiotoxic metabolites can accumulate.

ILLICIT USE

Because propoxyphene is an opioid narcotic, classic addictions and physical dependence can occur. Some opiate-abusing addicts use propoxyphene to help ease withdrawal symptoms from stronger narcotics. Recreational abuse of propoxy-

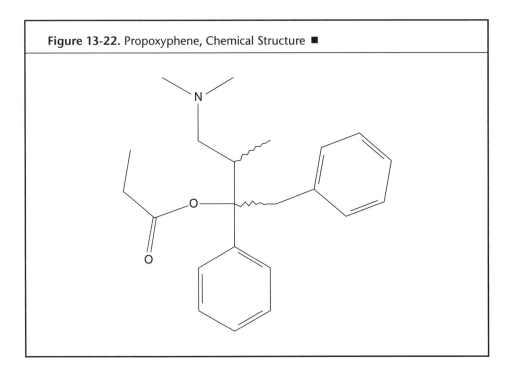

Figure 13-22. Propoxyphene, Chemical Structure ■

phene is typically in combination involving depressant drugs like carisoprodol and alprazolam.

METABOLISM AND EXCRETION

Propoxyphene's elimination half-life is approximately 12 hours. Its effect lasts 2–4 hours. Propoxyphene is metabolized primarily to norpropoxyphene, which is one-fourth to one-half as strong an analgesic as propoxyphene and has a half-life of 20–50 hours.

LABORATORY ANALYSIS

Propoxyphene screening is conducted with a propoxyphene-specific immunoassay. Such immunoassays have been available for many years, which may in part explain why laboratories often include propoxyphene in expanded drug test panels. Confirmation tests identify propoxyphene or its primary metabolite, norpropoxyphene. The inclusion of norpropoxyphene in confirmation testing lengthens the window of detection from 1–2 days to approximately 1 week. Typical cutoffs are 300 ng/mL for both screening and confirmation.

INTERPRETING RESULTS

Most people who test positive for propoxyphene will have a prescription for themselves or will claim to have borrowed someone else's prescription. MROs should be aware of the distinction between Propacet (propoxyphene) and Perco-cet (oxycodone), two trade names that sound alike but contain different ingredients.

Phencyclidine ■

Phencyclidine (PCP) is a synthetic chemical and hallucinogen. Figure 13-23 presents the chemical structure of phencyclidine. It is a Schedule II drug and, in the United States, is used as a drug standard.

PCP intoxication begins several minutes after smoking or injection and can begin up to 30 minutes after oral ingestion. Major effects decline over 4–6 hours. A return to "normal" may take up to 24 hours. PCP produces unpredictable side effects, such as agitation, excitability, and psychosis similar to clinical schizophrenia. The most common physical findings are nystagmus (horizontal, vertical, or rotatory), hypertension, and tachycardia. Severe impairment of mental and physical abilities can occur following single doses.

THERAPEUTIC USES

PCP was first synthesized in 1926. In the 1950s, physicians and veterinarians started administering it as a general anesthetic. PCP's use as a human anesthetic was discontinued in 1965 because, as the anesthetic wore off, psychotic reactions (i.e., "emergence delirium") were common. The drug remained in use as a veterinary tranquilizing agent until about 1978, when the commercial manufacture of PCP in the United States ceased.

Ketamine, an analog of PCP, is currently used in veterinary treatment. There are also reports of ketamine abuse, especially in Europe and Asia. Ketamine does not cross-react with PCP in initial or confirmation testing.

Figure 13-23. Phencyclidine, Chemical Structure ■

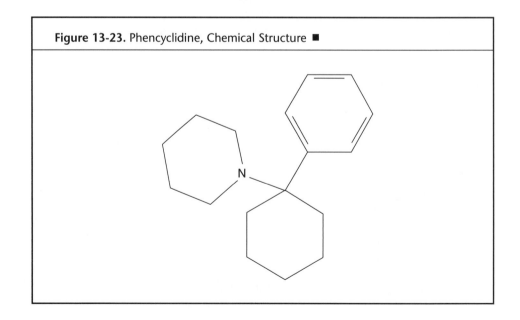

ILLICIT USES

PCP first became popular as a drug of abuse in the 1960s, and its use resurged in the late 1970s and 1980s and then declined. During the 1990s, it accounted for approximately 1% of all laboratory-positive drug tests; many of these were laboratory proficiency-testing samples. Illicit PCP is usually smoked but may be eaten, snorted, or injected intravenously. It is sometimes administered or mixed with other drugs such as cocaine and marijuana to produce more dramatic sensory distortions. PCP has a number of street names, most notably *Angel Dust*.

METABOLISM AND EXCRETION

PCP is well absorbed by any route. It is highly lipid soluble and accumulates in fat and brain tissue. Blood concentrations peak 1–4 hours after ingestion. About 10–15% of a PCP dose is excreted in the urine unchanged. The half-life is 7–16 hours. Urine PCP concentrations decrease rapidly during the first 9 days after use and then decrease more slowly. Most people who use PCP will have positive urine test results for less than 2 weeks; few will have positive results beyond 30 days [61]. PCP is a weak base. Urine acidification—for example, by drinking vinegar or cranberry juice—increases its elimination rate.

LABORATORY ANALYSIS

If the laboratory has detected PCP, the MRO informs the donor that the test identified PCP and this will be reported to the employer. Agents that cause false-positive PCP reactions on urine drug tests are rare. False-positive PCP immunoassay screens have been reported from use of dextromethorphan [62], diphenhydramine [63], ketamine [64], tramadol [65], and venlafaxine [66,67]. Use of these medications does not account for confirmed positive results for PCP.

INTERPRETING RESULTS

There are no therapeutic uses for PCP.

References ■

1. Ewing JA. Detecting alcoholism. The CAGE questionnaire. *JAMA* 1984;252:1905–07.
2. Society for Hair Testing. Consensus of the Society of Hair Testing on hair testing for chronic excessive alcohol consumption. Roma, Italy. June 16, 2009.
3. Caplan YH. Blood, urine and other fluids and tissue specimens for alcohol analyses. In: JC Garriott (ed), *Medicolegal Aspects of Alcohol*, 3rd ed. Tucson, AZ: Lawyers & Judges Publishing Company, 1996. Chapter 5.
4. Høiseth G, Bernard J, Karinene R, et al. A pharmacokinetic study of ethyl glucuronide in blood and urine: Applications to forensic toxicology. *For Sci Int* 2007;172:119–24.
5. Hegstad S, Johnson L, Mørland J, Christophersen A. Determination of ethylglucuronide in oral fluid by ultra-performance liquid chromatography-tandem mass spectrometry. *J Anal Toxicol* 2009;33:204–07.
6. Helander A, Olsson I, Dahl H. Postcollection synthesis of ethyl glucuronide by bacteria in urine may cause false identification of alcohol consumption. *Clin Chem* 2007;53:1855–57.
7. Helander A, Dahl H. Urinary tract infection: A risk factor for false-negative urinary ethyl glucuronide but not ethyl sulfate in the detection of recent alcohol consumption. *Clin Chem* 2005;51:1728–30.
8. Costantino A, DiGregorio E, Korn W, et al. The effect of the use of mouthwash on ethylglucuronide concentrations in urine. *J Anal Toxicol* 2006;30:659–62.

9. Rohrig T, Huber C, Goodson L, et al. Detection of ethylglucuronide in urine following the application of Germ-X. *J Anal Toxicol* 2006;30:703–4.
10. Rosano T, Lin J. Ethyl glucuronide excretion in humans following oral administration of and dermal exposure to ethanol. *J Anal Toxicol* 2008;32:594–600.
11. Center for Substance Abuse Treatment. The Role of Biomarkers in the Treatment of Alcohol Use Disorders. *Substance Abuse Treatment Advisory.* HHS Publication No. 06-4223. Volume 5, Issue 4, September 2006.
12. Jemionek J, Addison J, Past M. Low concentrations of methamphetamine detectable in urine in the presence of high concentrations of amphetamine. *J Anal Toxicol* 2009;33:170–03.
13. Stout P, Horn C, Klette K, et al. Occupational exposure to methamphetamine in workers preparing training aids for drug detection dogs. *J Anal Toxicol* 2006;30:551–53.
14. Ambre J. The urinary excretion of cocaine and metabolites in humans: A kinetic analysis of published data. *J Anal Toxicol* 1985;9:241–45.
15. Bosker W, Huestis M. Oral fluid testing for drugs of abuse. *Clin Chem* 2009;55:1910–31.
16. Cone EJ, Yousefilejad D, Hillsgrove MJ, et al. Passive inhalation of cocaine. *J Anal Toxicol* 1995;19:399–411.
17. ElSohly MA. Urinalysis and casual handling of marijuana and cocaine. *J Anal Toxicol* 1991;15:46.
18. Fitzmaurice L, Wasserman G, Knapp J, et al. TAC use and absorption of cocaine in a pediatric emergency department. *Ann Emergency Med* 1990;19:515–18.
19. Gelhausen J, Klette K, Given J. Urine analysis of laboratory personnel preparing cocaine training aids for a military working dog program. *J Anal Toxicol* 2001;25:637–40.
20. Gelhuausen J, Klette K, Stout P, Given J. Occupational cocaine exposure of crime laboratory personnel preparing training aids for a military working dog program. *J Anal Toxicol* 2003;27:453–58.
21. Cone EJ, Kato K, Hillsgrove M. Cocaine excretion in the semen of drug users. *J Anal Toxicol* 1996;20:139–40.
22. Wang W, Cone E. Testing human hair for drugs of abuse. IV. Environmental cocaine contamination and washing effects. *Forensic Sci Int* 1995;70:39–51.
23. Cairns T, Hill V, Schaffer M, et al. Removing and identifying drug contamination in the analysis of human hair. *Forensic Sci Int* 2004;145:97–108.
24. Schaffer M, Hill V, Cairns T. Hair analysis for cocaine: The requirement for effective wash procedures and effects of drug concentration and hair porosity in contamination and decontamination. *J Anal Toxicol* 2005;29:319–26.
25. Jenkins A, Oyler J, Cone E. Comparison of heroin and cocaine concentrations in saliva with concentrations in blood and plasma. *J Anal Toxicol* 1995;19:359–74.
26. Cone E, Oyler J, Darwin W. Cocaine deposition in saliva following intravenous, intranasal, and smoked administration. *J Anal Toxicol* 1997;19:359–74.
27. U.S. Food and Drug Administration. Herbal teas containing cocaine. (Import Alert No. 31-05). Rockville, MD. Revised October 10, 1992.
28. Jenkins A, Llosa T, Montoya I, Cone E. Identification and quantitation of alkaloids in coca tea. *Forensic Sci Int* 1996;77:179–89.
29. Siegel RK, ElSohly MA, Plowman T, et al. Cocaine in herbal tea. *JAMA* 1986;255:40.
30. ElSohly M, Stanford D, ElSohly H. Coca tea and urinalysis for cocaine metabolites. *J Anal Toxicol* 1986;10:256.
31. Floren AE, Small JW. Mate de Coca equals cocaine. *J Occup Med* 1993;35:95–96.
32. Mazor S, Mycyk M, Wills B, et al. Coca tea consumption causes positive urine cocaine assay. *Eur J Emerg Med* 2006;13:340–41.
33. ElSohly M. Quarterly report potency monitoring project. Report. University, MS: National Center for Natural Products Research.
34. Dackis C, Pottash A, Annitto W, Gold M. Persistence of urinary marijuana levels after supervised abstinence. *Am J Psychiatry* 1982;139:1196–98.
35. Ellis G, Mann M, Judson B, et al. Excretion patterns of cannabinoid metabolites after last use in a group of chronic users. *Clin Pharmacol Ther* 1985;38:572–78.
36. Smith-Kielland A. Urinary excretion of 11-nor-9-carboxy-delta-9-tetrahydrocannabinol: A case with an apparent long terminal half-life. *Scand J Clin Lab Invest* 2006;66:169–71.
37. Huestis MA, Cone EJ. Differentiating new marijuana use from residual drug excretion in occasional marijuana users. *J Anal Toxicol* 1998;22:445–54.
38. Smith M, Barnes A, Huestis M. Identifying new cannabis use with urine creatinine-normalized THCCOOH concentrations and time intervals between specimen collections. *J Anal Toxicol* 2009;33:185–89.
39. Perez-Reyes M, Guiseppi S, Macon AP, et al. Passive inhalation of marijuana smoke and urinary excretion of cannabinoids. *Clin Pharmacol Ther* 1983;34:36–41.
40. Law B, Mason PA, Moffat AC, et al. Passive inhalation of cannabis smoke. *J Pharm Pharmacol* 1984;36:578–81.
41. Cone EJ, Johnson RE, Darwin M, et al. Passive inhalation of marijuana smoke: Urinalysis and room air levels of delta THC. *J Anal Toxicol* 1987;11:89–96.

42. Substance Abuse and Mental Health Services Administration. *Manual for Federal Agency Workplace Drug Testing Programs.* Rockville, MD, Department of Health and Human Services 2004.
43. Pless P, Leson G. Assessing the impact of THC uptake from hemp oil cosmetics on workplace drug testing. Personal communication. Berkeley, CA: Leson Environmental Consulting. March 2001.
44. Cirimele V, Kintz P, Jamey C, et al. Are cannabinoids detected in hair after washing with Cannabio shampoo? *J Anal Toxicol* 1999;23:349–51.
45. Niedbala R, Kardos K, Fritch D, et al. Detection of marijuana use by oral fluid and urine analysis following single-dose administration of smoked and oral marijuana. *J Anal Toxicol* 2001;25:289–303.
46. Niedbala R, Kardos K, Salamone S, et al. Passive cannabis smoke exposure and oral fluid testing. *J Anal Toxicol* 2004;28:546–52.
47. Huestis M, Cone E. Relationship of delta^9-tetrahydrocannabinol concentration in oral fluid and plasma after controlled administration of smoked cannabis. *J Anal Toxicol* 2004;28:394–99.
48. Cone EJ, Johnson RE, Paul BD, et al. Marijuana-laced brownies: Behavioral effects, physiologic effects, and urinalysis in humans following ingestion. *J Anal Toxicol* 1988;12:169–75.
49. ElSohly MA, Jones AB. Drug testing in the workplace: Could a positive test for one of the mandated drugs be for reasons other than illicit use of the drug? *J Anal Toxicol* 1995;19:450–58.
50. Steinagle GC, Upfal M. Concentration of marijuana metabolites in the urine after ingestion of hemp seed tea. *J Occup Environ Med* 1999;41:510–13.
51. Gustafson RA, Levine B, Stout PR, et al. Urinary cannabinoid detection times after controlled oral administration of delta^9-tetrahydrocannabinol to humans. *Clin Chem* 2003;49:1114–24.
52. Holler J, Bosy T, Dunkley C, et al. Delta-9-tetrahydrocannabinol content of commercially available hemp products. *J Anal Toxicol* 2008;32:428–32.
53. Hegaard H, Kjaergaard H, Moller L, et al. Determination of a saliva cotinine cut-off to distinguish pregnant smokers from pregnant non-smokers. *Acta Obstet Gynecol Scand* 2007;86:401–06.
54. Semple S, Maccalman L, Naji A, et al. Bar workers' exposure to second-hand smoke: The effect of Scottish smoke-free legislation on occupational exposure. *Ann Occup Hyg* 2007;51:571–80.
55. Manchikanti L. National drug control policy and prescription drug abuse: Facts and fallacies. *Pain Physician* 2007;10:399–424.
56. West R, Crews B, Mikel C, et al. Anomalous observations of codeine in patients on morphine. *Ther Drug Monit* 2009;31:776–78.
57. Moore C, Feldman M, Harrison E, et al. Disposition of hydrocodone in hair. *J Anal Toxicol* 2006;30:353–59.
58. FMCSA. Frequently Asked Question 21 (FAQ)—Medical. Washington, DC. US Department of Transportation 2009.
59. International Narcotics Control Board. Narcotic Drugs: Estimated World Requirements for 2009; Statistics for 2007. New York: United Nations, 2009.
60. Jenkins A, Poirier J, Juhascik M. Cross-reactivity of naloxone with oxycodone immunoassays: Implications for individuals taking Suboxone. *Clin Chem* 2009;55:1434–36.
61. Simpson GM, Khajawall AM, Alatorre E, et al. Urinary phencyclidine excretion in chronic abusers. *J Toxicol Clin Toxicol* 1982;19:1051–59.
62. Budai B, Iskandar H. Dextromethorphan can produce false-positive phencyclidine testing with HPLC. *Am J Emerg Med* 2002;20:61–62.
63. Levine BS, Smith ML. Effects of diphenhydramine on immunoassay of phencyclidine in urine. *Clin Chem* 1990;36:1258.
64. Shannon M. Recent ketamine administration can produce a urine toxic screen which is falsely positive for phencyclidine [letter]. *Pediatr Emerg Care* 1998;14:180.
65. Hull M, Griggs D, Knoepp S, et al. Postmortem urine immunoassay showing false-positive phencyclidine reactivity in a case of fatal tramadol overdose. *Am J Forensic Med Pathol* 2006;27:359–62.
66. Sena S, Kazimi S, Wu A. False-positive phencyclidine immunoassay results caused by venlafaxine and O-desmethyl venlafaxine [letter]. *Clin Chem* 2002;48:676–77.
67. Bond G, Steele P, Uges D. Massive venlafaxine overdose resulted in a false positive Abbott AxSYM urine immunoassay for phencyclidine. *J Toxicol Clin Toxicol* 2003;41:999–1002.

Alcohol Testing ■

This chapter is about alcohol testing procedures. There is also information relevant to alcohol testing in sections of Chapter 6, "Specimen Collection":

1. Collection/Alcohol Test Site
2. Release and Consent Forms
3. Testing of Minors
4. On-Time Arrival for Testing
5. DOT and Non-DOT Tests at the Same Visit
6. Donor Identification
7. Refusal to Test

Breath Alcohol Technician, Screening Test Technician ■

Workplace alcohol testing is completed at the test site. The technician collects the specimen, completes the analysis, and reports the result. By comparison, urine specimen collectors just collect specimens, i.e., have a more limited role.

A breath alcohol technician (BAT) is authorized to perform both screening and confirmation tests. A screening test technician (STT) is authorized only to perform screening tests for alcohol. Before conducting tests regulated by the U.S. Department of Transportation (DOT), BATs and STTs must complete qualification training.

To avoid potential conflicts between supervisors and subordinates, an immediate supervisor should not perform an alcohol test on a donor who reports directly to him or her, unless no other technician is available and the supervisor is otherwise qualified to perform the test.

BAT AND STT TRAINING COURSES

The STT or the BAT who administers regulated alcohol tests must have qualification training and demonstrated proficiency in the alcohol testing device he or she will be using. To promote consistency in the training curriculum, DOT published a model training course for BATs and a similar course for STTs. The DOT curricula include questions and answers to reinforce the information. Trainers may use DOT's model training courses or their equivalent to train STTs and BATs to conduct DOT-mandated tests. Trainers may ask DOT to have their course reviewed for equivalency.

The qualification training for BATs and STTs per DOT must contain the following elements:

- Knowledge about Part 40 alcohol testing procedures.
- Instruction using the DOT model BAT or STT course or an equivalent.
- In-depth knowledge in the operation of the alcohol testing device to be used.
- Their responsibility for maintaining the integrity and credibility of the testing process, ensuring privacy of the donors being tested, and avoiding conduct or statements that could be viewed as offensive or inappropriate.

NRC's alcohol testing rule has similar requirements, but refers to knowledge about the NRC rule and not Part 40.

The course material may be taught in person, conducted by video, by computer and web-based programs, by video conference, or by other equivalent means. Trainers provide their students with certificate of completion. The federal government does not maintain or sponsor lists of qualified BATs or STTs.

BAT AND STT INSTRUCTORS

The instructor (trainer) must be a qualified BAT or STT who has demonstrated the necessary knowledge, skills, and abilities by:

- Regularly conducting DOT alcohol tests for a period of at least a year as a BAT or STT.
- Conducting Part 40 BAT or STT training for a year.
- Successfully completing a "train-the-trainer" course.

Some clinics train BATs in house by staff who are trained and experienced in conducting DOT alcohol tests. Some clinics send staff to training courses, or hire trainers to visit the clinics. Sources of training include BAT training companies, evidential breath testing device (EBT) manufacturers, law enforcement officers, and health and safety training consultants.

MOCK TESTS

After successfully completing qualification training, the student must complete seven consecutive error-free mock tests for initial BAT qualification or five consecutive error-free mock tests for initial STT qualification. The monitor decides what scenarios to use for these mock tests. The BAT student should successfully demonstrate that he or she can:

- Respond to the device's messages and commands or displays.
- Take appropriate actions when an error message or malfunction occurs within the device.
- Recognize that an air blank has been conducted.
- Identify and explain actions the technician will take when the device does not function properly.
- Explain when an external calibration check is required, if applicable to the device being used, and identify the procedures used to perform the check.

The mock tests must be conducted on the same device(s) the STT/BAT will use. If the device involves color changes, contrasts, or color readings, the technician must demonstrate that he or she can see the changes.

The mock tests are intended to portray a real event conducted with someone (for example, the instructor) acting as the test subject. The tests must be directly observed in real-time by the instructor or clearly able to be monitored in real-time that allows direct interaction between monitor and trainee. The proficiency monitor must also attest in writing that the mock collections were error-free. The use of a "checklist" during the mock tests is acceptable if the use of a checklist was part of the training the BAT or STT received and was to be used in real-life tests.

The proficiency monitor does not have to be the same person who taught the qualification training. However, the proficiency monitor must have the qualifications of an instructor.

RETRAINING

DOT requires that each BAT or STT go through refresher training every 5 years to remain eligible to conduct DOT alcohol tests. The content of the refresher training must include material equivalent to the initial training but updated as needed. The refresher training includes conducting error-free mock tests monitored by the trainer.

ERROR CORRECTION TRAINING

A BAT or STT who makes an error causing a DOT test to be canceled must undergo error correction training within 30 days of notification of the error. Error correction training is not required for errors related to equipment failure unless the failure is related to the BAT's failure to maintain the EBT. Error-correction training is also required if, in the event of equipment failure, the BAT does not try to accomplish the test with using another, alternative device, provided that another device is reasonably available.

The error-correction training focuses on the mistake(s) made and includes three error-free mock collections, at least two of which are related to the area in which the error was made. If a BAT or STT requires error-collection training, he or she may continue to perform DOT tests for up to 30 days prior to completion of the error correction training. However, the goal is to complete the error correction training as soon as practical after the error(s) occurred. The employer or service agent designated by the employer is responsible for notifying the alcohol testing site of the error and the retraining requirement and for ensuring that the training takes place.

Alcohol Test Devices ■

The National Highway Traffic Safety Administration (NHTSA) has established model specifications for alcohol test devices [1, 2]. These specifications include accuracy and precision for levels at 0.02 and above and noninterference by acetone. Acetone is an issue because people exhale acetone under certain conditions, such as fasting and diabetic ketoacidosis. Devices that meet screening or evidential breath test specifications are listed on the NHTSA conforming products lists (CPL).

Current CPLs are published periodically in the *Federal Register* and DOT posts them online. Employers that conduct DOT-regulated alcohol testing must use screening and evidential breath alcohol test devices that are listed on the CPL.

ALCOHOL SCREENING DEVICE

An alcohol screening device (ASD) analyzes a breath or oral fluid specimen for alcohol. A breath ASD is essentially an alcohol test device similar to an EBT but does not meet the accuracy requirements of an EBT and, in most cases, does not have a direct link to a printer. An oral fluid ASD provides a quick device using immunoassay technology similar to those used for on-site urine and oral fluid drug tests. Because confirmatory tests must be performed using EBTs, an EBT must be readily accessible in case a screening test result is 0.02 or greater. If an EBT is not available for use within 30 minutes to confirm the screening result, the employer is *not* in compliance with the DOT rule unless there is an unusual circumstance (for example, a remote location). Most test sites find it simplest to use EBTs for both screening and confirmatory tests.

The U.S. Coast Guard (USCG), which tests under authority of the Department of Homeland Security, only requires screening tests when testing after serious marine incidents. The screening test device used in this situation must appear on the CPL. This exception is allowed because the USCG believes it is not feasible to always get confirmation tests performed in off-shore settings.

EVIDENTIAL BREATH TEST DEVICE

An evidential breath test device (EBT) meets strict accuracy and precision requirements set by NTHSA and can directly print the result on paper. Without a functioning printer an EBT cannot be used for DOT confirmation tests. Each EBT uses one of the following technologies:

- *Fuel cell.* A fuel cell device uses a chemical oxidation process that correlates a release of electrons to an alcohol concentration. Fuel cell units used most often are compact and portable. They cost $1500–$4500.
- *Infrared spectrometry.* Infrared light passes through the breath sample in an infrared spectrometry unit. Alcohol, if present, absorbs the light at a characteristic wavelength in proportion to the alcohol concentration. These devices are generally larger and less portable than fuel cell devices. They cost $2500–$7000.
- *Gas chromatography.* A gas chromatography (GC) unit requires compressed gas as a carrier, is not portable, and costs approximately $7000. Because GC devices are expensive, not portable, complicated to operate, and offer little advantage over current fuel cell and infrared spectrometry devices, few workplace testing programs use GC devices.

Some EBTs can be purchased together with software that provides more clear and detailed instructions for conducting tests and provides more options for storing data and printing results. Most EBTs use stand-alone, small portable printers that print results on single- or triple-ply paper or on adhesive labels. Some impact printers are designed to print directly onto the alcohol testing form (ATF).

Results of breath alcohol analysis are expressed in terms of grams of alcohol per 2100 mL (or g/210 L) of breath. This corresponds to the equivalent and commonly used unit of measure for blood alcohol, grams per deciliter (g/dL). For example, a breath alcohol result of 0.04% (grams of alcohol per 2100 mL breath) corresponds with a blood alcohol concentration of 0.04 g/dL or 0.04 g/210 L.

The breath sample is not retained for potential future retests or split tests. In fuel cell devices, the breath sample that undergoes oxidation is quite small and its ethanol content is destroyed as part of the analysis. There are no commercially available products for retaining a breath sample unchanged. The Supreme Court has ruled that retention of the breath sample is unnecessary in forensic breath alcohol testing [3].

QUALITY ASSURANCE PLAN

The manufacturer of each ASD or EBT develops a quality assurance plan (QAP) for the device that describes the accuracy checks, tolerance ranges, maintenance requirements, and quality control procedures. NHTSA reviews the QAP when it considers listing a device on its CPL. A copy of the QAP should be kept at the test site where the ASD or EBT is used. Extra copies of the QAP can be obtained, as needed, from the manufacturer.

Each EBT's QAP includes external calibration check (accuracy check) requirements. An accuracy check is performed with a known alcohol standard in a liquid solution or compressed dry gas. The EBT's measured value is compared to the expected value and must be within the tolerance limits designated by the manufacturer's QAP, which is typically ±0.005 for workplace testing. Accuracy check requirements vary depending upon the QAP and the program guidelines or internal procedures of the test site. In general, the site should perform an accuracy check once a month and as soon as conveniently possible after a positive test. The post-positive accuracy check helps ensure the validity of each test and minimizes any potential timespan for discrepancy. If the EBT fails a check, it is taken out of service according to the manufacture's QAP. Also, every result of 0.02 or above obtained on the EBT since the last valid check is cancelled. The QAP and calibration records are usually scrutinized in the event of a challenged EBT result. DOT requires calibration logbook records to be kept with each device for a minimum of 2 years.

Alcohol Testing Form ■

A DOT breath ATF is used for each DOT alcohol test. The DOT ATF is a three-ply carbonless paper form that is published near the end of its Part 40 Procedures (see Appendix F). Look-alike forms that do not reference the federal rules are used for non-DOT tests.

In DOT-regulated testing, the employer (company) name and the designated employer representative (DER) name and phone number must be in Step 1 of the ATF. If the employer information is not preprinted in Step 1, the BAT writes it in. DOT also allows information needed for billing purposes and other information, such as bar codes and tracking numbers, to be affixed or printed on the ATF.

Alcohol Test Site ■

Alcohol test sites require little set-up other than to ensure the test device is fully functional. Alcohol tests are therefore easy to perform on site at the workplace. Each alcohol test should be conducted with reasonable visual and auditory privacy so that bystanders cannot know or infer the test results.

Alcohol Test Procedure ■

Alcohol tests should begin promptly once the donor arrives. Only one donor is tested at a time. The BAT explains the test procedure and shows the donor the instructions on the back of the ATF. The BAT completes Step 1 of the ATF and asks the donor to complete Step 2. If the donor refuses to sign Step 2, this is a refusal to test and the BAT documents the refusal to test on the ATF, then notifies the employer.

The alcohol test is initially performed using either an ASD or EBT. If the initial alcohol concentration is at or above 0.02, the test is repeated 15–30 minutes later using an EBT. The delay between the initial and repeat tests allows for the dispersion of any alcohol in the oral cavity that is not measured in the repeat test. During the 15–30 minute interval, the BAT tells the donor to not eat, drink, or belch, and to wait nearby within view of the BAT or another employer representative who will watch the donor to help ensure he or she complies. (If the donor does not comply, the BAT makes a note of this on the ATF and proceeds with confirmation testing.) The no eating/drinking/belching rule is intended to prevent the donor from introducing anything into his or her mouth that might elevate the confirmation result. Prior to the confirmation test, the BAT must ensure an air blank reading of zero is displayed, demonstrating that no alcohol is present in the EBT.

The BAT should complete the confirmation test prior to collecting a urine specimen or conducting other tasks in which the donor cannot remain under the direct observation of the BAT. If circumstances delay confirmatory testing beyond 30 minutes, the BAT still performs a confirmation test and not another screening test and notes why a delay occurred.

The BAT shows the donor the result as displayed on the EBT. The EBT prints the test result. The BAT ensures the results are affixed or directly printed on all three copies of the ATF, preferably in the designated space on the front of the ATF, either by a label that is tamper-evident or by affixing the printout to the ATF with tamper-evident tape. The BAT signs and dates Step 3 of the ATF. The result is expressed on these copies as a number, rather than as positive or negative. If the confirmation test result is 0.02 or higher, the BAT asks the donor to sign Step 4. If the donor refuses to sign Step 4, the BAT makes note of the refusal on the ATF (but this is not a refusal to test). The BAT then immediately sends (faxes) the ATF to the employer.

In non-DOT testing in which a laboratory performs the analysis (i.e., urine or blood testing), the result may be reported to the MRO or directly to the employer. If the MRO receives the result, he or she relays it to the employer without interpretation. Medical review of alcohol test results is not performed because the source of the result is clear (i.e., alcohol consumption) and there is no acceptable explanation for having an alcohol concentration above the policy's limit while on duty. DOT does not accept use of medicinal alcohol or tolerance to alcohol as a mitigating circumstance for an alcohol test result that violates the rules. Under the NRC rule, a donor with a positive breath alcohol test may ask for a blood alcohol test.

Shy Lung ■

SHY LUNG EVENT AT TEST SITE

The term *shy lung* refers to a situation where the donor does not provide a sufficient amount of breath to permit a valid breath test. The donor must be given a minimum of two attempts to provide an adequate sample. If the donor does not provide an adequate sample based on the EBT requirement, the BAT should:

1. Repeat the procedure if the BAT believes there is a strong likelihood of success with additional attempts.
2. Try to conduct the test in manual mode if the EBT has this capability.
3. Consider using an oral fluid device if the donor fails after two attempts, and the BAT is also a qualified STT. Breath will still be required if confirmation testing is necessary.

If the donor is unable to provide an adequate sample after at least two attempts, the technician records the circumstances—e.g., "Inadequate breath sample after three attempts"—on the ATF and immediately informs the DER. If the BAT believes the donor is purposefully *not* blowing adequately or forcefully into the breath testing device, then the BAT notes in Step 3, "Refusal to Test" and the DER must immediately take action.

EMPLOYER SENDS DONOR FOR SHY LUNG EVALUATION

The employer directs the donor to get a medical ("shy lung") evaluation by a physician acceptable to the employer within 5 business days. The 5-day time frame should be extended if the donor makes a good-faith effort but fails to get the evaluation within 5 days.

ARRANGING THE SHY LUNG EVALUATION

The physician who performs the evaluation must have sufficient expertise to deal effectively with the medical issues associated with inability to provide a sufficient amount of breath, should have some knowledge of workplace alcohol drug testing procedures, and should be neutral and objective. The physician should not delegate this exam to an advanced practitioner; the issues are too complex and the stakes are too high. Shy lung evaluations are rare. Most MROs should understand the context and be available and willing to perform shy lung evaluations.

EXAMINING PHYSICIAN'S REPORT

The evaluating physician communicates his or her determination directly to the DER. Unsupported claims of situational anxiety or hyperventilation are unacceptable explanations for shy lung. A preexisting psychological disorder may be an acceptable explanation if it has been medically documented before the test. If the physician states that there was a valid medical reason—for example, a severe asthma attack—for the insufficient amount of breath, the test is canceled. If the physician identifies no valid medical reason, the donor is deemed to have refused testing.

Insufficient Saliva Sample ■

An insufficient saliva sample refers to a situation where the donor does not provide sufficient saliva to activate the saliva screening device. The technician re-attempts the procedure with a new screening device. If the donor still cannot produce enough saliva to complete the test, the technician documents the fact on the ATF and notifies the DER. The DER then promptly tries to arrange a breath alcohol test.

Alcohol Test Errors ■

If the BAT or STT becomes aware of an event that will cause the test to be cancelled, he or she must try to correct the problem promptly, if practicable. This may require repeating the test, using a new ATF and, if needed, a new alcohol screening device or a different EBT. Some errors cannot be fixed; see the fatal flaws listed in Table 14-1. Some errors are potentially correctable by amending the ATF; see the correctable flaws listed in Table 14-1. If a valid test cannot be performed, the BAT or STT cancels the test and immediately informs the DER.

If the BAT, STT, employer or other service agent becomes aware of a correctable flaw that has not already been corrected, he or she must try to get it corrected. If the error is a fatal flaw, the test must be canceled. The BAT, STT, or other person who determines that cancellation is necessary must notify the DER within 48 hours of the cancellation.

A cancelled test is neither positive nor negative. A cancelled test does not count toward any required random rate or number of follow-up tests. A cancelled test, in DOT-regulated programs, is not cause for the employer to order a non-DOT test or a reasonable suspicion DOT test, or to take disciplinary action. If a test is cancelled and a negative test result is required, e.g., for pre-employment, return-to-duty, or follow-up purposes, the employer should retest the donor.

Reporting Results ■

For results equal to or greater than 0.02, the STT or BAT informs the employer immediately, usually by telephone and by later sending a copy of the result to the employer. For results below 0.02, the STT or BAT informs the employer directly or routes the reports through a C/TPA. The BAT notifies the DER within 48 hours of any test that has a fatal flaw. If the BAT does not initially report this information in writing, he or she must follow up the phoned-in report with Copy 1 of the ATF. In regulated testing, the ATF must not be routed to the DER by sending it with the urine specimen to the laboratory for forwarding to the employer; the ATF has donor identifiers on it and sending it to the laboratory would disclose the test subject's identity.

If the result is at or above 0.02%, the BAT should instruct the donor to remain at the testing site until the employer arranges transportation for the donor.

Table 14-1. Breath/Saliva Alcohol Test Flaws ■

Fatal Flaws

1. BAT/STT fails to both print his or her name and sign the ATF.

Saliva Screening Test:
2. The STT reads the result sooner or later than the time allotted by the manufacturer.
3. The ASD does not activate.
4. The ASD is used after its expiration date.

Screening or Confirmation Evidential Breath Test:
5. The test number or alcohol concentration displayed on the EBT is not the same as the test number or alcohol concentration on the printed result.

Confirmation Evidential Breath Test:
6. Minimum 15 minute waiting period prior to confirmation test is not observed.
7. EBT does not print a confirmation test result.
8. Air blank is not performed before a confirmation test.
9. The EBT fails the next external calibration check. In this situation, every result of 0.02 or above obtained on the EBT since the last valid external calibration check is cancelled.

Correctable Flaws

1. BAT/STT fails to sign the ATF.
2. BAT/STT fails to note donor's refusal to sign (Step 4) if confirmation result is greater than or equal to 0.02.
3. Use of a non-DOT ATF for a DOT authorized test, provided that the test device and procedure is otherwise consistent with DOT requirements. The BAT/STT corrects this by signing a statement acknowledging the error and the steps that have been taken to avoid repeating it.

Flaws That Are Neither Fatal Nor Need Immediate Correction

1. Use of a STT or BAT that has not completed training or retraining.
2. Claims that the donor was improperly selected for testing

The BAT should contact the DER and ask him/her what transportation arrangements will be made. If the result is at or above 0.08% and the donor drives his/her vehicle anyway, the BAT should notify the police. This advice is not in the DOT regulations but is based on individual responsibility to protect the donor and public safety.

Alcohol test results do not undergo medical review. The source of the alcohol—beverage, cough syrup, vanilla extract, or another substance—does not mitigate the policy violation that occurs when the alcohol concentration is at or above the employer's cutoff value. (Nonbeverage sources of alcohol are unlikely to significantly increase the alcohol concentration.)

When the test site performs an alcohol test result that provides immediate results, it normally reports the result directly to the employer, without interviewing the donor and without any interpretation. When an outside laboratory performs the alcohol analysis, e.g., urinalysis, the result may be reported to the MRO, who then reports it to the employer without interviewing the donor and without interpretation.

Supervisors and billing personnel with a "need to know" are permitted to have access to documentation of breath alcohol testing. The need to know must address a specific purpose and must be necessary for the employer's successful implementation of the workplace alcohol testing program.

Recordkeeping ■

Recordkeeping requirements under the DOT rule are as follows:

1 year—Records of alcohol tests with a concentration of less than 0.020 and cancelled alcohol tests

2 years—Documentation of the inspection, maintenance, and calibration of EBTs

5 years—Alcohol test results of 0.020 or greater, and documentation of refusals and follow-up alcohol tests

Upon written request, donors are entitled to obtain copies of any records about their alcohol tests.

Fitness-for-Duty Determination ■

Under DOT rules, alcohol testing is only conducted just before, during, or immediately after performing safety-sensitive job tasks. Measurement of the alcohol concentration is used to determine a person's fitness to perform safety-sensitive job tasks as well as to deter alcohol misuse and abuse. The NRC rules authorize licensees to conduct alcohol tests as a part of each donor's gaining access to a restricted site.

A commercial motor vehicle (CMV) driver is not required to undergo a physical examination and obtain a new medical examiner's certificate based solely on a violation of DOT's alcohol misuse prevention rule. If the substance abuse professional believes that alcoholism exists, the employer should then send the driver for an examination to determine qualification to drive. Current alcoholism is disqualifying from CMV operation [49 *CFR* 391.33(b)(13)].

References ■

1. National Highway Traffic Safety Administration. Department of Transportation. Highway safety programs; model specifications for devices to measure breath alcohol. *Federal Register* 1993; 58(Sept 17):48,705–10.
2. Department of Transportation, National Highway Traffic Safety Administration. Highway safety programs; model specifications for screening devices to measure alcohol in bodily fluids. *Federal Register* 1994;59(Aug 2):39,382–90.
3. *California v. Trombetta et al.* U.S. Supreme Court. 83-305. June 11, 1984.

Return-to-Duty Process ■

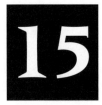

This chapter describes the process that must be completed before resuming safety-sensitive duties after a DOT positive test, refusal to test, or other violation of the DOT anti-drug and alcohol misuse prevention rules. Under Part 40, this requirement is triggered by prohibited alcohol- or drug-related conduct. It is not triggered by an admission of substance abuse, participation in a treatment program, or a charge of driving under the influence (DUI). The return-to-duty process consists of the following steps:

1. An initial evaluation and treatment recommendation(s) by a substance abuse professional (SAP).
2. Treatment.
3. A follow-up evaluation in which the SAP (a) determines whether the individual successfully complied with the treatment recommendations, and (b) provides recommendations to the employer about follow-up testing.
4. The employee's agreement to submit to follow-up testing as determined by the SAP.
5. A return-to-duty test.

The NRC follows this same process but uses the term *substance abuse expert* instead of SAP. Some nonregulated programs follow this process, too.

Responsibilities of the Substance Abuse Professional ■

A SAP is a person who evaluates employees who have test-program violations, recommends treatment, and determines if the employees have successfully completed recommended treatment.

The SAP is not just responsible for the welfare of the person seeking treatment. The SAP's first and foremost priority is public safety. The SAP also owes a duty to the employer and, in DOT-regulated testing, the DOT.

SAP Qualifications ■

To be a SAP under DOT rules, a person must have certain credentials, possess specific knowledge, complete training and pass an examination, and, every 3 years, complete continuing education.

Medical review officers (MROs) can serve as SAPs if they meet the SAP qualification requirements. The MRO's knowledge and experience in workplace drug testing and medical background provide a good basis for becoming a SAP. MROs should understand that SAP assessments, unlike interviews with drug test specimen donors, must be performed face-to-face. MROs can also help coordinate SAP services, including referrals to SAPs on behalf of employers.

SAP CREDENTIALS

Any of the following are acceptable credentials:

- Licensed physician (medical doctor [MD] or doctor of osteopathy [DO]).
- Licensed or certified psychologist, social worker, or certified employee assistance professional (EAP).
- State-licensed or certified marriage and family therapist.
- Drug and alcohol abuse counselor certified by the National Association of Alcohol and Drug Abuse Counselors Certification Commission (NAADAC) or the International Certification Reciprocity Consortium, or a master addictions counselor certified by the National Board for Certified Counselors and Affiliates.

SAP KNOWLEDGE

Many of those who serve as SAPs also provide drug and alcohol abuse counseling services. The SAP must be knowledgeable about, and have clinical experience in, the diagnosis and treatment of disorders related to drug and alcohol abuse. The SAP must also be knowledgeable about SAP functions, DOT drug and alcohol testing rules applicable to the employers for whom the SAP evaluates employees, and DOT's *Substance Abuse Professional Procedures Guidelines* [1]. The SAP should be knowledgeable about insurance coverage and the availability and quality of local treatment programs. The SAP should have some understanding about the procedures and reliability of workplace drug and alcohol testing. This helps keep perspective should the employee claim the test result was wrong.

SAP TRAINING AND EXAMINATION

A SAP must complete training and pass an examination on the training material. DOT requires that SAP training include the following subjects:

- The background, rationale, and coverage of DOT's testing program.
- Part 40 and DOT agency drug and alcohol testing rules.
- Key DOT alcohol testing requirements, including the testing process, the role of BATs and STTs, and problems in alcohol tests.
- SAP qualifications and prohibitions.
- The role of the SAP in the return-to-duty process.
- SAP consultation and communication with employers, MROs, and treatment providers.
- Reporting and recordkeeping requirements.

DOT requires that the SAP examination be given by a nationally recognized professional or training organization and comprehensively cover the subjects just listed. DOT requires these training or professional organizations to have their SAP examinations validated by a test-evaluation organization. DOT does not refer to "certification" of SAPs. Nevertheless, organizations that qualify SAPs give them "certificates" and SAPs call themselves "certified." DOT maintains a list of organizations offering SAP training or examinations and posts this list on its website.

DOT requires that SAPs complete at least 12 hours of continuing education units (CEUs) relevant to SAP duties every 3 years. Continuing education must include material on new drug and alcohol abuse evaluation technologies, current DOT interpretations and rule guidance, and DOT regulation changes and other information about developments related to the SAP functions in the DOT program. Continuing education must also include a documented assessment of how well the SAP learned the materials. There is no requirement that SAPs "recertify." Nevertheless, some SAP credentialing organizations market their training and examination programs for both initial and periodic certification. For example, the certificate that NAADAC issues to those who pass its SAP exam includes a 3-year "expiration" date. SAPs must maintain training and initial examination documentation and, upon request, provide it to DOT agencies and employers or service agents who use or contemplate using their services.

Referring the Employee to the SAP ■

If an applicant or employee has a DOT positive test or refusal to test, the employer is required to give that person a listing of SAPs readily available to the employee and acceptable to the employer. The list should have more than one SAP. The applicant or employee can select from that list and make arrangements for the initial evaluation. Employers find SAPs by asking for referrals from their consortium/third-party administrators (C/TPAs), MROs, or local occupational health providers, or by searching the Internet.

Only a fraction of donors who have positive results or refusals to test undergo SAP evaluations. Some employers fail to refer donors to SAPs. Some donors find it too expensive or otherwise problematic. SAP evaluations almost always involve employees rather than job applicants or ex-employees. The possibility of an employee's returning to an available job is a strong motivator; otherwise, the employee may find it easier to seek employment with an employer who is unaware of the positive result. (A similar situation occurs with split specimen testing, which is sometimes ordered by employees and rarely by applicants.)

Payment for SAP Services, Treatment, and Follow-Up Tests ■

Part 40 does not address who pays for SAP services. In many, if not most, cases, the employee pays the SAP out of pocket. This is expensive and not covered by health insurance of by many employers. Some SAPs require one up-front payment for the initial and follow-up visits. Some employees attend the initial evaluation and never complete treatment or return for a follow-up visit. However, the proportion of employees who follow through is greater when they pay for both visits up front.

Few employers pay for treatment. Employees with coverage can sometimes use their personal health insurance to help pay for clinical visits related to treatment.

Some employers require employees to pay for follow-up tests either directly (i.e., by paying at the time of specimen collection) or by deducting the employer's costs for follow-up testing from the employee's paycheck.

Initial SAP Evaluation ■

INITIAL EVALUATION PROTOCOL

The SAP should ask for a copy of the drug and/or alcohol test result or the refusal to test record prior to or at the time of the evaluation. This record offers the SAP clear documentation of what prompted the referral. The initial evaluation is intended to determine the extent of the person's substance abuse and the kind of education or treatment that is needed. The person is evaluated by a face-to-face clinical assessment. The face-to-face evaluation allows the SAP to observe the person's nonverbal cues such as facial expression, posture, ability to make eye contact, and reactions to questions during the evaluation. The evaluation should include a standard psychosocial assessment using interview questions and standardized testing tools. The more widely used standardized tests include the Michigan Alcoholism Screening Test, the Drug Abuse Screening Test, and the Alcohol Use Disorder Identification Test. The SAP should conduct a complete drug and alcohol use history, including onset of use, frequency, duration, amount used, and dates of last three uses. The SAP should ask the client about his or her family history of substance abuse. If the employee was referred due to a positive drug test result, the SAP should ask if the person used alcohol, too. A mental status exam should be completed because the SAP is responsible for appropriately assessing any coexisting mental health problems. If the employee appears intoxicated, the SAP may want to include a non-DOT drug or alcohol testing as part of the initial evaluation to corroborate and document the employee's intoxication.

The SAP's questions should be structured to evoke answers, not denials (for example, see Figure 15-1). A drug/alcohol test violation has been established before the person sees the SAP. Most people will admit to SAPs that they used drugs, although admissions of adulteration or substitution are relatively rare. (Inciden-

---

Figure 15-1. Interview Strategies ■

Do not ask:	Instead, ask:
"Do you ever use?"	"When is the last time you used?"
"Does it ever cause blackouts?"	"How often do have blackouts?"
"Does your spouse say anything?"	"What does your spouse say?"
Avoid questions that have yes/no answers.	

---

tally, these same people often deny any drug use during their interviews with MROs.) In many if not most cases, they will say it was a one-time, only-time drug use, i.e., they minimize the extent of their use. Denial is common among drug abusers and can be magnified by the person's desire to get back to work as soon and cheaply as possible. The SAP has some, albeit limited, resources to assess the extent of past drug misuse. These include speaking with the personal physician, family members, or other outside resources, with the person's consent. The SAP can also obtain information from the MRO, e.g., drug/metabolite concentrations, and the MRO's interview notes. If no history of repeated drug abuse is established, and if the person insists it was a one-time, only-time use, the SAP is more likely to recommend education and group meetings rather than more direct and extensive interventions. The latter may be overdone, and the person will get limited benefit from treatment that he or she resists.

The SAP should not be intimidated in regard to the treatment recommendations or the time frame for return-to-duty and should not be unduly influenced by the financial pressure an employee may experience. In determining recommendations for treatment, SAPs are prohibited from considering the employee's denial of drug/alcohol misuse, claims that the testing was unjust or inaccurate, or the SAP's personal opinions about the justification or rationale for drug and alcohol testing. If the employee tells the SAP there was a medical explanation for the test result, the SAP should perhaps suggest the employee contact the MRO to discuss this further.

INITIAL REPORT

The SAP provides the designated employer representative (DER) with a written initial evaluation report that includes the education or treatment recommendation(s). The SAP should also send this report to the employee to clearly inform him or her of the education or treatment recommendations. It is important to make specific and concrete recommendations, thereby preempting possible later confusion about whether treatment was completed. The report should identify a likely time frame for conducting the follow-up assessment. The SAP should not agree to a specific time for return to duty because completion of the process is not entirely within the SAP's control. The report should not reveal any personal or clinical information about the employee or his or her family. DOT discourages the SAP from use of "fill-in-the-blanks"/"check-the-boxes" preprinted forms.

The SAP sends the report directly to the DER. If a C/TPA is involved, the SAP can also send a copy to the C/TPA. If the employee has no job to return to, the SAP can just send the report to the employee and, if requested in the future, to the employee's subsequent DOT-covered employer. The SAP's report should be in letter format on the SAP's own letterhead and should be signed. (The SAP's "own letterhead" means the letterhead the SAP uses in his or her daily professional practice.) The SAP's report must also include the following identifiers: employee's name and social security number, employer's name and address, reason for the assessment (i.e., specific violation and date), date of the assessment, and SAP's telephone number. SAPs need no written authorizations from employees to conduct SAP evaluations, to confer with employers, to confer with MROs, to confer with appropriate education and treatment providers, or to provide SAP reports to employers.

Treatment ■

The SAP refers each person who has an initial evaluation to treatment for drug or alcohol misuse. This usually consists of outpatient education or counseling. Recommendations for inpatient treatment are the exception, but may be appropriate for people who have severe chemical dependency problems or for whom other treatment modalities have been unsuccessful. Inpatient treatment can cost $20,000 or more, and some employees have no health insurance coverage for this. In making a referral, the SAP should consider the employee's insurance coverage and ability to pay for care, the employer's policies regarding availability of leave for employees needing assistance, and the availability of education and treatment programs. Self-help groups such as Alcoholics Anonymous and Narcotics Anonymous are affordable and accessible and may be appropriate parts of treatment for some illicit drug users.

To ensure objectivity and avoid conflicts of interest, DOT rules prohibit SAPs from referring employees to education or treatment in which the SAP has a financial interest or from receiving referral fees. There are four exceptions to this prohibition. A SAP may refer a employee to *any* education or treatment provider if the provider is:

1. A public agency operated by a state, county, or municipality.
2. An employee, a person, or organization under contract to the employer to provide alcohol or drug treatment or education services.
3. The sole source of therapeutically appropriate treatment under the employee's health insurance program.
4. The sole source of therapeutically appropriate treatment available to the employee.

A SAP must be able to justify recommendations and show consistency in case the SAP's recommendations are challenged. The American Society of Addiction Medicine (ASAM) publishes placement criteria for treatment and discharge of people with substance abuse disorders [2]. The SAP may wish to consult the ASAM criteria or other references for help in making treatment recommendations.

The employee, and not the SAP, is responsible for arranging the treatment. The SAP should send the treatment provider a note explaining the purpose of the referral, asking for a report or copy of the records from treatment, and asking for suggestions for continuing care. The employee will need to complete a release authorizing the treatment provider to report information to the SAP.

Follow-up Evaluation ■

FOLLOW-UP EVALUATION PROTOCOL

The follow-up evaluation is intended to allow the SAP to determine if the employee has successfully complied with the SAP's treatment recommendations. The same SAP who conducted the initial evaluation should conduct the follow-up evaluation, unless that SAP is unavailable or the employee has moved away. The follow-up evaluation consists of a face-to-face interview and discussion with, or review of, documentation from the treatment program professional(s). Written information from the provider could include a progress report or discharge summary that addresses the person's attendance, attitude, level of participation, and other aspects of treatment and the employee's progress. An employee is usually ready to return to work once he or she has met the treatment program's goals. The risk of relapse is reduced when the person acknowledges addiction, commits to recovery, has support systems at work and at home, and removes or reduces inducements to use the substance of abuse.

The interview with the employee should focus on determining if the employee has complied with the initial recommendations. The follow-up assessment accomplishes more than just verifying attendance. The SAP should also try to assess the extent to which the employee understands substance abuse as an illness.

The SAP may want to include a POCT drug test as part of the follow-up evaluation. The SAP would not report this result to the employer, but would instead use this information to help corroborate that the employee is not using drugs and is unlikely to test positive on the return-to-duty test.

FOLLOW-UP REPORT

The SAP provides the DER with a written follow-up evaluation report that addresses compliance with education/treatment recommendations, and recommends the duration and type of follow-up testing. The SAP report states one of two determinations:

1. The employee *has* demonstrated successful compliance. This report also includes:
   - Follow-up testing plan. (See the "Follow-up Tests" section of this chapter.)
   - Continuing care recommendations (if any).
2. The employee *has not* demonstrated successful compliance. This report also includes:
   - The SAP's reasons for determining that the employee has not demonstrated successful compliance.
   - The date(s) of any further follow-up evaluation the SAP has scheduled.

The SAP sends this report directly to the DER. If a C/TPA is involved, the SAP can send a copy to the C/TPA, too. At the employee's direction, the SAP can provide the report to a future DOT-covered employer. If the employee is no longer employed, the SAP can give the report to the employee but only if the SAP first removes or redacts the follow-up testing recommendations, which must not be disclosed to the employee. The SAP's report should be in letter format on the SAP's own letterhead and should be signed. The SAP's report must also include the following identifiers: employee's name and social security number, employer's name and address, reason for the assessment (i.e., specific violation and date), date of the initial and follow-up assessments and synopsis of the treatment plan, name of the education/treatment service provider, inclusive dates of the employee's program participation, clinical characterization of the employee's program participation, and SAP's telephone number.

The SAP's determination of successful compliance is a prerequisite, not a guarantee, that the employer will return the employee to safety-sensitive duties. Once the SAP has determined that the employee has demonstrated successful compliance, the employer then decides whether to put the employee back to work in a safety-sensitive position.

Continuing Care Recommendations ■

If the SAP believes that ongoing treatment is needed to help an employee maintain sobriety or abstinence from drug use after the employee resumes safety-sensitive duties, the SAP includes these continuing care recommendations in the follow-up evaluation report. Among the more common continuing-care recommendations is attendance at Alcoholics Anonymous or Narcotics Anonymous meetings. The SAP or employee assistance program (EAP) can help monitor the employee's compliance with these continuing care recommendations. Monitoring attendance at meetings can be challenging and probably requires face-to-face encounters at which the SAP or EAP can ask the employee about the meeting and review handouts or other materials the employee has brought back from the meeting. An employee's failure to comply with continuing care recommendations may be cause for disciplinary action by the employer.

Return-to-Duty Test ■

Before the employer returns the employee to safety-sensitive duties, the employer must first ensure that the employee has a negative return-to-duty test result. Return-to-duty testing is conducted after the SAP has determined that the person has successfully complied with recommended treatment. A positive, adulterated, substituted, or refusal DOT return-to-duty test outcome is a Part 40 violation and triggers a referral to a SAP for an initial evaluation, i.e., the process starts all over again.

Chapter 3 has more information about return-to-duty testing.

Return to Duty Under USCG ■

Under the U.S. Coast Guard (USCG) rule, a mariner who has a drug test rule violation must complete the usual DOT process (i.e., SAP evaluations and education/treatment) along with the Coast Guard requirements for the return of the credential if one is held by the mariner.

For a mariner holding a Coast Guard–issued credential, the mariner should contact the MRO who verified the test as non-negative. That MRO can make a treatment recommendation or refer the mariner to the SAP for a treatment recommendation. After completion of the initial treatment program, the mariner must pass 12 tests over the next 12 months and must have a "return-to-work" letter from the MRO along with a letter from the SAP verifying the completion of recommended treatment. The mariner is required to pass a return-to-work drug test before returning to work in a safety-sensitive position. Before the mariner can return to work in a position that requires the holding of a Coast Guard–issued credential, the mariner has to complete the terms of the settlement agreement.

For personnel who do not have a credential, the mariner is required to complete the SAP recommendations and also to obtain a letter from the MRO.

In the MRO letter, the MRO states that the crew member is drug free and the risk of subsequent use is sufficiently low to justify return to work. The mariner will have to present the MRO letter to the administrative law judge for purposes of reinstating his or her Coast Guard credentials, i.e., his or her license. Once the mariner's license is renewed, the employer is responsible for conducting follow-up testing per the schedule recommended by the SAP and/or the MRO. It is highly recommended that the SAP and MRO communicate with each other on this process.

Follow-up Tests ■

DOT requires follow-up testing of any employee who has violated the DOT testing rules and has resumed safety-sensitive duties. Under the DOT rule, the SAP decides the type (i.e., drugs, alcohol, or both) and schedule (frequency and duration, but not the specific test dates) of follow-up testing. The schedule must include at least six tests during the first 12 months after return to duty. Follow-up testing under DOT can last up to 60 months. The follow-up testing plan may dictate changes in frequency over time, e.g., twelve tests in the first year and six tests in the second year. In establishing the plan, the SAP should consider the employee's drug of choice and how long it can be detected after use. Tests for cocaine and other short half-life drugs should be performed relatively frequently, for example, four times a month, initially. Tests for marijuana and other long half-life drugs can be performed less frequently, for example, twice a month, initially. The duration of testing depends on the person's past extent of use, degree of addiction, and other factors. While 1 year of testing may suffice for an occasional, recreational marijuana user, several years of testing are more appropriate for a person who abuses drugs that are more addictive, such as cocaine, prescription narcotics, or alcohol.

The employer determines the specific dates and times for follow-up tests based on the follow-up testing plan. The testing period begins when the employee resumes covered activities. Like random tests, follow-up tests should be unannounced, scheduled with no discernible pattern, and spread throughout the year. To help enhance deterrence, the employee is not entitled under the DOT rule to know the testing schedule recommended by the SAP. Follow-up testing requirements follow the employee to subsequent employers and through breaks in safety-sensitive service. Subsequent employers are supposed to obtain follow-up testing schedules from previous employers as part of the background history checks. If a follow-up test is cancelled for any reason, the employee must be retested and have a negative result to continue performing safety-sensitive duties. A positive, adulterated, substituted, or refusal follow-up test outcome triggers immediate removal from safety-sensitive duties and referral to a SAP for an initial evaluation.

Chapter 3 has more information about follow-up tests.

Return-to-Duty Agreement ■

The return-to-duty agreement should include mandatory compliance with SAP recommendations for continuing care. If the employee subsequently fails to comply, he or she may be subject to disciplinary action by the employer. Employers may but are not required to monitor continuing care for employees who have returned to work following a violation. The return-to-duty agreement should therefore include provisions for monitoring compliance with continuing care and include sanctions for failure to comply. Monitoring can be performed by the employer, or employer's agent, e.g., SAP or EAP. In addition to follow-up testing and random testing, an employer has other means available to ascertain an employee's alcohol- and drug-free performance and functions. The employer can meet regularly with the employee to discuss the employee's continuing sobriety and drug-free status. In addition, the employer can conduct reasonable suspicion testing if the employee exhibits signs of drug or alcohol use.

Changing SAP Recommendations ■

No one may change the SAP's evaluation or recommendations for assistance. The employer may not ask for or rely upon a second SAP's evaluation after a SAP has already evaluated the employee. A SAP may modify his or her own recommendations if new or additional information has been obtained.

Recordkeeping ■

SAPs must retain copies of evaluation records and reports to employers for at least 5 years. The SAP can give the employee copies of the reports to the employer, with any follow-up testing schedule(s) excluded. The SAP can give a copy of the employee's follow-up testing schedule to a prospective employer. Before doing so, the SAP should obtain a signed authorization from the employee/applicant and should confirm that the employee/applicant is actually trying to work for that particular employer. The latter step is a precaution to ensure that the testing schedule is not released to a third party that would give the schedule to the applicant/employee.

References ■

1. U.S. Department of Transportation. *The Substance Abuse Professional Guidelines.* Washington, DC: 2006.
2. Mee-Lee D, Gartner L, Miller M, et al. *Patient Placement Criteria,* 2nd ed. (PPC-2R). Annapolis Junction, MD: American Society of Addiction Medicine, 2001.

The Medical Review Officer Certification Council ■

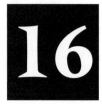

by Brian L. Compney, Executive Director, MROCC

The Council and Its Philosophy ■

Workplace drug testing is performed to discourage drug abuse and promote safety. School drug testing, particularly in athletic programs, is becoming more widespread to protect our youth. Courts use drug testing to detect use among those in trouble with the law. Certified laboratories process more than 20 million drug test specimens every year. More than 6000 medical review officers (MROs) review and evaluate these results. The Medical Review Officer Certification Council (MROCC) was incorporated in 1992 to set a professional standard of excellence for MROs. MROCC-certified physicians are uniquely qualified and provide an objective and verifiable assurance to clinics, companies, government agencies, and laboratories that they are competent and up-to-date in the latest techniques, regulatory changes, and clinical practices within this complex and rapidly evolving arena.

MROCC is a physician-based nonprofit organization governed by its board of directors, with representation from the American Academy of Clinical Toxicology and American College of Medical Toxicology, American College of Occupational and Environmental Medicine (ACOEM), American Society of Addiction Medicine (ASAM), College of American Pathologists, and the American Medical Association. MROCC offers certification to licensed physicians who have had appropriate training in the duties and responsibilities of the MRO. Since its inception, MROCC has certified more than 9000 physicians throughout the United States, Canada, and internationally. In 2008, MROCC newly certified 368 physicians and recertified 332 physicians.

In 2006 to address the growing number of non-physicians who assist MROs within workplace drug testing environments, MROCC developed a credentialing program for MRO assistants (MROAs). MROCC has certified more than 500 trained MROAs through its online examination. This online examination is based on federal regulation 49 *CFR* Part 40 as well as MROCC's "Competencies of the Medical Review Officer Assistantt" document.

MROCC's board of directors adheres to a philosophy that MRO and MROA certification extends beyond the mere receipt of a diploma and knowledge of the rules and regulations. Throughout its examination development and implementation process, MROCC strives to reflect a broad knowledge base that includes nonregulated testing, chemical dependency, and standards of practice.

MROCC's MRO certification is the ultimate mark of an MRO's competency and fulfills the requirement set forth in the U.S. Department of Transportation (DOT) 49 *CFR* Part 40 Rule:

> Following your completion of qualification training, you must satisfactorily complete an examination administered by a nationally-recognized MRO certification board or subspecialty board for medical practitioners in the field of medical review of DOT-mandated drug tests. The examination must comprehensively cover all the elements of qualification training.

Through its certification programs and continuing medical education (CME) opportunities, MROCC continues to promote and preserve the highest level of professional standards of training and care among MROs and MROAs.

The MRO Certification Examination ∎

MROCC offers two ways to take its MRO certification examination:

Onsite—following MRO training courses sponsored by ACOEM and ASAM.
Online—using a PC and Internet connection.

The onsite version offers physicians the convenience of taking a training course and examination at one time in a group setting. The online version is for those who have taken the training course and want extra time to review the course materials before taking the exam at a later date by PC and Internet connection. The online exam provides an immediate pass/fail determination when complete. Physicians who are recertifying with the online examination can save answers and log off and on at will until ready to submit the answers for scoring.

Prerequisites for Application ∎

All MROCC certification examinations are based upon the federal requirements developed by the DOT and Department of Health and Human Services for workplace drug testing programs. Each applicant for MRO certification must meet specific eligibility requirements, including:

1. graduation from an approved medical school or school of osteopathic medicine.
2. a current license to practice medicine (MD or DO) in a state, territory or possession of the United States or province of Canada, or in a geographical location outside the United States in which the physician resides and practices.
3. evidence of approved MRO training within the past 24 months (36 months for recertification). The training must offer a minimum of 12 Category 1 CME

credit hours and, for Initial certification, is limited to the onsite courses sponsored by ACOEM, ASAM, and AAMRO.

For recertification, the CME may also be obtained through MRO-specific self-assessment tools and distance learning activities offering Category 1 CME such as those offered by MROCC's CME programs.

Certification is time limited, in large part because the discipline changes over time. Certification is valid for a 6-year period, at which time recertification is required to remain in MROCC's online directory of currently certified MROs. Those physicians who opt to forego recertification remain in MROCC's database and are listed online within an archived directory of past certificate holders.

The Examination Blueprint and Content Areas ∎

The process of examination development has followed a comprehensive plan to ensure relevance, validity, and reliability. The examination items have been developed and critically reviewed by nationally recognized leaders in drug testing drawn from the fields of occupational medicine, addiction medicine, forensic chemistry and toxicology, and the legal profession. In addition, leading experts in educational measurement, evaluation, and psychometrics have provided guidance to the process.

Using both DOT's 49 *CFR* Part 40 rule as well as MROCC's "Competencies of the Medical Review Officer" document, the examination has been designed to measure the scope and knowledge and practical skills the MRO applies in fulfilling the professional responsibilities in the evaluation of workplace drug testing. The five areas covered on the MROCC examination are:

1. Substance Abuse

Although the skills of the MRO may be quite different from those of the addiction medicine specialist, the MRO must be knowledgeable about and have clinical experience in the field of substance abuse disorders. MROs may be called upon to be a general resource for substance use issues. General knowledge in the area of substance abuse will enable the MRO to:

1. recognize the public health implications of substance abuse.
2. recognize the clinical and behavioral signs of substance abuse and dependency disorders.
3. describe the natural history and epidemiology of alcohol and drug abuse.
4. interact effectively with assessment and treatment professionals in the management of individuals identified with alcohol or substance use disorders and workplace substance abuse prevention and control programs.
5. serve as a resource to the employer on issues of aftercare monitoring, return-to-work and medical qualifications for the performance of safety-sensitive duties.

2. Regulatory Issues

The MRO must be and remain knowledgeable about applicable rules including federal MRO guidelines and federal agency regulations that impact organizations for whom the MRO evaluates drug test results. The MRO is often called upon to assist clients in the implementation of legally defensible policies and programs. Therefore, the MRO must be able to advise organizations about both regulated and nonregulated drug and alcohol testing procedures. Knowledge in the area of regulatory issues and MRO responsibilities will enable the MRO to:

1. interact effectively with other program participants, including employees, employers, DERs, SAPs, TPAs, other health care workers, laboratories, and collection sites. Advise employers in the development and implementation of effective workplace substance abuse prevention program policies and procedures.
2. comply with applicable laws and federal regulations in the review, interpretation, and reporting of drug test results, including confidentiality, documentation, record maintenance and storage, and release of information.
3. develop a standard operating procedure for conducting an effective MRO interview that complies with applicable regulations.
4. recognize and address the major legal and regulatory issues that face the MRO, other service providers, and employers in the establishment and implementation of drug testing programs.
5. serve as an expert consultant or witness on matters involving drug testing.
6. adhere to and uphold the professional code of ethics relating to drug testing.
7. evaluate and help manage collector services, laboratory services, and other services in the program to ensure reliability, confidentiality, efficiency, appropriateness, and promptness of these services in response to the employer's needs.

3. Toxicology, Pharmacology, and Laboratory Issues

The MRO must be knowledgeable about the toxicology and pharmacology of drugs of abuse. Although the MRO is not a laboratory director, the MRO must know what goes on in the laboratory and how quality is assured. Knowledge in these areas will enable the MRO to:

1. recognize and describe the pharmaco/toxicokinetics of drugs of abuse and alcohol.
2. recognize both trade names and generic names for substances that are likely to appear in a drug screen, interfere with a drug test, or be presented to the MRO as a donor explanation for a positive drug test.
3. recognize the appropriate analytical methods for drug and alcohol screening and confirmation and properly interpret results, with consideration of limits of detection, sensitivity, specificity, limitations, interferences, cost, and availability.
4. advise clients regarding the use of various matrices and technologies for drug testing.
5. evaluate drug and alcohol testing services.
6. describe laboratory quality assurance, quality control, and certification requirements to an employer or other interested party.

7. efficiently transmit and receive drug test data and information while maintaining donor confidentiality.
8. evaluate laboratory findings relating to specimen validity.
9. recognize the basic types and mechanisms of action of performance-enhancing drugs.

4. Clinical Aspects

The MRO must be familiar with clinical issues related to drug and alcohol use and testing, including medical explanations for positive or indeterminate tests and medical qualifications for performance safety-sensitive duties. Knowledge in these clinical areas will enable the MRO to:

1. recognize clinical evidence of drug use and impairment.
2. evaluate alternative medical explanations for laboratory drug test results (including positive, substituted, adulterated, and invalid specimens).
3. evaluate the inability to produce urine specimens.
4. recognize and appropriately respond to conditions that may render an individual unfit or unqualified for duty, including: (1) unauthorized drug use, (2) authorized prescription, or over-the-counter drug use, (3) drug/alcohol addiction, and (4) illness.

5. Collection Procedures

Although the MRO does not routinely collect specimens, he or she must thoroughly understand collection procedures and chain of custody issues, as well as correctable and fatal flaws. Knowledge in the area of collections and procedures will enable the MRO to:

1. describe and apply appropriate procedures for urine specimen collections, including unwitnessed, witnessed, split specimen, and insufficient quantity collections.
2. describe and apply appropriate procedures for the use of custody and control forms.
3. identify and address procedural errors.
4. describe and apply appropriate procedures for alcohol testing.
5. serve as a consultant to breath alcohol technicians, saliva test technicians, and employers on alcohol testing procedures.

MRO Assistant Certification Program ■

Medical review officer assistants (MROAs) are non-physicians who assist the MRO within the drug testing review process. Under DOT and NRC regulations, the MRO assistant reports directly to the MRO and purely helps with the many administrative-type issues.

In addition to its MRO certification, the council offers a highly successful credentialing program for medical review officer assistants. This 3-year certification—awarded upon successful completion and passing of the MROA online examination—acknowledges competency in those practical skills the MRO assistant applies in fulfilling his or her professional responsibilities within the workplace drug testing arena.

The 40-question online certification examination (offered to individuals who have completed appropriate MRO assistant training or have adequate experience) consists of multiple choice items, distributed by content area according to the established MROA competencies, and intermingles recall (recognition), simple interpretation (analysis), and problem solving (evaluation) questions.

CME Activities and Monograph Series ■

Under DOT, MROs must obtain 12 hours of MRO-related CME every 3 years to remain in compliance. MROCC also requires these 12 hours of CME within the past 3 years for MROs who wish to recertify. Through a joint sponsorship with University Services, MROCC offers a variety of Category 1 CME activities that fulfill both DOT requirements and recertification prerequisites. University Services is accredited by the Pennsylvania Medical Society to provide CME for physicians.

Each of the MROCC monographs focuses on one specific MRO-related issue. Each offers a detailed overview and analysis of the topic and contains a self-assessment tool that provides up to 4 hours of Category 1 CME credit. As of the publication date of this manual, the titles in the current MROCC Monograph Series are:

1. *How to Collect a Specimen for Workplace Drug Testing Programs*
2. *Alternative Specimens for Workplace Drug Testing*
3. *Workplace Testing for Prescription Medicines*

Research Funding ■

In addition to its certification program, the MROCC has provided grants and awards to fund research projects that have direct relevance to the work of the MRO and continue to advance this field. Grants have been awarded for research on DNA typing of urine specimens, urine temperature and its effects on adulteration of specimens, and the concentration of marijuana metabolites in the urine following ingestion of hemp seed tea. MROCC also sponsored the development of this book, *The Medical Review Officer's Guide to Drug Testing*.

Information Sources ■

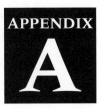

Books ■

Available on the U.S. Department of Health and Human Services (HHS) website (workplace.samhsa.gov/home.asp):

- HHS. *Urine Specimen Collection Handbook for Federal Agency Workplace Drug Testing Programs.* Rockville, MD, 2004.
- HHS. *Medical Review Officer Manual for Federal Agency Workplace Drug Testing Programs.* Rockville, MD, 2004.

Available on the U.S. Department of Transportation (DOT) website (www.dot.gov/ost/dapc):

- DOT. *Urine Specimen Collection Guidelines.* Washington, DC, December 2006.
- DOT. *Substance Abuse Professional Guidelines.* Washington, DC, August 2001.

Available from the U.S. Government Printing Office (GPO) (202-512-1800) and from the Transportation Safety Institute (405-949-0036, ext 323):

- Breath Alcohol Technician Training, Student Handbook. Stock # 050-000-00560-0.
- Instructor Training Curriculum, Breath Alcohol Technician Training. Stock # 050-000-00551-0.
- Instructor Training Curriculum, Screening Test Technician Training. Stock # 050-000-00559-3.

Available from the Institute for a Drug-Free Workplace (202-842-3914):

- deBernardo MA, Nieman MF. *Guide to State and Federal Drug-Testing Laws.* Washington, DC. Published annually. $225.

Newsletter ■

Available from the American College of Occupational and Environmental Medicine (ACOEM), Arlington Heights, IL (847-228-6850):

- Swotinsky RB (ed). *MRO Update.* (Ten issues per year. $210 for ACOEM members, $235 for nonmembers.)

Journal ■

Available from Preston Publications (847-647-2900):

- Goldberger B (ed). *Journal of Analytical Toxicology.* Niles, IL: Preston Publications. (Nine issues per year, $475 per year.)

Agency	Mailing Address	Internet Address	Telephone/Fax No.
Office of Drug & Alcohol Policy & Compliance	U.S. Department of Transportation W62-307 1200 New Jersey Avenue, SE Washington, DC 20590	www.dot.gov/ost/dapc/	tel. 202-366-3784 fax 202-366-3897
Federal Aviation Administration	Drug Abatement Division Room 803 (AAM-800) Independence Ave. SW Washington, DC 20591	www.faa.gov/avr/aam/adap/	tel. 202-267-8442 fax 202-267-5200
U.S. Coast Guard	Office of Investigation & Analysis Room 2406; 2100 2nd Street SW Washington, DC 20593-0001	www.uscg.mil/hq/g-m/moa/dapip.htm	tel. 202-372-1033 fax 202-372-1996
Federal Motor Carrier Safety Administration	Enforcement & Compliance Office Room 8314, 400 7th Street SW Washington, DC 20590	www.fmcsa.dot.gov/safetyprogs/drugs/drugs_alcohol.htm	tel. 202-366-2096 fax 202-366-7908
Federal Railroad Administration	Office of Safety 1200 New Jersey Avenue, SE W38-330 Washington, DC 20590	www.fra.dot.gov/us/content/504	tel. 202-493-6313 fax 202-493-6230
Federal Transit Administration	Office of Safety and Security TPM-30, Room E46 1200 New Jersey Ave., SE Washington, DC 20590	transit-safety.volpe.dot.gov/Safety/DATesting.asp	tel. 617-494-2395 fax 202-366-3394
Pipeline and Hazardous Materials Safety Administration	Office of Drug & Alcohol Policy & Investigations; PHMSA East Building, 2nd Floor PHP-1 1200 New Jersey Ave., SE Washington, DC 20590	http://ops.dot.gov/init/drug_alc/drug.htm	tel. 202-550-0629 fax 202-366-4566
Substance Abuse and Mental Health Services Administration	Division of Workplace Programs Room #2-1035; 1 Choke Cherry Rd. Rockville, MD 20857	dwp.samhsa.gov/DrugTesting/DTesting.aspx	tel. 240-276-2600 fax 240-276-2610
U.S. Nuclear Regulatory Commission	Office of Nuclear Reactor Regulation Div. of Reactor Program Mgmt. Washington, DC 20555	www.nrc.gov	tel. 301-415-2944 fax 301-415-1032

Professional Organizations ∎

Organization	Mailing Address	Internet Address	Telephone/Fax No.
American College of Occupational and Environmental Medicine (ACOEM)	25 Northwest Point Blvd., Suite 700 Elk Grove Village, IL 60007-1030	www.acoem.org	tel. 847-818-1800 fax 847-818-9266
American Society of Addiction Medicine (ASAM)	4601 North Park Drive Suite 101, Arcade Chevy Chase, MD 20815	www.asam.org	tel. 301-656-3920 fax 301-656-3815
Drug and Alcohol Testing Industry Association (DATIA)	1325 G Street, NW, Suite 500 Washington, DC 20005	www.datia.org	tel. 800-355-1257 fax 202-315-3579
Medical Review Officer Certification Council (MROCC)	836 Arlington Heights Road, #327 Elk Grove Village, IL 60007	www.mrocc.org	tel. 847-631-0599 fax 847-483-1282
National Association of Alcoholism and Drug Abuse Counselors (NAADAC)	901 N. Washington Street, Suite 600 Alexandria, VA 22314	www.naadac.org	tel. 703-741-7686 fax 703-741-7698
Substance Abuse Program Administrators Association (SAPAA)	1014 Whispering Oak Drive Bardstown, KY 40004	www.sapaa.com	tel. 800-672-7229 fax 281-664-3152

MRO Code of Ethics ■

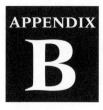

Medical Review Officers shall [1]:

- Behave in a professional manner as befits all activities of a physician, regardless of whether a true physician-patient relationship exists.
- Maintain the highest standards of practice and perform all professional functions with honesty and integrity.
- Handle and transmit laboratory results in an accurate, direct, precise, and confidential manner and strive for objectivity in dealing with all aspects of the drug testing system.
- Maintain scientific standards and appropriate application of science in the review process and refrain from any misrepresentation of the laboratory evidence or the scientific or technical basis of drug testing.
- Demonstrate a commitment to the development and maintenance of professional competence and personal scientific knowledge.
- Refrain from misuse of private information as may come to light in an interview with the donor. Employee or donor confidentiality is to be protected in so far as possible in all cases.
- Not currently misuse/abuse or be dependent on illegal drugs or alcohol, and not misuse/abuse prescription medications.

Reference ■

1. Board of Directors, Medical Review Officer Certification Council. *MRO Code of Ethics*. Schaumburg, IL: MROCC, October 2008.

Ethical Aspects of Drug Testing ■

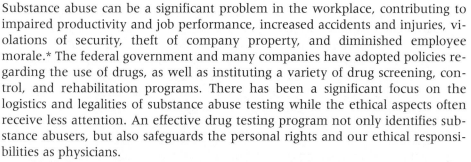

APPENDIX C

Substance abuse can be a significant problem in the workplace, contributing to impaired productivity and job performance, increased accidents and injuries, violations of security, theft of company property, and diminished employee morale.* The federal government and many companies have adopted policies regarding the use of drugs, as well as instituting a variety of drug screening, control, and rehabilitation programs. There has been a significant focus on the logistics and legalities of substance abuse testing while the ethical aspects often receive less attention. An effective drug testing program not only identifies substance abusers, but also safeguards the personal rights and our ethical responsibilities as physicians.

The following guidelines deal only with ethical issues involved in drug screening in the workplace. Other important considerations which must be addressed in the design and implementation of a drug screening program include biological factors concerning rates of absorption and elimination of drugs, technical factors relating to specificity and accuracy of analyses, legal safeguards, regulatory requirements, and employee relations concerns.

Appropriate constraints must be observed in order to ethically screen employees and prospective employees for the presence in their bodies of drugs and substances of abuse, including alcohol, that might affect ability to perform work in a safe manner.

ACOEM recommends strongly that employers obtain expert legal, medical and employee relations advice before making a decision to require screening of employees or applicants for drugs. Such experts also should be involved in the actual structuring and implementation of any program of screening of employees and applicants for drugs.

These guidelines are pertinent to drug testing done under the following circumstances: pre-placement assessment, job transfer evaluation, periodic mandatory medical surveillance, post-incident/accident, for reasonable suspicion/cause, and random testing of those in safety- and security-sensitive positions, special work fitness examinations, and monitoring of employees who are under treatment for drug abuse, including alcohol, as a condition of continuing employment.

---

*Board of Directors, American College of Occupational and Environmental Medicine. *Ethical Aspects of Drug Testing.* Elk Grove Village, IL: ACOEM, January 2006.

The following features should be included in any program for the screening of employees and prospective employees for drugs:

- A written company policy and procedure concerning substance abuse and screening should exist and be applied impartially.
- The reason for any requirement for the drug testing program should be clearly documented. Such reasons might involve safety for the individual, other employees, or the public; security needs; or requirements related to job performance.
- Affected employees and applicants should be informed in advance about the company's policy concerning drug use, misuse and screening. They should be made aware of their right to refuse such screening and the consequences of such refusal to their employment.
- Where special safety or security needs justify testing for the presence of drugs on an unannounced and random basis, employees should be made aware of all aspects of the drug testing program.
- Care should be taken to assure that such tests are done in a uniform and impartial manner for all employees in the affected group(s).
- Collection, transportation and analysis of the specimens and reporting of the results should meet stringent legal, technical, and ethical requirements. The process should be under the supervision of a licensed physician (MD/DO).
- A licensed physician (MD/DO) with appropriate qualifications should be designated as the medical review officer (MRO) and should evaluate positive results prior to a report being made to the employer. This may require the obtaining of supplemental information from the employee or applicant in order to ensure that a positive test does not represent appropriate use of prescription drugs, over-the-counter medication or other substances which could cause a positive test. MRO training should include the pharmacology of substance abuse, laboratory testing methodology and quality control, forensic toxicology, pertinent federal regulations, legal and ethical requirements, chemical dependency illness, employee assistance programs and rehabilitation.
- The affected employee or applicant should be advised of positive results by the physician and have the opportunity for explanation and discussion prior to the reporting of results to the employer, if feasible. The mechanism for accomplishing this should be clearly defined.
- Any report to the employer should provide only the information needed for work placement purposes or as required by government regulations. Identification to the employer of the particular drug(s) found and quantitative levels should not be done unless required by law. Reports to the employer should be made by a physician sensitive to the various considerations involved.

If carefully designed and carried out, programs for the screening of employees and applicants for drugs, including alcohol, serve to protect and improve employee health and safety in an ethically acceptable manner. Physicians are encouraged to refer to the Medical Review Officer Certification Council's *MRO Code of Ethics*.

Controlled Substances Act, Schedules I–V ■

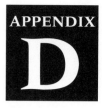

The drugs and drug products that come under the jurisdiction of the Controlled Substances Act are divided into five schedules. The more common drugs in each schedule are listed here. For a complete listing of all the controlled substances, see federal law 21 *CFR* §1308 or contact the Drug Enforcement Administration.

Schedule I substances are those that have no accepted medical use in the United States and have high abuse potential. Some examples of Schedule I drugs are heroin, LSD, marijuana, mescaline, methaqualone, MDMA, and peyote.

Schedule II substances have a high abuse potential with severe psychic or physical dependence liability. Some examples of Schedule II drugs are amobarbital, amphetamine (Dexedrine), cocaine, fentanyl (Sublimaze), hydromorphone (Dilaudid), meperidine (Demerol), methadone, methamphetamine (Desoxyn), methylphenidate (Ritalin), morphine, opium, oxycodone (Perodan, OxyContin, Roxicet, Tylox), oxymorphone (Numorphan), pentobarbital, phencyclidine, propoxyphene, and secobarbital. Amobarbital, codeine, secobarbital, and several other drugs appear in Schedule II at high doses and Schedule III at low doses.

Schedule III substances have an abuse potential less than those in Schedules I and II. Some examples of Schedule III drugs are anabolic steroids, benzphetamine, dronabinol (Marinol), hydrocodone (Vicodin, Lortab), and paregoric. Codeine appears in Schedule III when in combination with acetaminophen.

Schedule IV substances in this schedule have an abuse potential less than those listed in Schedule III and include such drugs as alprazolam (Xanax), barbital, chloral hydrate, chlordiazepoxide (Librium), clonazepam (Clonopin), clorazepate (Tranxene), dextropropoxyphene dosage forms (Darvon), diazepam (Valium), fenproporex, flurazepam (Dalmane), halazepam (Paxipam), lorazepam (Ativan), meprobamate (Equanil, Miltown), midazolam (Versed), oxazepam (Serax), paraldehyde, pentazocine (Talwin-NX), phenobarbital, phentermine, prazepam (Verstran), temazepam (Restoril), and triazolam (Halcion).

Schedule V substances have an abuse potential less than those listed in Schedule IV and consist primarily of preparations containing limited quantities of certain narcotic drugs generally for antitussive, antidiarrheal, and analgesic purposes. Schedule V products are available over-the-counter with restrictions; for example, they can be sold only by registered pharmacists, to individuals 18 years of age or older, and their sales must be recorded in bound ledgers.

Federal Drug Testing Custody and Control Form

Note: This is the revised form as proposed by the Substance Abuse and Mental Health Services (SAMHSA) in November 2009. SAMSHA planned to issue a final revision sometime in 2010.

FEDERAL DRUG TESTING CUSTODY AND CONTROL FORM

SPECIMEN ID NO. **0000001**

ACCESSION NO.

OMB No. 0930-0158

STEP 1: COMPLETED BY COLLECTOR OR EMPLOYER REPRESENTATIVE

A. Employer Name, Address, I.D. No.   B. MRO Name, Address, Phone No. and Fax No.

C. Donor SSN or Employee I.D. No. _____

D. Specify Testing Authority: ☐ HHS ☐ NRC ☐ DOT – Specify DOT Agency: ☐ FMCSA ☐ FAA ☐ FRA ☐ FTA ☐ PHMSA ☐ USCG

E. Reason for Test: ☐ Pre-employment ☐ Random ☐ Reasonable Suspicion/Cause ☐ Post Accident ☐ Return to Duty ☐ Follow-up ☐ Other (specify) _____

F. Drug Tests to be Performed: ☐ THC, COC, PCP, OPI, AMP ☐ THC & COC Only ☐ Other (specify) _____

G. Collection Site Address:

Collector Phone No. _____

Collector Fax No. _____

STEP 2: COMPLETED BY COLLECTOR (make remarks when appropriate) Collector reads specimen temperature within 4 minutes.

Temperature between 90° and 100° F? ☐ Yes ☐ No, Enter Remark | Collection: ☐ Split ☐ Single ☐ None Provided, Enter Remark | ☐ Observed, Enter Remark

REMARKS

STEP 3: Collector affixes bottle seal(s) to bottle(s). Collector dates seal(s). Donor initials seal(s). Donor completes STEP 5 on Copy 2 (MRO Copy)

STEP 4: CHAIN OF CUSTODY - INITIATED BY COLLECTOR AND COMPLETED BY TEST FACILITY

I certify that the specimen given to me by the donor identified in the certification section on Copy 2 of this form was collected, labeled, sealed and released to the Delivery Service noted in accordance with applicable Federal requirements.

	SPECIMEN BOTTLE(S) RELEASED TO:

X_____

Signature of Collector

AM / PM

(PRINT) Collector's Name (First, MI, Last) | Date (Mo/Day/Yr) | Time of Collection | Name of Delivery Service

RECEIVED AT IITF:
X_____

Signature of Accessioner

IITF Name and Address (if not above): | Primary Specimen Bottle Seal Intact | SPECIMEN BOTTLE(S) RELEASED TO:

☐ YES ☐ NO

If NO, Enter remark in Step 5A.

(PRINT) Accessioner's Name (First, MI, Last) | Date (Mo/Day/Yr)

TRANSFER FROM IITF TO LAB. I certify that the specimen identified on this form was handled using chain of custody procedures and resealed in accordance with applicable Federal requirements.

X_____

Signature | (PRINT) Name (First, MI, Last) | Date (Mo/Day/Yr) | Name of Delivery Service

SPECIMEN BOTTLE(S) RELEASED TO:

RECEIVED AT LAB:
X_____

Signature of Accessioner

Primary Specimen Bottle Seal Intact | SPECIMEN BOTTLE(S) RELEASED TO:

☐ YES ☐ NO

If NO, Enter remark in Step 5A.

(PRINT) Accessioner's Name (First, MI, Last) | Date (Mo/Day/Yr)

STEP 5A: PRIMARY SPECIMEN REPORT - COMPLETED BY TEST FACILITY

☐ NEGATIVE ☐ POSITIVE for: ☐ Marijuana Metabolite (Δ9-THCA) ☐ 6-Acetylmorphine ☐ Methamphetamine ☐ MDMA

☐ DILUTE ☐ Cocaine Metabolite (BZE) ☐ Morphine ☐ Amphetamine ☐ MDA

☐ PCP ☐ Codeine ☐ MDEA

☐ REJECTED ☐ ADULTERATED ☐ SUBSTITUTED ☐ INVALID RESULT

REMARKS: _____

Test Facility (if different from above) : _____

I certify that the specimen identified on this form was examined upon receipt, handled using chain of custody procedures, analyzed, and reported in accordance with applicable Federal requirements.

X_____

Signature of Certifying Technician/Scientist | (PRINT) Certifying Technician/Scientist's Name (First, MI, Last) | Date (Mo/Day/Yr)

STEP 5B: COMPLETED BY SPLIT TESTING LABORATORY

☐ SPLIT SPECIMEN TESTED; SEE LABORATORY REPORT _____

Split Testing Laboratory (Name, City, State)

0000001
SPECIMEN ID NO.   **A**

PLACE OVER CAP

0000001
SPECIMEN BOTTLE SEAL

Date (Mo/Day/Yr)
Donor's Initials

0000001 (SPLIT)
SPECIMEN ID NO.   **B**

PLACE OVER CAP

0000001
SPECIMEN BOTTLE SEAL

Date (Mo/Day/Yr)
Donor's Initials

COPY 1 - TEST FACILITY COPY

Version C

PRESS HARD - YOU ARE MAKING MULTIPLE COPIES

FEDERAL DRUG TESTING CUSTODY AND CONTROL FORM

SPECIMEN ID NO.   **0000001**

STEP 1: COMPLETED BY COLLECTOR OR EMPLOYER REPRESENTATIVE   ACCESSION NO.

A. Employer Name, Address, I.D. No.   B. MRO Name, Address, Phone No. and Fax No.

C. Donor SSN or Employee I.D. No. _____

D. Specify Testing Authority: ☐ HHS ☐ NRC   ☐ DOT – Specify DOT Agency: ☐ FMCSA ☐ FAA ☐ FRA ☐ FTA ☐ PHMSA ☐ USCG

E. Reason for Test: ☐ Pre-employment ☐ Random ☐ Reasonable Suspicion/Cause ☐ Post Accident ☐ Return to Duty ☐ Follow-up ☐ Other (specify) _____

F. Drug Tests to be Performed: ☐ THC, COC, PCP, OPI, AMP   ☐ THC & COC Only   ☐ Other (specify) _____

G. Collection Site Address:

Collector Phone No. _____

Collector Fax No. _____

STEP 2: COMPLETED BY COLLECTOR (make remarks when appropriate) Collector reads specimen temperature within 4 minutes.

Temperature between 90° and 100° F? ☐ Yes ☐ No, Enter Remark | Collection: ☐ Split ☐ Single | ☐ None Provided, Enter Remark | ☐ Observed, Enter Remark

REMARKS

STEP 3: Collector affixes bottle seal(s) to bottle(s). Collector dates seal(s). Donor initials seal(s). Donor completes STEP 5 on Copy 2 (MRO Copy)

STEP 4: CHAIN OF CUSTODY - INITIATED BY COLLECTOR AND COMPLETED BY TEST FACILITY

I certify that the specimen given to me by the donor identified in the certification section on Copy 2 of this form was collected, labeled, sealed and released to the Delivery Service noted in accordance with applicable Federal requirements.   SPECIMEN BOTTLE(S) RELEASED TO:

X_____
                    Signature of Collector   AM
_____   ___/___/___   _____   PM
(PRINT) Collector's Name (First, MI, Last)   Date (Mo/Day/Yr)   Time of Collection   Name of Delivery Service

STEP 5: COMPLETED BY DONOR

I certify that I provided my urine specimen to the collector; that I have not adulterated it in any manner; each specimen bottle used was sealed with a tamper-evident seal in my presence; and that the information provided on this form and on the label affixed to each specimen bottle is correct.

X_____   ___/___/___
         Signature of Donor   (PRINT) Donor's Name (First, MI, Last)   Date (Mo/Day/Yr)

Daytime Phone No. (____) _____   Evening Phone No. (____) _____   Date of Birth ___/___/___
                                                                                                              (Mo/Day/Yr)

After the Medical Review Officer receives the test results for the specimen identified by this form, he/she may contact you to ask about prescriptions and over-the-counter medications you may have taken. Therefore, you may want to make a list of those medications for your own records. THIS LIST IS NOT NECESSARY. If you choose to make a list, do so either on a separate piece of paper or on the back of your copy (Copy 5). – DO NOT PROVIDE THIS INFORMATION ON THE BACK OF ANY OTHER COPY OF THE FORM. TAKE COPY 5 WITH YOU.

STEP 6: COMPLETED BY MEDICAL REVIEW OFFICER - PRIMARY SPECIMEN

In accordance with applicable Federal requirements, my verification is:

☐ NEGATIVE   ☐ POSITIVE for: _____
            ☐ DILUTE

☐ REFUSAL TO TEST because – check reason(s) below: ☐ TEST CANCELLED
        ☐ ADULTERATED (adulterant/reason): _____
            ☐ SUBSTITUTED
                ☐ OTHER: _____

REMARKS: _____

X_____   ___/___/___
    Signature of Medical Review Officer   (PRINT) Medical Review Officer's Name (First, MI, Last)   Date (Mo/Day/Yr)

STEP 7: COMPLETED BY MEDICAL REVIEW OFFICER - SPLIT SPECIMEN

In accordance with applicable Federal requirements, my verification for the split specimen (if tested) is:

☐ RECONFIRMED for: _____   ☐ TEST CANCELLED

☐ FAILED TO RECONFIRM for: _____

REMARKS: _____

X_____   ___/___/___
    Signature of Medical Review Officer   (PRINT) Medical Review Officer's Name (First, MI, Last)   Date (Mo/Day/Yr)

COPY 2 - MEDICAL REVIEW OFFICER COPY

OMB No. 0930-0158

SPECIMEN ID NO. **0000001**

OMB No. 0930-0158

STEP 1: COMPLETED BY COLLECTOR OR EMPLOYER REPRESENTATIVE   ACCESSION NO.

A. Employer Name, Address, I.D. No.   B. MRO Name, Address, Phone No. and Fax No.

C. Donor SSN or Employee I.D. No. _____

D. Specify Testing Authority: ☐ HHS ☐ NRC ☐ DOT – Specify DOT Agency: ☐ FMCSA ☐ FAA ☐ FRA ☐ FTA ☐ PHMSA ☐ USCG

E. Reason for Test: ☐ Pre-employment ☐ Random ☐ Reasonable Suspicion/Cause ☐ Post Accident ☐ Return to Duty ☐ Follow-up ☐ Other (specify) _____

F. Drug Tests to be Performed: ☐ THC, COC, PCP, OPI, AMP ☐ THC & COC Only ☐ Other (specify) _____

G. Collection Site Address:

Collector Phone No. _____

Collector Fax No. _____

STEP 2: COMPLETED BY COLLECTOR (make remarks when appropriate) Collector reads specimen temperature within 4 minutes.

Temperature between 90° and 100° F? ☐ Yes ☐ No, Enter Remark | Collection: ☐ Split ☐ Single ☐ None Provided, Enter Remark ☐ Observed, Enter Remark

REMARKS

STEP 3: Collector affixes bottle seal(s) to bottle(s). Collector dates seal(s). Donor initials seal(s). Donor completes STEP 5 on Copy 2 (MRO Copy)

STEP 4: CHAIN OF CUSTODY - INITIATED BY COLLECTOR AND COMPLETED BY TEST FACILITY

I certify that the specimen given to me by the donor identified in the certification section on Copy 2 of this form was collected, labeled, sealed and released to the Delivery Service noted in accordance with applicable Federal requirements.

X_____   SPECIMEN BOTTLE(S) RELEASED TO:

Signature of Collector   AM / PM

(PRINT) Collector's Name (First, MI, Last)   Date (Mo/Day/Yr)   Time of Collection   Name of Delivery Service

STEP 5: COMPLETED BY DONOR

I certify that I provided my urine specimen to the collector; that I have not adulterated it in any manner; each specimen bottle used was sealed with a tamper-evident seal in my presence; and that the information provided on this form and on the label affixed to each specimen bottle is correct.

X_____

Signature of Donor   (PRINT) Donor's Name (First, MI, Last)   Date (Mo/Day/Yr)

Daytime Phone No. ( )   Evening Phone No. ( )   Date of Birth ___ / ___ / ___ (Mo/Day/Yr)

After the Medical Review Officer receives the test results for the specimen identified by this form, he/she may contact you to ask about prescriptions and over-the-counter medications you may have taken. Therefore, you may want to make a list of those medications for your own records. THIS LIST IS NOT NECESSARY. If you choose to make a list, do so either on a separate piece of paper or on the back of your copy (Copy 5). – DO NOT PROVIDE THIS INFORMATION ON THE BACK OF ANY OTHER COPY OF THE FORM. TAKE COPY 5 WITH YOU.

STEP 6: COMPLETED BY MEDICAL REVIEW OFFICER - PRIMARY SPECIMEN

In accordance with applicable Federal requirements, my verification is:

☐ NEGATIVE   ☐ POSITIVE for: _____

   ☐ DILUTE

☐ REFUSAL TO TEST because – check reason(s) below: ☐ TEST CANCELLED

   ☐ ADULTERATED (adulterant/reason): _____

     ☐ SUBSTITUTED

       ☐ OTHER: _____

REMARKS: _____

X_____

Signature of Medical Review Officer   (PRINT) Medical Review Officer's Name (First, MI, Last)   Date (Mo/Day/Yr)

STEP 7: COMPLETED BY MEDICAL REVIEW OFFICER - SPLIT SPECIMEN

In accordance with applicable Federal requirements, my verification for the split specimen (if tested) is:

☐ RECONFIRMED for: _____   ☐ TEST CANCELLED

   ☐ FAILED TO RECONFIRM for: _____

REMARKS: _____

X_____

Signature of Medical Review Officer   (PRINT) Medical Review Officer's Name (First, MI, Last)   Date (Mo/Day/Yr)

COPY 3 - COLLECTOR COPY

FEDERAL DRUG TESTING CUSTODY AND CONTROL FORM

SPECIMEN ID NO.   **0000001**

STEP 1: COMPLETED BY COLLECTOR OR EMPLOYER REPRESENTATIVE   ACCESSION NO.

A. Employer Name, Address, I.D. No.   B. MRO Name, Address, Phone No. and Fax No.

OMB No. 0930-0158

C. Donor SSN or Employee I.D. No. _____

D. Specify Testing Authority: ☐ HHS ☐ NRC ☐ DOT – Specify DOT Agency: ☐ FMCSA ☐ FAA ☐ FRA ☐ FTA ☐ PHMSA ☐ USCG

E. Reason for Test: ☐ Pre-employment ☐ Random ☐ Reasonable Suspicion/Cause ☐ Post Accident ☐ Return to Duty ☐ Follow-up ☐ Other (specify) _____

F. Drug Tests to be Performed: ☐ THC, COC, PCP, OPI, AMP ☐ THC & COC Only ☐ Other (specify) _____

G. Collection Site Address:

Collector Phone No. _____

Collector Fax No. _____

STEP 2: COMPLETED BY COLLECTOR (make remarks when appropriate) Collector reads specimen temperature within 4 minutes.

Temperature between 90° and 100° F? ☐ Yes ☐ No, Enter Remark Collection: ☐ Split ☐ Single ☐ None Provided, Enter Remark ☐ Observed, Enter Remark

REMARKS

STEP 3: Collector affixes bottle seal(s) to bottle(s). Collector dates seal(s). Donor initials seal(s). Donor completes STEP 5 on Copy 2 (MRO Copy)

STEP 4: CHAIN OF CUSTODY - INITIATED BY COLLECTOR AND COMPLETED BY TEST FACILITY

I certify that the specimen given to me by the donor identified in the certification section on Copy 2 of this form was collected, labeled, sealed and released to the Delivery Service noted in accordance with applicable Federal requirements.   SPECIMEN BOTTLE(S) RELEASED TO:

X _____

Signature of Collector   AM
                                                                    PM

_____ (PRINT) Collector's Name (First, MI, Last)   Date (Mo/Day/Yr)   Time of Collection   Name of Delivery Service

STEP 5: COMPLETED BY DONOR

I certify that I provided my urine specimen to the collector; that I have not adulterated it in any manner; each specimen bottle used was sealed with a tamper-evident seal in my presence; and that the information provided on this form and on the label affixed to each specimen bottle is correct.

X _____

Signature of Donor   (PRINT) Donor's Name (First, MI, Last)   Date (Mo/Day/Yr)

Daytime Phone No. (___) ____   Evening Phone No. (___) ____   Date of Birth ____
                                                                                    (Mo/Day/Yr)

After the Medical Review Officer receives the test results for the specimen identified by this form, he/she may contact you to ask about prescriptions and over-the-counter medications you may have taken. Therefore, you may want to make a list of those medications for your own records. THIS LIST IS NOT NECESSARY. If you choose to make a list, do so either on a separate piece of paper or on the back of your copy (Copy 5). – DO NOT PROVIDE THIS INFORMATION ON THE BACK OF ANY OTHER COPY OF THE FORM. TAKE COPY 5 WITH YOU.

STEP 6: COMPLETED BY MEDICAL REVIEW OFFICER - PRIMARY SPECIMEN

In accordance with applicable Federal requirements, my verification is:

☐ NEGATIVE   ☐ POSITIVE for: _____
  ☐ DILUTE

☐ REFUSAL TO TEST because – check reason(s) below: ☐ TEST CANCELLED
  ☐ ADULTERATED (adulterant/reason): _____
    ☐ SUBSTITUTED
      ☐ OTHER: _____

REMARKS: _____

X _____

Signature of Medical Review Officer   (PRINT) Medical Review Officer's Name (First, MI, Last)   Date (Mo/Day/Yr)

STEP 7: COMPLETED BY MEDICAL REVIEW OFFICER - SPLIT SPECIMEN

In accordance with applicable Federal requirements, my verification for the split specimen (if tested) is:

☐ RECONFIRMED for: _____   ☐ TEST CANCELLED

  ☐ FAILED TO RECONFIRM for: _____

REMARKS: _____

X _____

Signature of Medical Review Officer   (PRINT) Medical Review Officer's Name (First, MI, Last)   Date (Mo/Day/Yr)

COPY 4 - EMPLOYER COPY

FEDERAL DRUG TESTING CUSTODY AND CONTROL FORM

SPECIMEN ID NO. **0000001**

STEP 1: COMPLETED BY COLLECTOR OR EMPLOYER REPRESENTATIVE   ACCESSION NO.

A. Employer Name, Address, I.D. No.   B. MRO Name, Address, Phone No. and Fax No.

C. Donor SSN or Employee I.D. No. _____

D. Specify Testing Authority: ☐ HHS ☐ NRC   ☐ DOT – Specify DOT Agency: ☐ FMCSA ☐ FAA ☐ FRA ☐ FTA ☐ PHMSA ☐ USCG

E. Reason for Test: ☐ Pre-employment ☐ Random ☐ Reasonable Suspicion/Cause ☐ Post Accident ☐ Return to Duty ☐ Follow-up ☐ Other (specify) _____

F. Drug Tests to be Performed: ☐ THC, COC, PCP, OPI, AMP   ☐ THC & COC Only   ☐ Other (specify) _____

G. Collection Site Address:

Collector Phone No. _____

Collector Fax No. _____

STEP 2: COMPLETED BY COLLECTOR (make remarks when appropriate) Collector reads specimen temperature within 4 minutes.

| Temperature between 90° and 100° F? | ☐ Yes | ☐ No, Enter Remark | Collection: | ☐ Split | ☐ Single | ☐ None Provided, Enter Remark | ☐ Observed, Enter Remark |

REMARKS

STEP 3: Collector affixes bottle seal(s) to bottle(s). Collector dates seal(s). Donor initials seal(s). Donor completes STEP 5 on Copy 2 (MRO Copy)

STEP 4: CHAIN OF CUSTODY - INITIATED BY COLLECTOR AND COMPLETED BY TEST FACILITY

I certify that the specimen given to me by the donor identified in the certification section on Copy 2 of this form was collected, labeled, sealed and released to the Delivery Service noted in accordance with applicable Federal requirements.

| | SPECIMEN BOTTLE(S) RELEASED TO: |

X_____
Signature of Collector   AM
_____ PM
(PRINT) Collector's Name (First, MI, Last)   Date (Mo/Day/Yr)   Time of Collection   Name of Delivery Service

STEP 5: COMPLETED BY DONOR

I certify that I provided my urine specimen to the collector; that I have not adulterated it in any manner; each specimen bottle used was sealed with a tamper-evident seal in my presence; and that the information provided on this form and on the label affixed to each specimen bottle is correct.

X_____
Signature of Donor   (PRINT) Donor's Name (First, MI, Last)   Date (Mo/Day/Yr)

Daytime Phone No. (_____)   Evening Phone No. (_____)   Date of Birth _____/_____/_____
                                                                                                          (Mo/Day/Yr)

After the Medical Review Officer receives the test results for the specimen identified by this form, he/she may contact you to ask about prescriptions and over-the-counter medications you may have taken. Therefore, you may want to make a list of those medications for your own records. THIS LIST IS NOT NECESSARY. If you choose to make a list, do so either on a separate piece of paper or on the back of your copy (Copy 5). – DO NOT PROVIDE THIS INFORMATION ON THE BACK OF ANY OTHER COPY OF THE FORM. TAKE COPY 5 WITH YOU.

STEP 6: COMPLETED BY MEDICAL REVIEW OFFICER - PRIMARY SPECIMEN

In accordance with applicable Federal requirements, my verification is:

☐ NEGATIVE   ☐ POSITIVE for: _____
       ☐ DILUTE

☐ REFUSAL TO TEST because – check reason(s) below: ☐ TEST CANCELLED
       ☐ ADULTERATED (adulterant/reason): _____
              ☐ SUBSTITUTED
                     ☐ OTHER: _____

REMARKS: _____

X_____
Signature of Medical Review Officer   (PRINT) Medical Review Officer's Name (First, MI, Last)   Date (Mo/Day/Yr)

STEP 7: COMPLETED BY MEDICAL REVIEW OFFICER - SPLIT SPECIMEN

In accordance with applicable Federal requirements, my verification for the split specimen (if tested) is:

☐ RECONFIRMED for: _____   ☐ TEST CANCELLED

       ☐ FAILED TO RECONFIRM for: _____

REMARKS: _____

X_____
Signature of Medical Review Officer   (PRINT) Medical Review Officer's Name (First, MI, Last)   Date (Mo/Day/Yr)

COPY 5 - DONOR COPY

OMB No. 0930-0158

Instructions for Completing the Federal Drug Testing Custody and Control Form

When making entries use black or blue ink pen and press firmly

Collector ensures that the name and address of the HHS-certified Instrumented Initial Test Facility (IITF) or HHS-certified laboratory are on the top of the CCF and that the Specimen I.D. number on the top of the CCF matches the Specimen I.D. number on the labels/seals.

STEP 1:

- Collector ensures that the required information is in STEP 1. Collector enters a remark in STEP 2 if Donor refuses to provide his/her SSN or Employee I.D. number.

- Collector gives collection container to Donor and instructs Donor to provide a specimen. Collector notes any unusual behavior or appearance of Donor in the remarks line in STEP 2. If Donor conduct at any time during the collection process clearly indicates an attempt to tamper with the specimen, Collector notes the conduct in the remarks line in STEP 2 and takes action as required.

STEP 2:

- Collector checks specimen temperature within 4 minutes after receiving the specimen from Donor, and marks the appropriate temperature box in STEP 2. If temperature is outside the acceptable range, Collector enters a remark in STEP 2 and takes action as required.

- Collector inspects the specimen and notes any unusual findings in the remarks line in STEP 2 and takes action as required. Any specimen with unusual physical characteristics (e.g. unusual color, presence of foreign objects or material, unusual odor) cannot be sent to an IITF and must be sent to an HHS-certified laboratory for testing as required.

- Collector determines the volume of specimen in the collection container. If the volume is acceptable, Collector proceeds with the collection. If the volume is less than required by the Federal Agency, Collector takes action as required, and enters remarks in STEP 2. If no specimen is collected by the end of the collection process, Collector checks the *None Provided* box, enters a remark in STEP 2, discards Copy 1 and distributes remaining copies as required.

- Collector checks the Split or Single specimen collection box. If the collection is observed, Collector checks the Observed box and enters a remark in STEP 2.

STEP 3:

- Donor watches Collector pour the specimen from the collection container into the specimen bottle(s), place the cap(s) on the specimen bottle(s), and affix the label(s)/seal(s) on the specimen bottle(s).

- Collector dates the specimen bottle label(s)/seal(s) after placement on the specimen bottle(s).

- Donor initials the specimen bottle label(s)/seal(s) after placement on the specimen bottle(s).

- Collector turns to Copy 2 (Medical Review Officer Copy) and instructs Donor to read and complete the certification statement in STEP 5 (signature, printed name, date, phone numbers, and date of birth). If Donor refuses to sign the certification statement, Collector enters a remark in STEP 2 on Copy 1.

STEP 4:

- Collector completes STEP 4 on Copy 1 (signature, printed name, date, time of collection, and name of delivery service), places the sealed specimen bottle(s) and Copy 1 of the CCF in a leak-proof plastic bag, seals the bag, prepares the specimen package for shipment, and distributes the remaining CCF copies as required.

Privacy Act Statement: (For Federal Employees Only)

Submission of the information on the attached form is voluntary. However, incomplete submission of the information, refusal to provide a urine specimen, or substitution or adulteration of a specimen may result in delay or denial of your application for employment/appointment or may result in removal from the Federal service or other disciplinary action.

The authority for obtaining the urine specimen and identifying information contained herein is Executive Order 12564 ("Drug-Free Federal Workplace"), 5 U.S.C. Sec. 3301 (2), 5 U.S.C. Sec. 7301, and Section 503 of Public Law 100-71, 5 U.S.C. Sec. 7301 note. Under provisions of Executive Order 12564 and 5 U.S.C. 7301, test results may only be disclosed to agency officials on a need-to-know basis. This may include the agency Medical Review Officer (MRO), the administrator of the Employee Assistance Program, and a supervisor with authority to take adverse personnel action. This information may also be disclosed to a court where necessary to defend against a challenge to an adverse personnel action.

Submission of your SSN is not required by law and is voluntary. Your refusal to furnish your number will not result in the denial of any right, benefit, or privilege provided by law. Your SSN is solicited, pursuant to Executive Order 9397, for purposes of associating information in agency files relating to you and for purposes of identifying the specimen provided for testing. If you refuse to indicate your SSN, a substitute number or other identifier will be assigned, as required, to process the specimen.

Public Burden Statement:

An agency may not conduct or sponsor, and a person is not required to respond to, a collection of information unless it displays a currently valid OMB control number. The OMB control number for this project is 0930-0158. Public reporting burden for this collection of information is estimated to average: 5 minutes/donor; 4 minutes/collector; 3 minutes/test facility; and 3 minutes/Medical Review Officer. Send comments regarding this burden estimate or any other aspect of this collection of information, including suggestions for reducing this burden, to SAMHSA Reports Clearance Officer, 1 Choke Cherry Road, Room 7-1044, Rockville, Maryland, 20857.

DOT Procedures, 49 *CFR* Part 40 ■

PROCEDURES FOR TRANSPORTATION WORKPLACE DRUG AND
ALCOHOL TESTING PROGRAMS
(Updated as of August 31, 2009)

U.S. Department of Transportation,
Drug and Alcohol Policy and Compliance Office, 1200 New Jersey Avenue, SE,
Washington, DC 20590 (202) 366-3784

APPENDIX A TO PART 40—DOT STANDARDS FOR URINE COLLECTION KITS

APPENDIX B TO PART 40—DOT DRUG TESTING SEMI-ANNUAL LABORATORY REPORT TO EMPLOYERS

APPENDIX C TO PART 40—DOT DRUG TESTING SEMI-ANNUAL LABORATORY REPORT TO DOT

APPENDIX D TO PART 40—REPORT FORMAT: SPLIT SPECIMEN FAILURE TO RECONFIRM

APPENDIX E TO PART 40—SAP EQUIVALENCY REQUIREMENTS FOR CERTIFICATION ORGANIZATIONS

APPENDIX F TO PART 40—DRUG AND ALCOHOL TESTING INFORMATION THAT C/TPAS MAY TRANSMIT TO EMPLOYERS

APPENDIX G TO PART 40—ALCOHOL TESTING FORM

APPENDIX H TO PART 40—DOT DRUG AND ALCOHOL TESTING MANAGEMENT INFORMATION SYSTEM (MIS) DATA COLLECTION FORM

Authority: 49 U.S.C. 102, 301, 322, 5331, 20140, 31306, and 45101 et seq.

Source: 65 FR 79526, Dec. 19, 2000, unless otherwise noted.

SUBPART A—ADMINISTRATIVE PROVISIONS

§ 40.1   Who does this regulation cover?

(a) This part tells all parties who conduct drug and alcohol tests required by Department of Transportation (DOT) agency regulations how to conduct these tests and what procedures to use.

(b) This part concerns the activities of transportation employers, safety-sensitive transportation employees (including self-employed individuals, contractors and volunteers as covered by DOT agency regulations), and service agents.

(c) Nothing in this part is intended to supersede or conflict with the implementation of the Federal Railroad Administration's post-accident testing program (see 49 CFR 219.200).

§ 40.3   What do the terms used in this regulation mean?

In this part, the terms listed in this section have the following meanings:

Adulterated specimen. A urine specimen containing a substance that is not a normal constituent or containing an endogenous substance at a concentration that is not a normal physiological concentration.

Affiliate. Persons are affiliates of one another if, directly or indirectly, one controls or has the power to control the other, or a third party controls or has the power to control both. Indicators of control include, but are not limited to: interlocking management or ownership; shared interest among family members; shared facilities or equipment; or common use of employees. Following the issuance of a public interest exclusion, an organization having the same or similar management, ownership, or principal employees as the service agent concerning whom a public interest exclusion is in effect is regarded as an affiliate. This definition is used in connection with the public interest exclusion procedures of Subpart R of this part.

Air blank. In evidential breath testing devices (EBTs) using gas chromatography technology, a reading of the device's internal standard. In all other EBTs, a reading of ambient air containing no alcohol.

Alcohol. The intoxicating agent in beverage alcohol, ethyl alcohol or other low molecular weight alcohols, including methyl or isopropyl alcohol.

Alcohol concentration. The alcohol in a volume of breath expressed in terms of grams of alcohol per 210 liters of breath as indicated by a breath test under this part.

Alcohol confirmation test. A subsequent test using an EBT, following a screening test with a result of 0.02 or greater, that provides quantitative data about the alcohol concentration.

Alcohol screening device (ASD). A breath or saliva device, other than an EBT, that is approved by the National Highway Traffic Safety Administration (NHTSA) and placed on a conforming products list (CPL) for such devices.

Alcohol screening test. An analytic procedure to determine whether an employee may have a prohibited concentration of alcohol in a breath or saliva specimen.

Alcohol testing site. A place selected by the employer where employees present themselves for the purpose of providing breath or saliva for an alcohol test.

Alcohol use. The drinking or swallowing of any beverage, liquid mixture or preparation (including any medication), containing alcohol.

Aliquot. A fractional part of a specimen used for testing. It is taken as a sample representing the whole specimen.

Blind specimen or blind performance test specimen. A specimen submitted to a laboratory for quality control testing purposes, with a fictitious identifier, so that the laboratory cannot distinguish it from an employee specimen.

Breath Alcohol Technician (BAT). A person who instructs and assists employees in the alcohol testing process and operates an evidential breath testing device.

Cancelled test. A drug or alcohol test that has a problem identified that cannot be or has not been corrected, or which this part otherwise requires to be cancelled. A cancelled test is neither a positive nor a negative test.

Chain of custody. The procedure used to document the handling of the urine specimen from the time the employee gives the specimen to the collector until the specimen is destroyed. This procedure uses the Federal Drug Testing Custody and Control Form (CCF).

Collection container. A container into which the employee urinates to provide the specimen for a drug test.

Collection site. A place selected by the employer where employees present themselves for the purpose of providing a urine specimen for a drug test.

Collector. A person who instructs and assists employees at a collection site, who receives and makes an initial inspection of the specimen provided by those employees, and who initiates and completes the CCF.

Confirmatory drug test. A second analytical procedure to identify the presence of a specific drug or metabolite which is independent of the initial test and which uses a different technique and chemical principle from that of the initial test in order to ensure reliability and accuracy. (Gas chromatography/mass spectrometry (GC/MS) is the only authorized confirmation method for cocaine, marijuana, opiates, amphetamines, and phencyclidine).

Confirmatory validity test. A second test performed on a different aliquot of the original urine specimen to further support a validity test result.

Confirmed drug test. A confirmation test result received by an MRO from a laboratory.

Consortium/Third-party administrator (C/TPA). A service agent that provides or coordinates the provision of a variety of drug and alcohol testing services to employers. C/TPAs typically perform administrative tasks concerning the operation of the employers' drug and alcohol testing programs. This term includes, but is not limited to, groups of employers who join together to administer, as a single entity, the DOT drug and alcohol testing programs of its members. C/TPAs are not "employers" for purposes of this part.

Continuing education. Training for medical review officers (MROs) and substance abuse professionals (SAPs) who have completed qualification training and are performing MRO or SAP functions, designed to keep MROs and SAPs current on changes and developments in the DOT drug and alcohol testing program.

Designated employer representative (DER). An employee authorized by the employer to take immediate action(s) to remove employees from safety-sensitive duties, or cause employees to be removed from these covered duties, and to make required decisions in the testing and evaluation processes. The DER also receives test results and other communications for the employer, consistent with the requirements of this part. Service agents cannot act as DERs.

Dilute specimen. A urine specimen with creatinine and specific gravity values that are lower than expected for human urine.

DOT, The Department, DOT agency. These terms encompass all DOT agencies, including, but not limited to, the United States Coast Guard (USCG), the Federal Aviation Administration (FAA), the Federal Railroad Administration (FRA), the Federal Motor Carrier Safety Administration (FMCSA), the Federal Transit Administration (FTA), the National Highway Traffic Safety Administration (NHTSA), the Pipeline and Hazardous Materials Safety Administration (PHMSA), and the Office of the Secretary (OST). These terms include any designee of a DOT agency.

Drugs. The drugs for which tests are required under this part and DOT agency regulations are marijuana, cocaine, amphetamines, phencyclidine (PCP), and opiates.

Employee. Any person who is designated in a DOT agency regulation as subject to drug testing and/or alcohol testing. The term includes individuals currently performing safety-sensitive functions designated in DOT agency regulations and applicants for employment subject to pre-employment testing. For purposes of drug testing under this part, the term employee has the same meaning as the term "donor" as found on CCF and related guidance materials produced by the Department of Health and Human Services.

Employer. A person or entity employing one or more employees (including an individual who is self-employed) subject to DOT agency regulations requiring compliance with this part. The term includes an employer's officers, representatives, and management personnel. Service agents are not employers for the purposes of this part.

Error Correction Training. Training provided to BATs, collectors, and screening test technicians (STTs) following an error that resulted in the cancellation of a drug or alcohol test. Error correction training must be provided in person or by a means that provides real-time observation and interaction between the instructor and trainee.

Evidential Breath Testing Device (EBT). A device approved by NHTSA for the evidential testing of breath at the .02 and .04 alcohol concentrations, placed on NHTSA's Conforming Products List (CPL) for "Evidential Breath Measurement Devices" and identified on the CPL as conforming with the model specifications available from NHTSA's Traffic Safety Program.

HHS. The Department of Health and Human Services or any designee of the Secretary, Department of Health and Human Services.

Initial drug test (also known as a Screening drug test). An immunoassay test to eliminate "negative" urine specimens from further consideration and to identify the presumptively positive specimens that require confirmation or further testing.

Initial validity test. The first test used to determine if a urine specimen is adulterated, diluted, or substituted.

Invalid result. The result reported by a laboratory for a urine specimen that contains an unidentified adulterant, contains an unidentified interfering substance, has an abnormal physical characteristic, or has an endogenous substance at an abnormal concentration that prevents the laboratory from completing testing or obtaining a valid drug test result.

Laboratory. Any U.S. laboratory certified by HHS under the National Laboratory Certification Program

as meeting the minimum standards of Subpart C of the HHS Mandatory Guidelines for Federal Workplace Drug Testing Programs; or, in the case of foreign laboratories, a laboratory approved for participation by DOT under this part. (The HHS Mandatory Guidelines for Federal Workplace Drug Testing Programs are available on the internet at http://www.health.org/workpl.htm or from the Division of Workplace Programs, 1 Choke Cherry Road, Room 2-1035, Rockville, MD 20857)

Limit of Detection (LOD). The lowest concentration at which an analyte can be reliably shown to be present under defined conditions.

Medical Review Officer (MRO). A person who is a licensed physician and who is responsible for receiving and reviewing laboratory results generated by an employer's drug testing program and evaluating medical explanations for certain drug test results.

Non-negative specimen. A urine specimen that is reported as adulterated, substituted, positive (for drug(s) or drug metabolite(s)), and/or invalid.

Office of Drug and Alcohol Policy and Compliance (ODAPC). The office in the Office of the Secretary, DOT, that is responsible for coordinating drug and alcohol testing program matters within the Department and providing information concerning the implementation of this part.

Oxidizing adulterant. A substance that acts alone or in combination with other substances to oxidize drugs or drug metabolites to prevent the detection of the drug or drug metabolites, or affects the reagents in either the initial or confirmatory drug test.

Primary specimen. In drug testing, the urine specimen bottle that is opened and tested by a first laboratory to determine whether the employee has a drug or drug metabolite in his or her system; and for the purpose of validity testing. The primary specimen is distinguished from the split specimen, defined in this section.

Qualification Training. The training required in order for a collector, BAT, MRO, SAP, or STT to be qualified to perform their functions in the DOT drug and alcohol testing program. Qualification training may be provided by any appropriate means (e.g., classroom instruction, internet application, CD–ROM, video).

Refresher Training. The training required periodically for qualified collectors, BATs, and STTs to review basic requirements and provide instruction concerning changes in technology (e.g., new testing methods that may be authorized) and amendments, interpretations, guidance, and issues concerning this part and DOT agency drug and alcohol testing regulations. Refresher training can be provided by any appropriate means (e.g., classroom instruction, internet application, CD–ROM, video).

Screening Drug Test. See Initial drug test definition above.

Screening Test Technician (STT). A person who instructs and assists employees in the alcohol testing process and operates an ASD.

Secretary. The Secretary of Transportation or the Secretary's designee.

Service agent. Any person or entity, other than an employee of the employer, who provides services specified under this part to employers and/or employees in connection with DOT drug and alcohol testing requirements. This includes, but is not limited to, collectors, BATs and STTs, laboratories, MROs, substance abuse professionals, and C/TPAs. To act as service agents, persons and organizations must meet the qualifications set forth in applicable sections of this part. Service agents are not employers for purposes of this part.

Shipping container. A container that is used for transporting and protecting urine specimen bottles and associated documents from the collection site to the laboratory.

Specimen bottle. The bottle that, after being sealed and labeled according to the procedures in this part, is used to hold the urine specimen during transportation to the laboratory.

Split specimen. In drug testing, a part of the urine specimen that is sent to a first laboratory and retained unopened, and which is transported to a second laboratory in the event that the employee requests that it be tested following a verified positive test of the primary specimen or a verified adulterated or substituted test result.

Stand-down. The practice of temporarily removing an employee from the performance of safety-sensitive functions based only on a report from a laboratory to the MRO of a confirmed positive test for a drug or drug metabolite, an adulterated test, or a substituted test, before the MRO has completed verification of the test result.

Substance Abuse Professional (SAP). A person who evaluates employees who have violated a DOT drug and alcohol regulation and makes recommendations concerning education, treatment, follow-up testing, and aftercare.

Substituted specimen. A urine specimen with creatinine and specific gravity values that are so diminished or so divergent that they are not consistent with normal human urine.

Verified test. A drug test result or validity testing result from an HHS-certified laboratory that has undergone review and final determination by the MRO.

[65 FR 79526, Dec. 19, 2000, as amended at 66 FR 41950, Aug. 9, 2001; 71 FR 49384, August 23, 2006; 71 FR 55347, Sept. 22, 2006; 73 FR 35969, June 25, 2008]

§ 40.5 Who issues authoritative interpretations of this regulation?

ODAPC and the DOT Office of General Counsel (OGC) provide written interpretations of the provisions of this part. These written DOT interpretations are the only official and authoritative interpretations concerning the provisions of this part. DOT agencies may incorporate ODAPC/OGC interpretations in written guidance they issue concerning drug and alcohol testing matters. Only Part 40 interpretations issued after August 1, 2001, are considered valid.

§ 40.7 How can you get an exemption from a requirement in this regulation?

(a) If you want an exemption from any provision of this part, you must request it in writing from the Office of the Secretary of Transportation, under the provisions and standards of 49 CFR part 5. You must send requests for an exemption to the following address: Department of Transportation, Deputy Assistant General Counsel for Regulation and Enforcement, 1200 New Jersey Avenue, SE, Washington, DC 20590.

(b) Under the standards of 49 CFR part 5, we will grant the request only if the request documents special or exceptional circumstances, not likely to be generally applicable and not contemplated in connection with the rulemaking that established this part, that make your compliance with a specific provision of this part impracticable.

(c) If we grant you an exemption, you must agree to take steps we specify to comply with the intent of the provision from which an exemption is granted.

(d) We will issue written responses to all exemption requests.

[65 FR 79526, Dec. 19, 2000, as amended at 73 FR 33329, June 12, 2008]

SUBPART B—EMPLOYER RESPONSIBILITIES

§ 40.11 What are the general responsibilities of employers under this regulation?

(a) As an employer, you are responsible for meeting all applicable requirements and procedures of this part.

(b) You are responsible for all actions of your officials, representatives, and agents (including service agents) in carrying out the requirements of the DOT agency regulations.

(c) All agreements and arrangements, written or unwritten, between and among employers and service agents concerning the implementation of DOT drug and alcohol testing requirements are deemed, as a matter of law, to require compliance with all applicable provisions of this part and DOT agency drug and alcohol testing regulations. Compliance with these provisions is a material term of all such agreements and arrangements.

§ 40.13 How do DOT drug and alcohol tests relate to non-DOT tests?

(a) DOT tests must be completely separate from non-DOT tests in all respects.

(b) DOT tests must take priority and must be conducted and completed before a non-DOT test is begun. For example, you must discard any excess urine left over from a DOT test and collect a separate void for the subsequent non-DOT test.

(c) Except as provided in paragraph (d) of this section, you must not perform any tests on DOT urine or breath specimens other than those specifically authorized by this part or DOT agency regulations. For example, you may not test a DOT urine specimen for additional drugs, and a laboratory is prohibited from making a DOT urine specimen available for a DNA test or other types of specimen identity testing.

(d) The single exception to paragraph (c) of this section is when a DOT drug test collection is conducted as part of a physical examination required by DOT agency regulations. It is permissible to conduct required medical tests related to this physical examination (e.g., for glucose) on any urine remaining in the collection container after the drug test urine specimens have been sealed into the specimen bottles.

(e) No one is permitted to change or disregard the results of DOT tests based on the results of non-DOT tests. For example, as an employer you must not disregard a verified positive DOT drug test result because the employee presents a negative test result from a blood or urine specimen collected by the employee's physician or a DNA test result purporting to question the identity of the DOT specimen.

(f) As an employer, you must not use the CCF or the ATF in your non-DOT drug and alcohol testing programs. This prohibition includes the use of the DOT forms with references to DOT programs and agencies crossed out. You also must always use the CCF and ATF for all your DOT-mandated drug and alcohol tests.

§ 40.15 May an employer use a service agent to meet DOT drug and alcohol testing requirements?

(a) As an employer, you may use a service agent to perform the tasks needed to comply with this part and DOT agency drug and alcohol testing regulations, consistent with the requirements of Subpart Q and other applicable provisions of this part.

(b) As an employer, you are responsible for ensuring that the service agents you use meet the qualifications set forth in this part (e.g., §40.121 for MROs). You may require service agents to show you documentation that they meet the requirements of this part (e.g., documentation of MRO qualifications required by §40.121(e)).

(c) You remain responsible for compliance with all applicable requirements of this part and other DOT drug and alcohol testing regulations, even when you use a service agent. If you violate this part or other DOT drug and alcohol testing regulations because a service agent has not provided services as our rules require, a DOT agency can subject you to sanctions. Your good faith use of a service agent is not a defense in an enforcement action initiated by a DOT agency in which your alleged noncompliance with this part or a DOT agency drug and alcohol regulation may have resulted from the service agent's conduct.

(d) As an employer, you must not permit a service agent to act as your DER.

§ 40.17 Is an employer responsible for obtaining information from its service agents?

Yes, as an employer, you are responsible for obtaining information required by this part from your service agents. This is true whether or not you choose to use a C/TPA as an intermediary in transmitting information to you. For example, suppose an applicant for a safety-sensitive job takes a pre-employment drug test, but there is a significant delay in your receipt of the test result from an MRO or C/TPA. You must not assume that "no news is good news" and permit the applicant to perform safety-sensitive duties before receiving the result. This is a violation of the Department's regulations.

§ 40.19 [Reserved]

§ 40.21 May an employer stand down an employee before the MRO has completed the verification process?

(a) As an employer, you are prohibited from standing employees down, except consistent with a waiver a DOT agency grants under this section.

(b) You may make a request to the concerned DOT agency for a waiver from the prohibition of paragraph (a) of this section. Such a waiver, if granted, permits you to stand an employee down following the MRO's receipt of a laboratory report of a confirmed positive test for a drug or drug metabolite, an adulterated test, or a substituted test pertaining to the employee.

(1) For this purpose, the concerned DOT agency is the one whose drug and alcohol testing rules apply to the majority of the covered employees in your organization. The concerned DOT agency uses its applicable procedures for considering requests for waivers.

(2) Before taking action on a waiver request, the concerned DOT agency coordinates with other DOT agencies that regulate the employer's other covered employees.

(3) The concerned DOT agency provides a written response to each employer that petitions for a waiver, setting forth the reasons for the agency's decision on the waiver request.

(c) Your request for a waiver must include, as a minimum, the following elements:

(1) Information about your organization:

(i) Your determination that standing employees down is necessary for safety in your organization and a statement of your basis for it, including any data on safety problems or incidents that could have been prevented if a stand-down procedure had been in place;

(ii) Data showing the number of confirmed laboratory positive, adulterated, and substituted test results for your employees over the two calendar years preceding your waiver request, and the number and percentage of those test results that were verified positive, adulterated, or substituted by the MRO;

(iii) Information about the work situation of the employees subject to stand-down, including a description of the size and organization of the unit(s) in which the employees work, the process through which employees will be informed of the stand-down, whether there is an in-house MRO, and whether your organization has a medical disqualification or stand-down policy for employees in situations other than drug and alcohol testing; and

(iv) A statement of which DOT agencies regulate your employees.

(2) Your proposed written company policy concerning stand-down, which must include the following elements:

(i) Your assurance that you will distribute copies of your written policy to all employees that it covers;

(ii) Your means of ensuring that no information about the confirmed positive, adulterated, or substituted test result or the reason for the employee's temporary removal from performance of safety-sensitive functions becomes available, directly or indirectly, to anyone in your organization (or subsequently to another employer) other than the employee, the MRO and the DER;

(iii) Your means of ensuring that all covered employees in a particular job category in your organization are treated the same way with respect to stand-down;

(iv) Your means of ensuring that a covered employee will be subject to stand-down only with respect to the actual performance of safety-sensitive duties;

(v) Your means of ensuring that you will not take any action adversely affecting the employee's pay and benefits pending the completion of the MRO's verification process. This includes continuing to pay the employee during the period of the stand-down in the same way you would have paid him or her had he or she not been stood down;

(vi) Your means of ensuring that the verification process will commence no later than the time an employee is temporarily removed from the performance of safety-sensitive functions and that the period of stand-down for any employee will not exceed five days, unless you are informed in writing by the MRO that a longer period is needed to complete the verification process; and

(vii) Your means of ensuring that, in the event that the MRO verifies the test negative or cancels it—

(A) You return the employee immediately to the performance of safety-sensitive duties;

(B) The employee suffers no adverse personnel or financial consequences as a result; and

(C) You maintain no individually identifiable record that the employee had a confirmed laboratory positive, adulterated, or substituted test result (i.e., you maintain a record of the test only as a negative or cancelled test).

(d) The Administrator of the concerned DOT agency, or his or her designee, may grant a waiver request only if he or she determines that, in the context of your organization, there is a high probability that the procedures you propose will effectively enhance safety and protect the interests of employees in fairness and confidentiality.

(1) The Administrator, or his or her designee, may impose any conditions he or she deems appropriate on the grant of a waiver.

(2) The Administrator, or his or her designee, may immediately suspend or revoke the waiver if he or she determines that you have failed to protect effectively the interests of employees in fairness and confidentiality, that you have failed to comply with the requirements of this section, or that you have failed to comply with any other conditions the DOT agency has attached to the waiver.

(e) You must not stand employees down in the absence of a waiver, or inconsistent with the terms of your waiver. If you do, you are in violation of this part and DOT agency drug testing regulations, and you are subject to enforcement action by the DOT agency just as you are for other violations of this part and DOT agency rules.

§ 40.23 What actions do employers take after receiving verified test results?

(a) As an employer who receives a verified positive drug test result, you must immediately remove the employee involved from performing safety-sensitive functions. You must take this action upon receiving the initial report of the verified positive test result. Do not wait to receive the written report or the result of a split specimen test.

(b) As an employer who receives a verified adulterated or substituted drug test result, you must consider this a refusal to test and immediately remove the employee involved from performing safety-sensitive functions. You must take this action on receiving the initial report of the verified adulterated or substituted test result. Do not wait to receive the written report or the result of a split specimen test.

(c) As an employer who receives an alcohol test result of 0.04 or higher, you must immediately remove the employee involved from performing safety-sensitive functions. If you receive an alcohol test result of 0.02–0.039, you must temporarily remove the employee involved from performing safety-sensitive functions, as provided in applicable DOT agency regulations. Do not wait to receive the written report of the result of the test.

(d) As an employer, when an employee has a verified positive, adulterated, or substituted test result, or has otherwise violated a DOT agency drug and alcohol regulation, you must not return the employee to the performance of safety-sensitive functions until or unless the employee successfully completes the return-to-duty process of Subpart O of this part.

(e) As an employer who receives a drug test result indicating that the employee's specimen was dilute, take action as provided in §40.197.

(f) As an employer who receives a drug test result indicating that the employee's urine specimen test was cancelled because it was invalid and that a second collection must take place under direct observation—

(1) You must immediately direct the employee to provide a new specimen under direct observation.

(2) You must not attach consequences to the finding that the test was invalid other than collecting a new specimen under direct observation.

(3) You must not give any advance notice of this test requirement to the employee.

(4) You must instruct the collector to note on the CCF the same reason (e.g. random test, post-accident test) as for the original collection.

(5) You must ensure that the collector conducts the collection under direct observation.

(g) As an employer who receives a cancelled test result when a negative result is required (e.g., pre-employment, return-to-duty, or follow-up test), you must direct the employee to provide another specimen immediately.

(h) As an employer, you may also be required to take additional actions required by DOT agency regulations (e.g., FAA rules require some positive drug tests to be reported to the Federal Air Surgeon).

(i) As an employer, you must not alter a drug or alcohol test result transmitted to you by an MRO, BAT, or C/TPA.

[65 FR 79526, Dec. 19, 2000, as amended at 71 FR 49384, Aug. 23, 2006; 73 FR 35970, June 25, 2008]

§ 40.25 Must an employer check on the drug and alcohol testing record of employees it is intending to use to perform safety-sensitive duties?

(a) Yes, as an employer, you must, after obtaining an employee's written consent, request the information about the employee listed in paragraph (b) of this section. This requirement applies only to employees seeking to begin performing safety-sensitive duties for you for the first time (i.e., a new hire, an employee transfers into a safety-sensitive position). If the employee refuses to provide this written consent, you must not permit the employee to perform safety-sensitive functions.

(b) You must request the information listed in this paragraph (b) from DOT-regulated employers who have employed the employee during any period during the two years before the date of the employee's application or transfer:

(1) Alcohol tests with a result of 0.04 or higher alcohol concentration;

(2) Verified positive drug tests;

(3) Refusals to be tested (including verified adulterated or substituted drug test results);

(4) Other violations of DOT agency drug and alcohol testing regulations; and

(5) With respect to any employee who violated a DOT drug and alcohol regulation, documentation of the employee's successful completion of DOT return-to-duty requirements (including follow-up tests). If the previous employer does not have information about the return-do-duty process (e.g., an employer who did not hire an employee who tested positive on a pre-employment test), you must seek to obtain this information from the employee.

(c) The information obtained from a previous employer includes any drug or alcohol test information obtained from previous employers under this section or other applicable DOT agency regulations.

(d) If feasible, you must obtain and review this information before the employee first performs safety-sensitive functions. If this is not feasible, you must obtain and review the information as soon as possible. However, you must not permit the employee to perform safety-sensitive functions after 30 days from the date on which the employee first performed safety-sensitive functions, unless you have obtained or made and documented a good faith effort to obtain this information.

(e) If you obtain information that the employee has violated a DOT agency drug and alcohol regulation, you must not use the employee to perform safety-sensitive functions unless you also obtain information that the employee has subsequently complied with the return-to-duty requirements of Subpart O of this part and DOT agency drug and alcohol regulations.

(f) You must provide to each of the employers from whom you request information under paragraph (b) of this section written consent for the release of the information cited in paragraph (a) of this section.

(g) The release of information under this section must be in any written form (e.g., fax, e-mail, letter) that ensures confidentiality. As the previous employer, you must maintain a written record of the information released, including the date, the party to whom it was released, and a summary of the information provided.

(h) If you are an employer from whom information is requested under paragraph (b) of this section, you must, after reviewing the employee's specific, written consent, immediately release the requested information to the employer making the inquiry.

(i) As the employer requesting the information required under this section, you must maintain a written, confidential record of the information you obtain or of the good faith efforts you made to obtain the information. You must retain this information for three years from the date of the employee's first performance of safety-sensitive duties for you.

(j) As the employer, you must also ask the employee whether he or she has tested positive, or refused to test, on any pre-employment drug or alcohol test administered by an employer to which the employee applied for, but did not obtain, safety-sensitive transportation work covered by DOT agency drug and alcohol testing rules during the past two years. If the employee admits that he or she had a positive test or a refusal to test, you must not use the employee to perform safety-sensitive functions for you, until and unless the employee documents successful completion of the return-to-duty process (see paragraphs (b)(5) and (e) of this section).

§ 40.26 What form must an employer use to report Management Information System (MIS) data to a DOT agency?

As an employer, when you are required to report MIS data to a DOT agency, you must use the form and instructions at appendix H to part 40. You must submit the MIS report in accordance with rule requirements (e.g., dates for submission; selection of companies required to submit, and method of reporting) established by the DOT agency regulating your operation.

[68 FR 43952, July 25, 2003]

§ 40.27 May an employer require an employee to sign a consent or release in connection with the DOT drug and alcohol testing program?

No, as an employer, you must not require an employee to sign a consent, release, waiver of liability, or indemnification agreement with respect to any part of the drug or alcohol testing process covered by this part (including, but not limited to, collections, laboratory testing, MRO and SAP services).

[66 FR 41950, Aug. 9, 2001]

§ 40.29 Where is other information on employer responsibilities found in this regulation?

You can find other information on the responsibilities of employers in the following sections of this part:

§40.3—Definition.

§40.35—Information about DERs that employers must provide collectors.

§40.45—Modifying CCFs, Use of foreign-language CCFs.

§40.47—Use of non-Federal forms for DOT tests or Federal CCFs for non-DOT tests.

§40.67—Requirements for direct observation.

§§40.103–40.105—Blind specimen requirements.

§40.173—Responsibility to ensure test of split specimen.

§40.193—Action in "shy bladder" situations.

§40.197—Actions following report of a dilute specimen.

§40.207—Actions following a report of a cancelled drug test.

§40.209—Actions following and consequences of non-fatal flaws in drug tests.

§40.215—Information about DERs that employers must provide BATs and STTs.

§40.225—Modifying ATFs; use of foreign-language ATFs.

§40.227—Use of non-DOT forms for DOT tests or DOT ATFs for non-DOT tests.

§40.235 (c) and (d)—responsibility to follow instructions for ASDs.

§40.255 (b)—receipt and storage of alcohol test information.

§40.265 (c)–(e)—actions in "shy lung" situations.

§40.267—Cancellation of alcohol tests.

§40.271—Actions in "correctable flaw" situations in alcohol tests.

§40.273—Actions following cancelled tests in alcohol tests.

§40.275—Actions in "non-fatal flaw" situations in alcohol tests.

§§40.287–40.289—Responsibilities concerning SAP services.

§§40.295–40.297—Prohibition on seeking second SAP evaluation or changing SAP recommendation.

§40.303—Responsibilities concerning aftercare recommendations.

§40.305—Responsibilities concerning return-to-duty decision.

§40.309—Responsibilities concerning follow-up tests.

§40.321—General confidentiality requirement.

§40.323—Release of confidential information in litigation.

§40.331—Other circumstances for the release of confidential information.

§40.333—Record retention requirements.

§40.345—Choice of who reports drug testing information to employers.

[65 FR 79526, Dec. 19, 2000. Redesignated at 66 FR 41950, Aug. 9, 2001]

SUBPART C—URINE COLLECTION PERSONNEL

§ 40.31   Who may collect urine specimens for DOT drug testing?

(a) Collectors meeting the requirements of this subpart are the only persons authorized to collect urine specimens for DOT drug testing.

(b) A collector must meet training requirements of §40.33.

(c) As the immediate supervisor of an employee being tested, you may not act as the collector when that employee is tested, unless no other collector is available and you are permitted to do so under DOT agency drug and alcohol regulations.

(d) You must not act as the collector for the employee being tested if you work for a HHS-certified laboratory (e.g., as a technician or accessioner) and could link the employee with a urine specimen, drug testing result, or laboratory report.

§ 40.33   What training requirements must a collector meet?

To be permitted to act as a collector in the DOT drug testing program, you must meet each of the requirements of this section:

(a) <u>Basic information</u>. You must be knowledgeable about this part, the current "DOT Urine Specimen Collection Procedures Guidelines," and DOT agency regulations applicable to the employers for whom you perform collections, and you must keep current on any changes to these materials. The DOT Urine Specimen Collection Procedures Guidelines document is available from ODAPC (Department of Transportation, 1200 New Jersey Avenue, SE, Washington DC, 20590, 202–366–3784, or on the ODAPC web site (http://www.dot.gov/ost/dapc).

(b) <u>Qualification training</u>. You must receive qualification training meeting the requirements of this paragraph. Qualification training must provide instruction on the following subjects:

(1) All steps necessary to complete a collection correctly and the proper completion and transmission of the CCF;

(2) "Problem" collections (e.g., situations like "shy bladder" and attempts to tamper with a specimen);

(3) Fatal flaws, correctable flaws, and how to correct problems in collections; and

(4) The collector's responsibility for maintaining the integrity of the collection process, ensuring the privacy of employees being tested, ensuring the security of the specimen, and avoiding conduct or statements that could be viewed as offensive or inappropriate;

(c) <u>Initial Proficiency Demonstration</u>. Following your completion of qualification training under paragraph (b) of this section, you must demonstrate proficiency in collections under this part by completing five consecutive error-free mock collections.

(1) The five mock collections must include two uneventful collection scenarios, one insufficient quantity of urine scenario, one temperature out of range scenario, and one scenario in which the employee refuses to sign the CCF and initial the specimen bottle tamper-evident seal.

(2) Another person must monitor and evaluate your performance, in person or by a means that provides real-time observation and interaction between the instructor and trainee, and attest in writing that the mock collections are "error-free." This person must be a qualified collector who has demonstrated necessary knowledge, skills, and abilities by—

(i) Regularly conducting DOT drug test collections for a period of at least a year;

(ii) Conducting collector training under this part for a year; or

(iii) Successfully completing a "train the trainer" course.

(d) <u>Schedule for qualification training and initial proficiency demonstration</u>. The following is the schedule for qualification training and the initial proficiency demonstration you must meet:

(1) If you became a collector before August 1, 2001, and you have already met the requirements of paragraphs (b) and (c) of this section, you do not have to meet them again.

(2) If you became a collector before August 1, 2001, and have yet to meet the requirements of paragraphs (b) and (c) of this section, you must do so no later than January 31, 2003.

(3) If you become a collector on or after August 1, 2001, you must meet the requirements of paragraphs (b) and (c) of this section before you begin to perform collector functions.

(e) <u>Refresher training</u>. No less frequently than every five years from the date on which you satisfactorily complete the requirements of paragraphs (b) and (c) of this section, you must complete refresher training that meets all the requirements of paragraphs (b) and (c) of this section.

(f) Error Correction Training. If you make a mistake in the collection process that causes a test to be cancelled (i.e., a fatal or uncorrected flaw), you must undergo error correction training. This training must occur within 30 days of the date you are notified of the error that led to the need for retraining.

(1) Error correction training must be provided and your proficiency documented in writing by a person who meets the requirements of paragraph (c)(2) of this section.

(2) Error correction training is required to cover only the subject matter area(s) in which the error that caused the test to be cancelled occurred.

(3) As part of the error correction training, you must demonstrate your proficiency in the collection procedures of this part by completing three consecutive error-free mock collections. The mock collections must include one uneventful scenario and two scenarios related to the area(s) in which your error(s) occurred. The person providing the training must monitor and evaluate your performance and attest in writing that the mock collections were "error-free."

(g) Documentation. You must maintain documentation showing that you currently meet all requirements of this section. You must provide this documentation on request to DOT agency representatives and to employers and C/TPAs who are using or negotiating to use your services.

[65 FR 79526, Dec 19, 2000; 66 FR 3885, Jan. 17, 2001, as amended at 66 FR 41950, Aug. 9, 2001; 73 FR 33329, June 12, 2008]

§ 40.35 What information about the DER must employers provide to collectors?

As an employer, you must provide to collectors the name and telephone number of the appropriate DER (and C/TPA, where applicable) to contact about any problems or issues that may arise during the testing process.

§ 40.37 Where is other information on the role of collectors found in this regulation?

You can find other information on the role and functions of collectors in the following sections of this part:

§40.3—Definition.

§40.43—Steps to prepare and secure collection sites.

§§40.45–40.47—Use of CCF.

§§40.49–40.51—Use of collection kit and shipping materials.

§§40.61–40.63—Preliminary steps in collections.

§40.65—Role in checking specimens.

§40.67—Role in directly observed collections.

§40.69—Role in monitored collections.

§40.71—Role in split specimen collections.

§40.73—Chain of custody completion and finishing the collection process.

§40.103—Processing blind specimens.

§40.191—Action in case of refusals to take test.

§40.193—Action in "shy bladder" situations.

§§40.199–40.205—Collector errors in tests, effects, and means of correction.

SUBPART D—COLLECTION SITES, FORMS, EQUIPMENT AND SUPPLIES USED IN DOT URINE COLLECTIONS

§ 40.41 Where does a urine collection for a DOT drug test take place?

(a) A urine collection for a DOT drug test must take place in a collection site meeting the requirements of this section.

(b) If you are operating a collection site, you must ensure that it meets the security requirements of §40.43.

(c) If you are operating a collection site, you must have all necessary personnel, materials, equipment, facilities and supervision to provide for the collection, temporary storage, and shipping of urine specimens to a laboratory, and a suitable clean surface for writing.

(d) Your collection site must include a facility for urination described in either paragraph (e) or paragraph (f) of this section.

(e) The first, and preferred, type of facility for urination that a collection site may include is a single-toilet room, having a full-length privacy door, within which urination can occur.

(1) No one but the employee may be present in the room during the collection, except for the observer in the event of a directly observed collection.

(2) You must have a source of water for washing hands, that, if practicable, should be external to the closed room where urination occurs. If an external source is not available, you may meet this requirement by securing all sources of water and other substances that could be used for adulteration and substitution (e.g., water faucets, soap dispensers) and providing moist towelettes outside the closed room.

(f) The second type of facility for urination that a collection site may include is a multistall restroom.

(1) Such a site must provide substantial visual privacy (e.g., a toilet stall with a partial-length door) and meet all other applicable requirements of this section.

(2) If you use a multi-stall restroom, you must either—

(i) Secure all sources of water and other substances that could be used for adulteration and substitution (e.g., water faucets, soap dispensers) and place bluing agent in all toilets or secure the toilets to prevent access; or

(ii) Conduct all collections in the facility as monitored collections (see §40.69 for procedures). This is the only circumstance in which you may conduct a monitored collection.

(3) No one but the employee may be present in the multistall restroom during the collection, except for the monitor in the event of a monitored collection or the observer in the event of a directly observed collection.

(g) A collection site may be in a medical facility, a mobile facility (e.g., a van), a dedicated collection facility, or any other location meeting the requirements of this section.

§ 40.43 What steps must operators of collection sites take to protect the security and integrity of urine collections?

(a) Collectors and operators of collection sites must take the steps listed in this section to prevent unauthorized access that could compromise the integrity of collections.

(b) As a collector, you must do the following before each collection to deter tampering with specimens:

(1) Secure any water sources or otherwise make them unavailable to employees (e.g., turn off water inlet, tape handles to prevent opening faucets);

(2) Ensure that the water in the toilet is blue;

(3) Ensure that no soap, disinfectants, cleaning agents, or other possible adulterants are present;

(4) Inspect the site to ensure that no foreign or unauthorized substances are present;

(5) Tape or otherwise secure shut any movable toilet tank, or put bluing in the tank;

(6) Ensure that undetected access (e.g., through a door not in your view) is not possible;

(7) Secure areas and items (e.g., ledges, trash receptacles, paper towel holders, under-sink areas) that appear suitable for concealing contaminants; and

(8) Recheck items in paragraphs (b)(1) through (7) of this section following each collection to ensure the site's continued integrity.

(c) If the collection site uses a facility normally used for other purposes, like a public rest room or hospital examining room, you must, as a collector, also ensure before the collection that:

(1) Access to collection materials and specimens is effectively restricted; and

(2) The facility is secured against access during the procedure to ensure privacy to the employee and prevent distraction of the collector. Limited-access signs must be posted.

(d) As a collector, you must take the following additional steps to ensure security during the collection process:

(1) To avoid distraction that could compromise security, you are limited to conducting a collection for only one employee at a time. However, during the time one employee is in the period for drinking fluids in a "shy bladder" situation (see §40.193(b)), you may conduct a collection for another employee.

(2) To the greatest extent you can, keep an employee's collection container within view of both you and the employee between the time the employee has urinated and the specimen is sealed.

(3) Ensure you are the only person in addition to the employee who handles the specimen before it is poured into the bottles and sealed with tamper-evident seals.

(4) In the time between when the employee gives you the specimen and when you seal the specimen, remain within the collection site.

(5) Maintain personal control over each specimen and CCF throughout the collection process.

(e) If you are operating a collection site, you must implement a policy and procedures to prevent unauthorized personnel from entering any part of the site in which urine specimens are collected or stored.

(1) Only employees being tested, collectors and other collection site workers, DERs, employee and employer representatives authorized by the employer (e.g., employer policy, collective bargaining agreement), and DOT agency representatives are authorized persons for purposes of this paragraph (e).

(2) Except for the observer in a directly observed collection or the monitor in the case of a monitored collection, you must not permit anyone to enter the urination facility in which employees provide specimens.

(3) You must ensure that all authorized persons are under the supervision of a collector at all times when permitted into the site.

(4) You or the collector may remove any person who obstructs, interferes with, or causes a delay in the collection process.

(f) If you are operating a collection site, you must minimize the number of persons handling specimens.

§ 40.45 What form is used to document a DOT urine collection?

(a) The Federal Drug Testing Custody and Control Form (CCF) must be used to document every urine collection required by the DOT drug testing program. The CCF must be a five-part carbonless manifold form. You may view this form on the Department's web site (http://www.dot.gov/ost/dapc) or the HHS web site (http://www.workplace.samhsa.gov).

(b) You must not use a non-Federal form or an expired Federal form to conduct a DOT urine collection.

As a laboratory, C/TPA or other party that provides CCFs to employers, collection sites, or other customers, you must not provide copies of an expired Federal form to these participants. You must also affirmatively notify these participants that they must not use an expired Federal form (e.g., that beginning August 1, 2001, they may not use the old 7-part Federal CCF for DOT urine collections).

(c) As a participant in the DOT drug testing program, you are not permitted to modify or revise the CCF except as follows:

(1) You may include, in the area outside the border of the form, other information needed for billing or other purposes necessary to the collection process.

(2) The CCF must include the names, addresses, telephone numbers and fax numbers of the employer and the MRO, which may be preprinted, typed, or handwritten. The MRO information must include the specific physician's name and address, as opposed to only a generic clinic, health care organization, or company name. This information is required, and it is prohibited for an employer, collector, service agent or any other party to omit it. In addition, a C/TPA's name, address, fax number, and telephone number may be included, but is not required. The employer may use a C/TPA's address in place of its own, but must continue to include its name, telephone number, and fax number.

(3) As an employer, you may add the name of the DOT agency under whose authority the test occurred as part of the employer information.

(4) As a collector, you may use a CCF with your name, address, telephone number, and fax number preprinted, but under no circumstances may you sign the form before the collection event.

(d) Under no circumstances may the CCF transmit personal identifying information about an employee (other than a social security number (SSN) or other employee identification (ID) number) to a laboratory.

(e) As an employer, you may use an equivalent foreign-language version of the CCF approved by ODAPC. You may use such a non-English language form only in a situation where both the employee and collector understand and can use the form in that language.

[65 FR 79526, Dec. 19, 2000, as amended at 66 FR 41950, Aug. 9, 2001]

§ 40.47 May employers use the CCF for non-Federal collections or non-Federal forms for DOT collections?

(a) No, as an employer, you are prohibited from using the CCF for non-Federal urine collections. You are also prohibited from using non-Federal forms for DOT urine collections. Doing either subjects you to enforcement action under DOT agency regulations.

(b) (1) In the rare case where the collector, either by mistake or as the only means to conduct a test

under difficult circumstances (e.g., post-accident or reasonable suspicion test with insufficient time to obtain the CCF), uses a non-Federal form for a DOT collection, the use of a non-Federal form does not present a reason for the laboratory to reject the specimen for testing or for an MRO to cancel the result.

(2) The use of the non-Federal form is a "correctable flaw." As an MRO, to correct the problem you must follow the procedures of §40.205(b)(2).

[65 FR 79526, Dec. 19, 2000, as amended at 66 FR 41950, Aug. 9, 2001]

§ 40.49 What materials are used to collect urine specimens?

For each DOT drug test, you must use a collection kit meeting the requirements of Appendix A of this part.

§ 40.51 What materials are used to send urine specimens to the laboratory?

(a) Except as provided in paragraph (b) of this section, you must use a shipping container that adequately protects the specimen bottles from shipment damage in the transport of specimens from the collection site to the laboratory.

(b) You are not required to use a shipping container if a laboratory courier hand-delivers the specimens from the collection site to the laboratory.

SUBPART E—URINE SPECIMEN COLLECTIONS

§ 40.61 What are the preliminary steps in the collection process?

As the collector, you must take the following steps before actually beginning a collection:

(a) When a specific time for an employee's test has been scheduled, or the collection site is at the employee's work site, and the employee does not appear at the collection site at the scheduled time, contact the DER to determine the appropriate interval within which the DER has determined the employee is authorized to arrive. If the employee's arrival is delayed beyond that time, you must notify the DER that the employee has not reported for testing. In a situation where a C/TPA has notified an owner/operator or other individual employee to report for testing and the employee does not appear, the C/TPA must notify the employee that he or she has refused to test (see §40.191(a)(1)).

(b) Ensure that, when the employee enters the collection site, you begin the testing process without undue delay. For example, you must not wait because the employee says he or she is not ready or is unable to urinate or because an authorized employer or employee representative is delayed in arriving.

(1) If the employee is also going to take a DOT alcohol test, you must, to the greatest extent practica-

ble, ensure that the alcohol test is completed before the urine collection process begins.

Example to Paragraph (b)(1): An employee enters the test site for both a drug and an alcohol test. Normally, the collector would wait until the BAT had completed the alcohol test process before beginning the drug test process. However, there are some situations in which an exception to this normal practice would be reasonable. One such situation might be if several people were waiting for the BAT to conduct alcohol tests, but a drug testing collector in the same facility were free. Someone waiting might be able to complete a drug test without unduly delaying his or her alcohol test. Collectors and BATs should work together, however, to ensure that post-accident and reasonable suspicion alcohol tests happen as soon as possible (e.g., by moving the employee to the head of the line for alcohol tests).

(2) If the employee needs medical attention (e.g., an injured employee in an emergency medical facility who is required to have a post-accident test), do not delay this treatment to collect a specimen.

(3) You must not collect, by catheterization or other means, urine from an unconscious employee to conduct a drug test under this part. Nor may you catheterize a conscious employee. However, you must inform an employee who normally voids through self-catheterization that the employee is required to provide a specimen in that manner.

(4) If, as an employee, you normally void through self-catheterization, and decline to do so, this constitutes a refusal to test.

(c) Require the employee to provide positive identification. You must see a photo ID issued by the employer (other than in the case of an owner-operator or other self-employed individual) or a Federal, state, or local government (e.g., a driver's license). You may not accept faxes or photocopies of identification. Positive identification by an employer representative (not a co-worker or another employee being tested) is also acceptable. If the employee cannot produce positive identification, you must contact a DER to verify the identity of the employee.

(d) If the employee asks, provide your identification to the employee. Your identification must include your name and your employer's name, but does not have to include your picture, address, or telephone number.

(e) Explain the basic collection procedure to the employee, including showing the employee the instructions on the back of the CCF.

(f) Direct the employee to remove outer clothing (e.g., coveralls, jacket, coat, hat) that could be used to conceal items or substances that could be used to tamper with a specimen. You must also direct the employee to leave these garments and any briefcase, purse, or other personal belongings with you or in a mutually agreeable location. You must advise the employee that failure to comply with your directions constitutes a refusal to test.

(1) If the employee asks for a receipt for any belongings left with you, you must provide one.

(2) You must allow the employee to keep his or her wallet.

(3) You must not ask the employee to remove other clothing (e.g., shirts, pants, dresses, underwear), to remove all clothing, or to change into a hospital or examination gown (unless the urine collection is being accomplished simultaneously with a DOT agency-authorized medical examination).

(4) You must direct the employee to empty his or her pockets and display the items in them to ensure that no items are present which could be used to adulterate the specimen. If nothing is there that can be used to adulterate a specimen, the employee can place the items back into his or her pockets. As the employee, you must allow the collector to make this observation.

(5) If, in your duties under paragraph (f)(4) of this section, you find any material that could be used to tamper with a specimen, you must:

(i) Determine if the material appears to be brought to the collection site with the intent to alter the specimen, and, if it is, conduct a directly observed collection using direct observation procedures (see §40.67); or

(ii) Determine if the material appears to be inadvertently brought to the collection site (e.g., eye drops), secure and maintain it until the collection process is completed and conduct a normal (i.e., unobserved) collection.

(g) You must instruct the employee not to list medications that he or she is currently taking on the CCF. (The employee may make notes of medications on the back of the employee copy of the form for his or her own convenience, but these notes must not be transmitted to anyone else.)

§ 40.63 What steps does the collector take in the collection process before the employee provides a urine specimen?

As the collector, you must take the following steps before the employee provides the urine specimen:

(a) Complete Step 1 of the CCF.

(b) Instruct the employee to wash and dry his or her hands at this time. You must tell the employee not to wash his or her hands again until after delivering the specimen to you. You must not give the employee any further access to water or other materials that could be used to adulterate or dilute a specimen.

(c) Select, or allow the employee to select, an individually wrapped or sealed collection container from collection kit materials. Either you or the employee, with both of you present, must unwrap or break the seal of the collection container. You must not unwrap or break the seal on any specimen bottle at this time. You must not allow the employee to take anything from the collection kit into the room used for urination except the collection container.

(d) Direct the employee to go into the room used for urination, provide a specimen of at least 45 mL, not flush the toilet, and return to you with the specimen as soon as the employee has completed the void.

(1) Except in the case of an observed or a monitored collection (see §§40.67 and 40.69), neither you nor anyone else may go into the room with the employee.

(2) As the collector, you may set a reasonable time limit for voiding.

(e) You must pay careful attention to the employee during the entire collection process to note any conduct that clearly indicates an attempt to tamper with a specimen (e.g., substitute urine in plain view or an attempt to bring into the collection site an adulterant or urine substitute). If you detect such conduct, you must require that a collection take place immediately under direct observation (see §40.67) and note the conduct and the fact that the collection was observed in the "Remarks" line of the CCF (Step 2). You must also, as soon as possible, inform the DER and collection site supervisor that a collection took place under direct observation and the reason for doing so.

§ 40.65   What does the collector check for when the employee presents a specimen?

As a collector, you must check the following when the employee gives the collection container to you:

(a) Sufficiency of specimen. You must check to ensure that the specimen contains at least 45 mL of urine.

(1) If it does not, you must follow "shy bladder" procedures (see §40.193(b)).

(2) When you follow "shy bladder" procedures, you must discard the original specimen, unless another problem (i.e., temperature out of range, signs of tampering) also exists.

(3) You are never permitted to combine urine collected from separate voids to create a specimen.

(4) You must discard any excess urine.

(b) Temperature. You must check the temperature of the specimen no later than four minutes after the employee has given you the specimen.

(1) The acceptable temperature range is 32–38 °C/ 90–100 °F.

(2) You must determine the temperature of the specimen by reading the temperature strip attached to the collection container.

(3) If the specimen temperature is within the acceptable range, you must mark the "Yes" box on the CCF (Step 2).

(4) If the specimen temperature is outside the acceptable range, you must mark the "No" box and enter in the "Remarks" line (Step 2) your findings about the temperature.

(5) If the specimen temperature is outside the acceptable range, you must immediately conduct a new collection using direct observation procedures (see §40.67).

(6) In a case where a specimen is collected under direct observation because of the temperature being out of range, you must process both the original specimen and the specimen collected using direct observation and send the two sets of specimens to the laboratory. This is true even in a case in which the original specimen has insufficient volume but the temperature is out of range. You must also, as soon as possible, inform the DER and collection site supervisor that a collection took place under direct observation and the reason for doing so.

(7) In a case where the employee refuses to provide another specimen (see §40.191(a)(3)) or refuses to provide another specimen under direct observation (see §40.191(a)(4)), you must notify the DER. As soon as you have notified the DER, you must discard any specimen the employee has provided previously during the collection procedure.

(c) Signs of tampering. You must inspect the specimen for unusual color, presence of foreign objects or material, or other signs of tampering (e.g., if you notice any unusual odor).

(1) If it is apparent from this inspection that the employee has tampered with the specimen (e.g., blue dye in the specimen, excessive foaming when shaken, smell of bleach), you must immediately conduct a new collection using direct observation procedures (see §40.67).

(2) In a case where a specimen is collected under direct observation because of showing signs of tampering, you must process both the original specimen and the specimen collected using direct observation and send the two sets of specimens to the laboratory. This is true even in a case in which the original specimen has insufficient volume but it shows signs of tampering. You must also, as soon as possible, inform the DER and collection site supervisor that a collection took place under direct observation and the reason for doing so.

(3) In a case where the employee refuses to provide a specimen under direct observation (see §40.191(a)(4)), you must discard any specimen the employee provided previously during the collection procedure. Then you must notify the DER as soon as practicable.

[65 FR 79526, Dec. 19, 2000, as amended at 66 FR 41950, Aug. 9, 2001]

§ 40.67 When and how is a directly observed collection conducted?

(a) As an employer, you must direct an immediate collection under direct observation with no advance notice to the employee, if:

(1) The laboratory reported to the MRO that a specimen is invalid, and the MRO reported to you that there was not an adequate medical explanation for the result;

(2) The MRO reported to you that the original positive, adulterated, or substituted result had to be cancelled because the test of the split specimen could not be performed; or

(3) The laboratory reported to the MRO that the specimen was negative-dilute with a creatinine concentration greater than or equal to 2 mg/dL but less than or equal to 5 mg/dL, and the MRO reported the specimen to you as negative-dilute and that a second collection must take place under direct observation (see §40.197(b)(1)).

(b) As an employer, you must direct a collection under direct observation of an employee if the drug test is a return-to-duty test or a follow-up test.

(c) As a collector, you must immediately conduct a collection under direct observation if:

(1) You are directed by the DER to do so (see paragraphs (a) and (b) of this section); or

(2) You observed materials brought to the collection site or the employee's conduct clearly indicates an attempt to tamper with a specimen (see §§40.61(f)(5)(i) and 40.63(e)); or

(3) The temperature on the original specimen was out of range (see §40.65(b)(5)); or (4) The original specimen appeared to have been tampered with (see §40.65(c)(1)).

(d)(1) As the employer, you must explain to the employee the reason for a directly observed collection under paragraph (a) or (b) of this section.

(2) As the collector, you must explain to the employee the reason, if known, under this part for a directly observed collection under paragraphs (c)(1) through (3) of this section.

(e) As the collector, you must complete a new CCF for the directly observed collection.

(1) You must mark the "reason for test" block (Step 1) the same as for the first collection.

(2) You must check the "Observed, (Enter Remark)" box and enter the reason (see §40.67(b)) in the "Remarks" line (Step 2).

(f) In a case where two sets of specimens are being sent to the laboratory because of suspected tampering with the specimen at the collection site, enter on the "Remarks" line of the CCF (Step 2) for each specimen a notation to this effect (e.g., collection 1 of 2, or 2 of 2) and the specimen ID number of the other specimen.

(g) As the collector, you must ensure that the observer is the same gender as the employee. You must never permit an opposite gender person to act as the observer. The observer can be a different person from the collector and need not be a qualified collector.

(h) As the collector, if someone else is to observe the collection (e.g., in order to ensure a same gender observer), you must verbally instruct that person to follow procedures at paragraphs (i) and (j) of this section. If you, the collector, are the observer, you too must follow these procedures.

(i) As the observer, you must request the employee to raise his or her shirt, blouse, or dress/skirt, as appropriate, above the waist; and lower clothing and underpants to show you, by turning around, that they do not have a prosthetic device. After you have determined that the employee does not have such a device, you may permit the employee to return clothing to its proper position for observed urination.

(j) As the observer, you must watch the employee urinate into the collection container. Specifically, you are to watch the urine go from the employee's body into the collection container.

(k) As the observer but not the collector, you must not take the collection container from the employee, but you must observe the specimen as the employee takes it to the collector.

(l) As the collector, when someone else has acted as the observer, you must include the observer's name in the "Remarks" line of the CCF (Step 2).

(m) As the employee, if you decline to allow a directly observed collection required or permitted under this section to occur, this is a refusal to test.

(n) As the collector, when you learn that a directly observed collection should have been collected but was not, you must inform the employer that it must direct the employee to have an immediate recollection under direct observation.

[65 FR 79526, Dec. 19, 2000, as amended at 66 FR 41950, Aug. 9, 2001; 68 FR 31626, May 28, 2003; 69 FR 64867, Nov. 9, 2004; 73 FR 35970, June 25, 2008; 73 FR 70283, November 20, 2008; 74 FR 37949, July 30, 2009]

§ 40.69 How is a monitored collection conducted?

(a) As the collector, you must secure the room being used for the monitored collection so that no one except the employee and the monitor can enter it until after the collection has been completed.

(b) As the collector, you must ensure that the monitor is the same gender as the employee, unless the monitor is a medical professional (e.g., nurse, doctor, physician's assistant, technologist, or technician licensed or certified to practice in the jurisdiction in which the collection takes place). The monitor can be a different person from the collector and need not be a qualified collector.

(c) As the collector, if someone else is to monitor the collection (e.g., in order to ensure a same-gender monitor), you must verbally instruct that person to follow the procedures of paragraphs (d) and (e) of this section. If you, the collector, are the monitor, you must follow these procedures.

(d) As the monitor, you must not watch the employee urinate into the collection container. If you hear sounds or make other observations indicating an attempt to tamper with a specimen, there must be an additional collection under direct observation (see §§40.63(e), 40.65(c), and 40.67(b)).

(e) As the monitor, you must ensure that the employee takes the collection container directly to the collector as soon as the employee has exited the enclosure.

(f) As the collector, when someone else has acted as the monitor, you must note that person's name in the "Remarks" line of the CCF (Step 2).

(g) As the employee being tested, if you decline to permit a collection authorized under this section to be monitored, it is a refusal to test.

[65 FR 79526, Dec. 19, 2000, as amended at 66 FR 41951, Aug. 9, 2001]

§ 40.71 How does the collector prepare the specimens?

(a) All collections under DOT agency drug testing regulations must be split specimen collections.

(b) As the collector, you must take the following steps, in order, after the employee brings the urine specimen to you. You must take these steps in the presence of the employee.

(1) Check the box on the CCF (Step 2) indicating that this was a split specimen collection.

(2) You, not the employee, must first pour at least 30 mL of urine from the collection container into one specimen bottle, to be used for the primary specimen.

(3) You, not the employee, must then pour at least 15 mL of urine from the collection container into the second specimen bottle to be used for the split specimen.

(4) You, not the employee, must place and secure (i.e., tighten or snap) the lids/caps on the bottles.

(5) You, not the employee, must seal the bottles by placing the tamper-evident bottle seals over the bottle caps/lids and down the sides of the bottles.

(6) You, not the employee, must then write the date on the tamper-evident bottle seals.

(7) You must then ensure that the employee initials the tamper-evident bottle seals for the purpose of certifying that the bottles contain the specimens he or she provided. If the employee fails or refuses to do so,

you must note this in the "Remarks" line of the CCF (Step 2) and complete the collection process.

(8) You must discard any urine left over in the collection container after both specimen bottles have been appropriately filled and sealed. There is one exception to this requirement: you may use excess urine to conduct clinical tests (e.g., protein, glucose) if the collection was conducted in conjunction with a physical examination required by a DOT agency regulation. Neither you nor anyone else may conduct further testing (such as adulteration testing) on this excess urine and the employee has no legal right to demand that the excess urine be turned over to the employee.

[65 FR 79526, Dec. 19, 2000, as amended at 66 FR 41951, Aug. 9, 2001]

§ 40.73 How is the collection process completed?

(a) As the collector, you must do the following things to complete the collection process. You must complete the steps called for in paragraphs (a)(1) through (a)(7) of this section in the employee's presence.

(1) Direct the employee to read and sign the certification statement on Copy 2 (Step 5) of the CCF and provide date of birth, printed name, and day and evening contact telephone numbers. If the employee refuses to sign the CCF or to provide date of birth, printed name, or telephone numbers, you must note this in the "Remarks" line (Step 2) of the CCF, and complete the collection. If the employee refuses to fill out any information, you must, as a minimum, print the employee's name in the appropriate place.

(2) Complete the chain of custody on the CCF (Step 4) by printing your name (note: you may pre-print your name), recording the time and date of the collection, signing the statement, and entering the name of the delivery service transferring the specimen to the laboratory,

(3) Ensure that all copies of the CCF are legible and complete.

(4) Remove Copy 5 of the CCF and give it to the employee.

(5) Place the specimen bottles and Copy 1 of the CCF in the appropriate pouches of the plastic bag.

(6) Secure both pouches of the plastic bag.

(7) Advise the employee that he or she may leave the collection site.

(8) To prepare the sealed plastic bag containing the specimens and CCF for shipment you must:

(i) Place the sealed plastic bag in a shipping container (e.g., standard courier box) designed to minimize the possibility of damage during shipment. (More than one sealed plastic bag can be placed into a single shipping container if you are doing multiple collections.)

(ii) Seal the container as appropriate.

(iii) If a laboratory courier hand-delivers the specimens from the collection site to the laboratory, prepare the sealed plastic bag for shipment as directed by the courier service.

(9) Send Copy 2 of the CCF to the MRO and Copy 4 to the DER. You must fax or otherwise transmit these copies to the MRO and DER within 24 hours or during the next business day. Keep Copy 3 for at least 30 days, unless otherwise specified by applicable DOT agency regulations.

(b) As a collector or collection site, you must ensure that each specimen you collect is shipped to a laboratory as quickly as possible, but in any case within 24 hours or during the next business day.

[65 FR 79526, Dec. 19, 2000, as amended at 71 FR 49384, Aug. 23, 2006]

SUBPART F—DRUG TESTING LABORATORIES

§ 40.81   What laboratories may be used for DOT drug testing?

(a) As a drug testing laboratory located in the U.S., you are permitted to participate in DOT drug testing only if you are certified by HHS under the National Laboratory Certification Program (NLCP) for all testing required under this part.

(b) As a drug testing laboratory located in Canada or Mexico which is not certified by HHS under the NLCP, you are permitted to participate in DOT drug testing only if:

(1) The DOT, based on a written recommendation from HHS, has approved your laboratory as meeting HHS laboratory certification standards or deemed your laboratory fully equivalent to a laboratory meeting HHS laboratory certification standards for all testing required under this part; or

(2) The DOT, based on a written recommendation from HHS, has recognized a Canadian or Mexican certifying organization as having equivalent laboratory certification standards and procedures to those of HHS, and the Canadian or Mexican certifying organization has certified your laboratory under those equivalent standards and procedures.

(c) As a laboratory participating in the DOT drug testing program, you must comply with the requirements of this part. You must also comply with all applicable requirements of HHS in testing DOT specimens, whether or not the HHS requirements are explicitly stated in this part.

(d) If DOT determines that you are in noncompliance with this part, you could be subject to PIE proceedings under Subpart R of this part. If the Department issues a PIE with respect to you, you are ineligible to participate in the DOT drug testing program even if you continue to meet the requirements of paragraph (a) or (b) of this section.

§ 40.83   How do laboratories process incoming specimens?

As the laboratory, you must do the following when you receive a DOT specimen:

(a) You are authorized to receive only the laboratory copy of the CCF. You are not authorized to receive other copies of the CCF nor any copies of the alcohol testing form.

(b) You must comply with applicable provisions of the HHS Guidelines concerning accessioning and processing urine drug specimens.

(c) You must inspect each specimen and CCF for the following "fatal flaws:"

(1) The specimen ID numbers on the specimen bottle and the CCF do not match;

(2) The specimen bottle seal is broken or shows evidence of tampering, unless a split specimen can be redesignated (see paragraph (h) of this section);

(3) The collector's printed name and signature are omitted from the CCF; and

(4) There is an insufficient amount of urine in the primary bottle for analysis, unless the specimens can be redesignated (see paragraph (h) of this section).

(d) When you find a specimen meeting the criteria of paragraph (c) of this section, you must document your findings and stop the testing process. Report the result in accordance with §40.97(a)(3).

(e) You must inspect each CCF for the presence of the collector's signature on the certification statement in Step 4 of the CCF. Upon finding that the signature is omitted, document the flaw and continue the testing process.

(1) In such a case, you must retain the specimen for a minimum of 5 business days from the date on which you initiated action to correct the flaw.

(2) You must then attempt to correct the flaw by following the procedures of §40.205(b)(1).

(3) If the flaw is not corrected, report the result as rejected for testing in accordance with §40.97(a)(3).

(f) If you determine that the specimen temperature was not checked and the "Remarks" line did not contain an entry regarding the temperature being outside of range, you must then attempt to correct the problem by following the procedures of §40.208.

(1) In such a case, you must continue your efforts to correct the problem for five business days, before you report the result.

(2) When you have obtained the correction, or five business days have elapsed, report the result in accordance with §40.97(a).

(g) If you determine that a CCF that fails to meet the requirements of §40.45(a) (e.g., a non-Federal form or an expired Federal form was used for the collection), you must attempt to correct the use of the improper form by following the procedures of §40.205(b)(2).

(1) In such a case, you must retain the specimen for a minimum of 5 business days from the date on which you initiated action to correct the problem.

(2) If the problem(s) is not corrected, you must reject the test and report the result in accordance with §40.97(a)(3).

(h) If the CCF is marked indicating that a split specimen collection was collected and if the split specimen does not accompany the primary, has leaked, or is otherwise unavailable for testing, you must still test the primary specimen and follow appropriate procedures outlined in §40.175(b) regarding the unavailability of the split specimen for testing.

(1) The primary specimen and the split specimen can be redesignated (i.e., Bottle B is redesignated as Bottle A, and vice-versa) if:

(i) The primary specimen appears to have leaked out of its sealed bottle and the laboratory believes a sufficient amount of urine exists in the split specimen to conduct all appropriate primary laboratory testing; or

(ii) The primary specimen is labeled as Bottle B, and the split specimen as Bottle A; or

(iii) The laboratory opens the split specimen instead of the primary specimen, the primary specimen remains sealed, and the laboratory believes a sufficient amount of urine exists in the split specimen to conduct all appropriate primary laboratory testing; or

(iv) The primary specimen seal is broken but the split specimen remains sealed and the laboratory believes a sufficient amount of urine exists in the split specimen to conduct all appropriate primary laboratory testing.

(2) In situations outlined in paragraph (g)(1) of this section, the laboratory shall mark through the "A" and write "B," then initial and date the change. A corresponding change shall be made to the other bottle by marking through the "B" and writing "A," and initialing and dating the change.

(i) A notation shall be made on Copy 1 of the CCF (Step 5a) and on any laboratory internal chain of custody documents, as appropriate, for any fatal or correctable flaw.

[65 FR 79526, Dec. 19, 2000, as amended at 66 FR 41951, Aug. 9, 2001; 71 FR 49384, Aug. 23, 2006; 73 FR 35970, June 25, 2008]

§ 40.85   What drugs do laboratories test for?

As a laboratory, you must test for the following five drugs or classes of drugs in a DOT drug test. You must not test "DOT specimens" for any other drugs.

(a) Marijuana metabolites.

(b) Cocaine metabolites.

(c) Amphetamines.

(d) Opiate metabolites.

(e) Phencyclidine (PCP).

§ 40.87   What are the cutoff concentrations for initial and confirmation tests?

(a) As a laboratory, you must use the cutoff concentrations displayed in the following table for initial and confirmation drug tests. All cutoff concentrations are expressed in nanograms per milliliter (ng/mL). The table follows:

Type of Drug or Metabolite	Initial Test	Confirmation Test
(1) Marijuana metabolites	50	
(i) Delta-9-tetrahydro-cannabinol-9-carboxylic acid (THC)		15
(2) Cocaine metabolites (Benzoylecgonine)	300	150
(3) Phencyclidine (PCP)	25	25
(4) Amphetamines	1000	
(i) Amphetamine		500
(ii) Methamphetamine		500 (Specimen must also contain amphetamine at a concentration of greater than or equal to 200 ng/mL
(5) Opiate metabolites	2000	
(i) Codeine		2000
(ii) Morphine		2000
(iii) 6-acetylmorphine		10 Test for 6-AM in the specimen. Conduct this test only when specimen contains morphine at a concentration greater than or equal to 2000 ng/mL.

(b) On an initial drug test, you must report a result below the cutoff concentration as negative. If the result is at or above the cutoff concentration, you must conduct a confirmation test.

(c) On a confirmation drug test, you must report a result below the cutoff concentration as negative and a result at or above the cutoff concentration as confirmed positive.

(d) You must report quantitative values for morphine or codeine at 15,000 ng/mL or above.

§ 40.89   What is validity testing, and are laboratories required to conduct it?

(a) Specimen validity testing is the evaluation of the specimen to determine if it is consistent with normal human urine. The purpose of validity testing is to determine whether certain adulterants or foreign substances were added to the urine, if the urine was diluted, or if the specimen was substituted.

(b) As a laboratory, you must conduct validity testing.

[65 FR 79526, Dec. 19, 2000, as amended at 66 FR 41951, Aug. 9, 2001; 73 FR 35970, June 25, 2008]

§ 40.91 What validity tests must laboratories conduct on primary specimens?

As a laboratory, when you conduct validity testing under §40.89, you must conduct it in accordance with the requirements of this section.

(a) You must determine the creatinine concentration on each primary specimen. You must also determine its specific gravity if you find the creatinine concentration to be less than 20 mg/dL.

(b) You must determine the pH of each primary specimen.

(c) You must perform one or more validity tests for oxidizing adulterants on each primary specimen.

(d) You must perform additional validity tests on the primary specimen when the following conditions are observed:

(1) Abnormal physical characteristics;

(2) Reactions or responses characteristic of an adulterant obtained during initial or confirmatory drug tests (e.g., non-recovery of internal standards, unusual response); or

(3) Possible unidentified interfering substance or adulterant.

(e) If you determine that the specimen is invalid and HHS guidelines direct you to contact the MRO, you must contact the MRO and together decide if testing the primary specimen by another HHS certified laboratory would be useful in being able to report a positive or adulterated test result.

[65 FR 79526, Dec. 19, 2000, as amended at 69 FR 64867, Nov.9, 2004]

§ 40.93 What criteria do laboratories use to establish that a specimen is dilute or substituted?

(a) As a laboratory you must consider the primary specimen to be dilute when:

(1) The creatinine concentration is greater than or equal to 2mg/dL but less than 20 mg/dL, and

(2) The specific gravity is greater than 1.0010 but less than 1.0030 on a single aliquot.

(b) As a laboratory you must consider the primary specimen to be substituted when the creatinine concentration is less than 2 mg/dL and the specific gravity is less than or equal to 1.0010 or greater than or equal to 1.0200 on both the initial and confirmatory creatinine tests and on both the initial and confirmatory specific gravity tests on two separate aliquots.

[65 FR 79526, Dec. 19, 2000, as amended at 69 FR 64867, Nov.9, 2004]

§ 40.95 What are the adulterant cutoff concentrations for initial and confirmation tests?

(a) As a laboratory, you must use the cutoff concentrations for the initial and confirmation adulterant testing as required by the HHS Mandatory Guidelines and you must use two separate aliquots—one for the initial test and another for the confirmation test.

(b) As a laboratory, you must report results at or above the cutoffs (or for pH, at or above or below the values, as appropriate) as adulterated and provide the numerical value that supports the adulterated result.

[65 FR 79526, Dec. 19, 2000, as amended at 73 FR 35970, June 25, 2008]

§ 40.96 What criteria do laboratories use to establish that a specimen is invalid?

(a) As a laboratory, you must use the invalid test result criteria for the initial and confirmation testing as required by the HHS Mandatory Guidelines and you must use two separate aliquots—one for the initial test and another for the confirmation test.

(b) As a laboratory, for a specimen having an invalid result for one of the reasons outlined in the HHS Mandatory Guidelines, you must contact the MRO to discuss whether sending the specimen to another HHS certified laboratory for testing would be useful in being able to report a positive or adulterated result.

(c) As a laboratory, you must report invalid results in accordance with the invalid test result criteria as required by the HHS Guidelines and provide the numerical value that support the invalid result. For pH, report at or above or below the values, as appropriate.

(d) As a laboratory, you must report the reason a test result is invalid.

[73 FR 35970, June 25, 2008]

§ 40.97 What do laboratories report and how do they report it?

(a) As a laboratory, you must report the results for each primary specimen. The result of a primary specimen will fall into one of the following three categories. However, as a laboratory, you must report the actual results (and not the categories):

(1) <u>Category 1: Negative Results</u>. As a laboratory, when you find a specimen to be negative, you must report the test result as being one of the following, as appropriate:

(i) Negative, or

(ii) Negative-dilute, with numerical values for creatinine and specific gravity.

(2) <u>Category 2: Non-negative Results</u>. As a laboratory, when you find a specimen to be non-negative,

you must report the test result as being one or more of the following, as appropriate:

(i) Positive, with drug(s)/metabolite(s) noted;

(ii) Positive-dilute, with drug(s)/metabolite(s) noted, with numerical values for creatinine and specific gravity;

(iii) Adulterated, with adulterant(s) noted, with confirmatory test values (when applicable), and with remarks(s);

(iv) Substituted, with confirmatory test values for creatinine and specific gravity; or

(v) Invalid result, with remark(s). Laboratories will report actual values for pH results.

(3) Category 3: Rejected for Testing. As a laboratory, when you reject a specimen for testing, you must report the result as being Rejected for Testing, with remark(s).

(b) As a laboratory, you must report laboratory results directly, and only, to the MRO at his or her place of business. You must not report results to or through the DER or a service agent (e.g., C/TPA).

(1) Negative results: You must fax, courier, mail, or electronically transmit a legible image or copy of the fully-completed Copy 1 of the CCF which has been signed by the certifying scientist, or you may provide the laboratory results report electronically (i.e., computer data file).

(i) If you elect to provide the laboratory results report, you must include the following elements, as a minimum, in the report format:

(A) Laboratory name and address;

(B) Employer's name (you may include I.D. or account number);

(C) Medical review officer's name;

(D) Specimen I.D. number;

(E) Donor's SSN or employee I.D. number, if provided;

(F) Reason for test, if provided;

(G) Collector's name and telephone number;

(H) Date of the collection;

(I) Date received at the laboratory;

(J) Date certifying scientist released the results;

(K) Certifying scientist's name;

(L) Results (e.g., positive, adulterated) as listed in paragraph (a) of this section; and

(M) Remarks section, with an explanation of any situation in which a correctable flaw has been corrected.

(ii) You may release the laboratory results report only after review and approval by the certifying scientist. It must reflect the same test result information as contained on the CCF signed by the certifying scientist. The information contained in the laboratory re-

sults report may not contain information that does not appear on the CCF.

(iii) The results report may be transmitted through any means that ensures accuracy and confidentiality. You, as the laboratory, together with the MRO, must ensure that the information is adequately protected from unauthorized access or release, both during transmission and in storage.

(2) Non-negative and Rejected for Testing results: You must fax, courier, mail, or electronically transmit a legible image or copy of the fully-completed Copy 1 of the CCF that has been signed by the certifying scientist. In addition, you may provide the electronic laboratory results report following the format and procedures set forth in paragraphs (b)(1)(i) and (ii) of this section.

(c) In transmitting laboratory results to the MRO, you, as the laboratory, together with the MRO, must ensure that the information is adequately protected from unauthorized access or release, both during transmission and in storage. If the results are provided by fax, the fax connection must have a fixed telephone number accessible only to authorized individuals.

(d) You must transmit test results to the MRO in a timely manner, preferably the same day that review by the certifying scientist is completed.

(e)(1) You must provide quantitative values for confirmed positive drug test results to the MRO when the MRO requests you to do so in writing. The MRO's request may be either a general request covering all such results you send to the MRO or a specific case-by-case request.

(2) You must provide numerical values that support the adulterated (when applicable) or substituted result, without a request from the MRO.

(3) You must also provide the MRO numerical values for creatinine and specific gravity for the negative-dilute test result, without a request from the MRO.

(f) You must provide quantitative values for confirmed opiate results for morphine or codeine at 15,000 ng/mL or above, even if the MRO has not requested quantitative values for the test result.

[65 FR 79526, Dec. 19, 2000, as amended at 66 FR 41951, Aug. 9, 2001; 68 FR 31626, May 28, 2003; 69 FR 64867, Nov.9, 2004; 73 FR 35970, June 25, 2008]

§ 40.99 How long does the laboratory retain specimens after testing?

(a) As a laboratory testing the primary specimen, you must retain a specimen that was reported with positive, adulterated, substituted, or invalid results for a minimum of one year.

(b) You must keep such a specimen in secure, long-term, frozen storage in accordance with HHS requirements.

(c) Within the one-year period, the MRO, the employee, the employer, or a DOT agency may request in writing that you retain a specimen for an additional period of time (e.g., for the purpose of preserving evidence for litigation or a safety investigation). If you receive such a request, you must comply with it. If you do not receive such a request, you may discard the specimen at the end of the year.

(d) If you have not sent the split specimen to another laboratory for testing, you must retain the split specimen for an employee's test for the same period of time that you retain the primary specimen and under the same storage conditions.

(e) As the laboratory testing the split specimen, you must meet the requirements of paragraphs (a) through (d) of this section with respect to the split specimen.

§ 40.101 What relationship may a laboratory have with an MRO?

(a) As a laboratory, you may not enter into any relationship with an MRO that creates a conflict of interest or the appearance of a conflict of interest with the MRO's responsibilities for the employer. You may not derive any financial benefit by having an employer use a specific MRO.

(b) The following are examples of relationships between laboratories and MROs that the Department regards as creating conflicts of interest, or the appearance of such conflicts. This following list of examples is not intended to be exclusive or exhaustive:

(1) The laboratory employs an MRO who reviews test results produced by the laboratory;

(2) The laboratory has a contract or retainer with the MRO for the review of test results produced by the laboratory;

(3) The laboratory designates which MRO the employer is to use, gives the employer a slate of MROs from which to choose, or recommends certain MROs;

(4) The laboratory gives the employer a discount or other incentive to use a particular MRO;

(5) The laboratory has its place of business co-located with that of an MRO or MRO staff who review test results produced by the laboratory; or

(6) The laboratory permits an MRO, or an MRO's organization, to have a financial interest in the laboratory.

§ 40.103 What are the requirements for submitting blind specimens to a laboratory?

(a) As an employer or C/TPA with an aggregate of 2000 or more DOT-covered employees, you must send blind specimens to laboratories you use. If you have an aggregate of fewer than 2000 DOT-covered employees, you are not required to provide blind specimens.

(b) To each laboratory to which you send at least 100 specimens in a year, you must transmit a number of blind specimens equivalent to one percent of the specimens you send to that laboratory, up to a maximum of 50 blind specimens in each quarter (i.e., January–March, April–June, July–September, October–December). As a C/TPA, you must apply this percentage to the total number of DOT-covered employees' specimens you send to the laboratory. Your blind specimen submissions must be evenly spread throughout the year. The following examples illustrate how this requirement works:

Example 1 to Paragraph (b). You send 2500 specimens to Lab X in Year 1. In this case, you would send 25 blind specimens to Lab X in Year 1. To meet the even distribution requirement, you would send 6 in each of three quarters and 7 in the other.

Example 2 to Paragraph (b). You send 2000 specimens to Lab X and 1000 specimens to Lab Y in Year 1. In this case, you would send 20 blind specimens to Lab X and 10 to Lab Y in Year 1. The even distribution requirement would apply in a similar way to that described in Example 1.

Example 3 to Paragraph (b). Same as Example 2, except that you also send 20 specimens to Lab Z. In this case, you would send blind specimens to Labs X and Y as in Example 2. You would not have to send any blind specimens to Lab Z, because you sent fewer than 100 specimens to Lab Z.

Example 4 to Paragraph (b). You are a C/TPA sending 2000 specimens to Lab X in Year 1. These 2000 specimens represent 200 small employers who have an average of 10 covered employees each. In this case you—not the individual employers—send 20 blind specimens to Lab X in Year 1, again ensuring even distribution. The individual employers you represent are not required to provide any blind specimens on their own.

Example 5 to Paragraph (b). You are a large C/TPA that sends 40,000 specimens to Lab Y in Year 1. One percent of that figure is 400. However, the 50 blind specimen per quarter "cap" means that you need send only 50 blind specimens per quarter, rather than the 100 per quarter you would have to send to meet the one percent rate. Your annual total would be 200, rather than 400, blind specimens.

(c) Approximately 75 percent of the specimens you submit must be negative (i.e., containing no drugs, nor adulterated or substituted). Approximately 15 percent must be positive for one or more of the five drugs involved in DOT tests, and approximately 10 percent must either be adulterated with a substance cited in HHS guidance or substituted (i.e., having specific gravity and creatinine meeting the criteria of §40.93(b)).

(1) All negative, positive, adulterated, and substituted blind specimens you submit must be certified by

the supplier and must have supplier-provided expiration dates.

(2) Negative specimens must be certified by immunoassay and GC/MS to contain no drugs.

(3) Drug positive blind specimens must be certified by immunoassay and GC/MS to contain a drug(s)/metabolite(s) between 1.5 and 2 times the initial drug test cutoff concentration.

(4) Adulterated blind specimens must be certified to be adulterated with a specific adulterant using appropriate confirmatory validity test(s).

(5) Substituted blind specimens must be certified for creatinine concentration and specific gravity to satisfy the criteria for a substituted specimen using confirmatory creatinine and specific gravity tests, respectively.

(d) You must ensure that each blind specimen is indistinguishable to the laboratory from a normal specimen.

(1) You must submit blind specimens to the laboratory using the same channels (e.g., via a regular collection site) through which employees' specimens are sent to the laboratory.

(2) You must ensure that the collector uses a CCF, places fictional initials on the specimen bottle label/seal, indicates for the MRO on Copy 2 that the specimen is a blind specimen, and discards Copies 4 and 5 (employer and employee copies).

(3) You must ensure that all blind specimens include split specimens.

[65 FR 79526, Dec. 19, 2000, as amended at 73 FR 35971, June 25, 2008]

§ 40.105 What happens if the laboratory reports a result different from that expected for a blind specimen?

(a) If you are an employer, MRO, or C/TPA who submits a blind specimen, and if the result reported to the MRO is different from the result expected, you must investigate the discrepancy.

(b) If the unexpected result is a false negative, you must provide the laboratory with the expected results (obtained from the supplier of the blind specimen), and direct the laboratory to determine the reason for the discrepancy.

(c) If the unexpected result is a false positive, adulterated, or substituted result, you must provide the laboratory with the expected results (obtained from the supplier of the blind specimen), and direct the laboratory to determine the reason for the discrepancy. You must also notify ODAPC of the discrepancy by telephone (202-366-3784) or e-mail (addresses are listed on the ODAPC website, http://www.dot.gov/ost/dapc). ODAPC will notify HHS who will take appropriate action.

[65 FR 79526, Dec. 19, 2000, as amended at 73 FR 35971, June 25, 2008]

§ 40.107 Who may inspect laboratories?

As a laboratory, you must permit an inspection, with or without prior notice, by ODAPC, a DOT agency, or a DOT-regulated employer that contracts with the laboratory for drug testing under the DOT drug testing program, or the designee of such an employer.

§ 40.109 What documentation must the laboratory keep, and for how long?

(a) As a laboratory, you must retain all records pertaining to each employee urine specimen for a minimum of two years.

(b) As a laboratory, you must also keep for two years employer-specific data required in §40.111.

(c) Within the two-year period, the MRO, the employee, the employer, or a DOT agency may request in writing that you retain the records for an additional period of time (e.g., for the purpose of preserving evidence for litigation or a safety investigation). If you receive such a request, you must comply with it. If you do not receive such a request, you may discard the records at the end of the two-year period.

§ 40.111 When and how must a laboratory disclose statistical summaries and other information it maintains?

(a) As a laboratory, you must transmit an aggregate statistical summary, by employer, of the data listed in Appendix B to this part to the employer on a semi-annual basis.

(1) The summary must not reveal the identity of any employee.

(2) In order to avoid sending data from which it is likely that information about an employee's test result can be readily inferred, you must not send a summary if the employer has fewer than five aggregate tests results.

(3) The summary must be sent by January 20 of each year for July 1 through December 31 of the prior year.

(4) The summary must also be sent by July 20 of each year for January 1 through June 30 of the current year.

(b) When the employer requests a summary in response to an inspection, audit, or review by a DOT agency, you must provide it unless the employer had fewer than five aggregate test results. In that case, you must send the employer a report indicating that not enough testing was conducted to warrant a summary. You may transmit the summary or report by hard copy, fax, or other electronic means.

(c) You must also release information to appropriate parties as provided in §§40.329 and 40.331.

(d) As a laboratory, you must transmit an aggregate statistical summary of the data listed in Appendix C to this part to DOT on a semi-annual basis. The summary must be sent by January 31 of each year for July 1 through December 31 of the prior year; it must be sent by July 31 of each year for January 1 through June 30 of the current year.

[65 FR 79526, Dec. 19, 2000, as amended at 73 FR 35971, June 25, 2008]

§ 40.113   Where is other information concerning laboratories found in this regulation?

You can find more information concerning laboratories in several sections of this part:

§40.3—Definition.

§40.13—Prohibition on making specimens available for other purposes.

§40.31—Conflicts of interest concerning collectors.

§40.47—Laboratory rejections of test for improper form.

§40.125—Conflicts of interest concerning MROs.

§40.175—Role of first laboratory in split specimen tests.

§40.177—Role of second laboratory in split specimen tests (drugs).

§40.179—Role of second laboratory in split specimen tests (adulterants).

§40.181—Role of second laboratory in split specimen tests (substitution).

§§40.183–40.185—Transmission of split specimen test results to MRO.

§§40.201–40.205—Role in correcting errors.

§40.329—Release of information to employees.

§40.331—Limits on release of information.

§40.355—Role with respect to other service agents.

SUBPART G—MEDICAL REVIEW OFFICERS AND THE VERIFICATION PROCESS

§ 40.121   Who is qualified to act as an MRO?

To be qualified to act as an MRO in the DOT drug testing program, you must meet each of the requirements of this section:

(a) Credentials. You must be a licensed physician (Doctor of Medicine or Osteopathy). If you are a licensed physician in any U.S., Canadian, or Mexican jurisdiction and meet the other requirements of this section, you are authorized to perform MRO services with respect to all covered employees, wherever they are located. For example, if you are licensed as an M.D. in one state or province in the U.S., Canada, or Mexico, you are not limited to performing MRO functions in that state or province, and you may perform MRO functions for employees in other states or provinces without becoming licensed to practice medicine in the other jurisdictions.

(b) Basic knowledge. You must be knowledgeable in the following areas:

(1) You must be knowledgeable about and have clinical experience in controlled substances abuse disorders, including detailed knowledge of alternative medical explanations for laboratory confirmed drug test results.

(2) You must be knowledgeable about issues relating to adulterated and substituted specimens as well as the possible medical causes of specimens having an invalid result.

(3) You must be knowledgeable about this part, the DOT MRO Guidelines, and the DOT agency regulations applicable to the employers for whom you evaluate drug test results, and you must keep current on any changes to these materials. The DOT MRO Guidelines document is available from ODAPC (Department of Transportation, 1200 New Jersey Avenue, SE, Washington DC, 20590, 202–366–3784, or on the ODAPC web site (http://www.dot.gov/ost/dapc).

(c) Qualification training. You must receive qualification training meeting the requirements of this paragraph (c).

(1) Qualification training must provide instruction on the following subjects:

(i) Collection procedures for urine specimens;

(ii) Chain of custody, reporting, and recordkeeping;

(iii) Interpretation of drug and validity tests results;

(iv) The role and responsibilities of the MRO in the DOT drug testing program;

(v) The interaction with other participants in the program (e.g., DERs, SAPs); and

(vi) Provisions of this part and DOT agency rules applying to employers for whom you review test results, including changes and updates to this part and DOT agency rules, guidance, interpretations, and policies affecting the performance of MRO functions, as well as issues that MROs confront in carrying out their duties under this part and DOT agency rules.

(2) Following your completion of qualification training under paragraph (c)(1) of this section, you must satisfactorily complete an examination administered by a nationally-recognized MRO certification board or subspecialty board for medical practitioners in the field of medical review of DOT-mandated drug tests. The examination must comprehensively cover all the elements of qualification training listed in paragraph (c)(1) of this section.

(3) The following is the schedule for qualification training you must meet:

(i) If you became an MRO before August 1, 2001, and have already met the qualification training requirement, you do not have to meet it again.

(ii) If you became an MRO before August 1, 2001, but have not yet met the qualification training requirement, you must do so no later than January 31, 2003.

(iii) If you become an MRO on or after August 1, 2001, you must meet the qualification training requirement before you begin to perform MRO functions.

(d) <u>Continuing Education</u>. During each three-year period from the date on which you satisfactorily complete the examination under paragraph (c)(2) of this section, you must complete continuing education consisting of at least 12 professional development hours (e.g., Continuing Education Medical Units) relevant to performing MRO functions.

(1) This continuing education must include material concerning new technologies, interpretations, recent guidance, rule changes, and other information about developments in MRO practice, pertaining to the DOT program, since the time you met the qualification training requirements of this section.

(2) Your continuing education activities must include assessment tools to assist you in determining whether you have adequately learned the material.

(3) If you are an MRO who completed the qualification training and examination requirements prior to August 1, 2001, you must complete your first increment of 12 CEU hours before August 1, 2004.

(e) <u>Documentation</u>. You must maintain documentation showing that you currently meet all requirements of this section. You must provide this documentation on request to DOT agency representatives and to employers and C/TPAs who are using or negotiating to use your services.

[65 FR 79526, Dec. 19, 2000, as amended at 66 FR 41951, Aug. 9, 2001; 73 FR 33329, June 12, 2008]

§ 40.123 What are the MRO's responsibilities in the DOT drug testing program?

As an MRO, you have the following basic responsibilities:

(a) Acting as an independent and impartial "gatekeeper" and advocate for the accuracy and integrity of the drug testing process.

(b) Providing a quality assurance review of the drug testing process for the specimens under your purview. This includes, but is not limited to:

(1) Ensuring the review of the CCF on all specimen collections for the purposes of determining whether there is a problem that may cause a test to be cancelled (see §§40.199–40.203). As an MRO, you are not required to review laboratory internal chain of custody documentation. No one is permitted to cancel a test because you have not reviewed this documentation;

(2) Providing feedback to employers, collection sites and laboratories regarding performance issues where necessary; and

(3) Reporting to and consulting with the ODAPC or a relevant DOT agency when you wish DOT assistance in resolving any program issue. As an employer or service agent, you are prohibited from limiting or attempting to limit the MRO's access to DOT for this purpose and from retaliating in any way against an MRO for discussing drug testing issues with DOT.

(c) You must determine whether there is a legitimate medical explanation for confirmed positive, adulterated, substituted, and invalid drug tests results from the laboratory.

(d) While you provide medical review of employees' test results, this part does not deem that you have established a doctor-patient relationship with the employees whose tests you review.

(e) You must act to investigate and correct problems where possible and notify appropriate parties (e.g., HHS, DOT, employers, service agents) where assistance is needed, (e.g., cancelled or problematic tests, incorrect results, problems with blind specimens).

(f) You must ensure the timely flow of test results and other information to employers.

(g) You must protect the confidentiality of the drug testing information.

(h) You must perform all your functions in compliance with this part and other DOT agency regulations.

§ 40.125 What relationship may an MRO have with a laboratory?

As an MRO, you may not enter into any relationship with an employer's laboratory that creates a conflict of interest or the appearance of a conflict of interest with your responsibilities to that employer. You may not derive any financial benefit by having an employer use a specific laboratory. For examples of relationships between laboratories and MROs that the Department views as creating a conflict of interest or the appearance of such a conflict, see §40.101(b).

§ 40.127 What are the MRO's functions in reviewing negative test results?

As the MRO, you must do the following with respect to negative drug test results you receive from a laboratory, prior to verifying the result and releasing it to the DER:

(a) Review Copy 2 of the CCF to determine if there are any fatal or correctable errors that may require you to initiate corrective action or to cancel the test (see §§40.199 and 40.203).

(b) Review the negative laboratory test result and ensure that it is consistent with the information contained on the CCF.

(c) Before you report a negative test result, you must have in your possession the following documents:

(1) Copy 2 of the CCF, a legible copy of it, or any other CCF copy containing the employee's signature; and

(2) A legible copy (fax, photocopy, image) of Copy 1 of the CCF or the electronic laboratory results report that conveys the negative laboratory test result.

(d) If the copy of the documentation provided to you by the collector or laboratory appears unclear, you must request that the collector or laboratory send you a legible copy.

(e) On Copy 2 of the CCF, place a check mark in the "Negative" box (Step 6), provide your name, and sign, initial, or stamp and date the verification statement.

(f) Report the result in a confidential manner (see §§40.163–40.167).

(g) Staff under your direct, personal supervision may perform the administrative functions of this section for you, but only you can cancel a test. If you cancel a laboratory-confirmed negative result, check the "Test Cancelled" box (Step 6) on Copy 2 of the CCF, make appropriate annotation in the "Remarks" line, provide your name, and sign, initial or stamp and date the verification statement.

(1) On specimen results that are reviewed by your staff, you are responsible for assuring the quality of their work.

(2) You are required to personally review at least 5 percent of all CCFs reviewed by your staff on a quarterly basis, including all results that required a corrective action. However, you need not review more than 500 negative results in any quarter.

(3) Your review must, as a minimum, include the CCF, negative laboratory test result, any accompanying corrective documents, and the report sent to the employer. You must correct any errors that you discover. You must take action as necessary to ensure compliance by your staff with this part and document your corrective action. You must attest to the quality assurance review by initialing the CCFs that you review.

(4) You must make these CCFs easily identifiable and retrievable by you for review by DOT agencies.

[65 FR 79526, Dec. 19, 2000, as amended at 66 FR 41951, Aug. 9, 2001]

§ 40.129 What are the MRO's functions in reviewing laboratory confirmed non-negative drug test results?

(a) As the MRO, you must do the following with respect to confirmed positive, adulterated, substituted, or invalid drug tests you receive from a laboratory, before you verify the result and release it to the DER:

(1) Review Copy 2 of the CCF to determine if there are any fatal or correctable errors that may require you to cancel the test (see §§40.199 and 40.203). Staff under your direct, personal supervision may conduct this administrative review for you, but only you may verify or cancel a test.

(2) Review Copy 1 of the CCF and ensure that it is consistent with the information contained on Copy 2, that the test result is legible, and that the certifying scientist signed the form. You are not required to review any other documentation generated by the laboratory during their analysis or handling of the specimen (e.g., the laboratory internal chain of custody).

(3) If the copy of the documentation provided to you by the collector or laboratory appears unclear, you must request that the collector or laboratory send you a legible copy.

(4) Except in the circumstances spelled out in §40.133, conduct a verification interview. This interview must include direct contact in person or by telephone between you and the employee. You may initiate the verification process based on the laboratory results report.

(5) Verify the test result, consistent with the requirements of §§ 40.135 through 40.145, 40.159, and 40.160, as:

(i) Negative; or

(ii) Cancelled; or

(iii) Positive, and/or refusal to test because of adulteration or substitution.

(b) Before you report a verified negative, positive, test cancelled, refusal to test because of adulteration or substitution, you must have in your possession the following documents:

(1) Copy 2 of the CCF, a legible copy of it, or any other CCF copy containing the employee's signature; and

(2) A legible copy (fax, photocopy, image) of Copy 1 of the CCF, containing the certifying scientist's signature.

(c) With respect to verified positive test results, place a check mark in the "Positive" box (Step 6) on Copy 2 of the CCF, indicate the drug(s)/metabolite(s) detected on the "Remarks" line, sign and date the verification statement.

(d) If you cancel a laboratory confirmed positive, adulterated, substituted, or invalid drug test report, check the "test cancelled" box (Step 6) on Copy 2 of the CCF, make appropriate annotation in the "Remarks" line, sign, provide your name, and date the verification statement.

(e) Report the result in a confidential manner (see §§40.163–40.167).

(f) With respect to adulteration or substitution test results, check the "refusal to test because:" box (Step 6) on Copy 2 of the CCF, check the "Adulterated" or "Substituted" box, as appropriate, make appropriate annotation in the "Remarks" line, sign and date the verification statement.

(g) As the MRO, your actions concerning reporting confirmed positive, adulterated, or substituted results to the employer before you have completed the verification process are also governed by the stand-down provisions of §40.21.

(1) If an employer has a stand-down policy that meets the requirements of §40.21, you may report to the DER that you have received an employee's laboratory confirmed positive, adulterated, or substituted test result, consistent with the terms of the waiver the employer received. You must not provide any further details about the test result (e.g., the name of the drug involved).

(2) If the employer does not have a stand-down policy that meets the requirements of §40.21, you must not inform the employer that you have received an employee's laboratory confirmed positive, adulterated, or substituted test result until you verify the test result. For example, as an MRO employed directly by a company, you must not tell anyone on the company's staff or management that you have received an employee's laboratory confirmed test result.

[65 FR 79526, Dec. 19, 2000, as amended at 66 FR 41952, Aug. 9, 2001; 73 FR 35971, June 25, 2008]

§ 40.131 How does the MRO or DER notify an employee of the verification process after receiving laboratory confirmed non-negative drug test results?

(a) When, as the MRO, you receive a confirmed positive, adulterated, substituted, or invalid test result from the laboratory, you must contact the employee directly (i.e., actually talk to the employee), on a confidential basis, to determine whether the employee wants to discuss the test result. In making this contact, you must explain to the employee that, if he or she declines to discuss the result, you will verify the test as positive or as a refusal to test because of adulteration or substitution, as applicable.

(b) As the MRO, staff under your personal supervision may conduct this initial contact for you.

(1) This staff contact must be limited to scheduling the discussion between you and the employee and explaining the consequences of the employee's declining to speak with you (i.e., that the MRO will verify the test without input from the employee). If the employee declines to speak with you, the staff person must document the employee's decision, including the date and time.

(2) A staff person must not gather any medical information or information concerning possible explanations for the test result.

(3) A staff person may advise an employee to have medical information (e.g., prescriptions, information forming the basis of a legitimate medical explanation for a confirmed positive test result) ready to present at the interview with the MRO.

(4) Since you are required to speak personally with the employee, face-to-face or on the phone, your staff must not inquire if the employee wishes to speak with you.

(c) As the MRO, you or your staff must make reasonable efforts to reach the employee at the day and evening telephone numbers listed on the CCF. Reasonable efforts include, as a minimum, three attempts, spaced reasonably over a 24-hour period, to reach the employee at the day and evening telephone numbers listed on the CCF. If you or your staff cannot reach the employee directly after making these efforts, you or your staff must take the following steps:

(1) Document the efforts you made to contact the employee, including dates and times. If both phone numbers are incorrect (e.g., disconnected, wrong number), you may take the actions listed in paragraph (c)(2) of this section without waiting the full 24-hour period.

(2) Contact the DER, instructing the DER to contact the employee.

(i) You must simply direct the DER to inform the employee to contact you.

(ii) You must not inform the DER that the employee has a confirmed positive, adulterated, substituted, or invalid test result.

(iii) You must document the dates and times of your attempts to contact the DER, and you must document the name of the DER you contacted and the date and time of the contact.

(d) As the DER, you must attempt to contact the employee immediately, using procedures that protect, as much as possible, the confidentiality of the MRO's request that the employee contact the MRO. If you successfully contact the employee (i.e., actually talk to the employee), you must document the date and time of the contact, and inform the MRO. You must inform the employee that he or she should contact the MRO immediately. You must also inform the employee of the consequences of failing to contact the MRO within the next 72 hours (see §40.133(a)(2)).

(1) As the DER, you must not inform anyone else working for the employer that you are seeking to contact the employee on behalf of the MRO.

(2) If, as the DER, you have made all reasonable efforts to contact the employee but failed to do so, you may place the employee on temporary medically unqualified status or medical leave. Reasonable efforts include, as a minimum, three attempts, spaced reasonably over a 24-hour period, to reach the employee at the day and evening telephone numbers listed on the CCF.

(i) As the DER, you must document the dates and times of these efforts.

(ii) If, as the DER, you are unable to contact the employee within this 24-hour period, you must leave a message for the employee by any practicable means (e.g., voice mail, e-mail, letter) to contact the MRO and inform the MRO of the date and time of this attempted contact.

[65 FR 79526, Dec. 19, 2000, as amended at 66 FR 41952, Aug. 9, 2001; 68 FR 31626, May 28, 2003; 69 FR 64867, Nov.9, 2004; 73 FR 35971, June 25, 2008]

§ 40.133   Without interviewing the employee, under what circumstances may the MRO verify a test result as positive, or as a refusal to test because of adulteration or substitution, or as cancelled because the test was invalid?

(a) As the MRO, you normally may verify a confirmed positive test (for any drug or drug metabolite, including opiates), or as a refusal to test because of adulteration or substitution, only after interviewing the employee as provided in §§40.135–40.145. However, there are three circumstances in which you may verify such a result without an interview:

(1) You may verify a test result as a positive or refusal to test, as applicable, if the employee expressly declines the opportunity to discuss the test with you. You must maintain complete documentation of this occurrence, including notation of informing, or attempting to inform, the employee of the consequences of not exercising the option to speak with you.

(2) You may verify a test result as a positive or refusal to test, as applicable, if the DER has successfully made and documented a contact with the employee and instructed the employee to contact you and more than 72 hours have passed since the time the DER contacted the employee.

(3) You may verify a test result as a positive or refusal to test, as applicable, if neither you nor the DER, after making and documenting all reasonable efforts, has been able to contact the employee within ten days of the date on which the MRO receives the confirmed test result from the laboratory.

(b) As the MRO, you may verify an invalid test result as cancelled (with instructions to recollect immediately under direct observation) without interviewing the employee, as provided at § 40.159:

(1) If the employee expressly declines the opportunity to discuss the test with you;

(2) If the DER has successfully made and documented a contact with the employee and instructed the employee to contact you and more than 72 hours have passed since the time the DER contacted the employee; or

(3) If neither you nor the DER, after making and documenting all reasonable efforts, has been able to contact the employee within ten days of the date on which you received the confirmed invalid test result from the laboratory.

(c) As the MRO, after you verify a test result as a positive or as a refusal to test under this section, you must document the date and time and reason, following the instructions in § 40.163. For a cancelled test due to an invalid result under this section, you must follow the instructions in § 40.159(a)(5).

(d) As the MRO, after you have verified a test result under this section and reported the result to the DER, you must allow the employee to present information to you within 60 days of the verification to document that serious illness, injury, or other circumstances unavoidably precluded contact with the MRO and/or DER in the times provided. On the basis of such information, you may reopen the verification, allowing the employee to present information concerning whether there is a legitimate medical explanation of the confirmed test result.

[65 FR 79526, Dec. 19, 2000, as amended at 73 FR 35971, June 25, 2008]

§ 40.135   What does the MRO tell the employee at the beginning of the verification interview?

(a) As the MRO, you must tell the employee that the laboratory has determined that the employee's test result was positive, adulterated, substituted, or invalid, as applicable. You must also tell the employee of the drugs for which his or her specimen tested positive, or the basis for the finding of adulteration or substitution.

(b) You must explain the verification interview process to the employee and inform the employee that your decision will be based on information the employee provides in the interview.

(c) You must explain that, if further medical evaluation is needed for the verification process, the employee must comply with your request for this evaluation and that failure to do so is equivalent of expressly declining to discuss the test result.

(d) As the MRO, you must warn an employee who has a confirmed positive, adulterated, substituted or invalid test that you are required to provide to third parties drug test result information and medical information affecting the performance of safety-sensitive duties that the employee gives you in the verification process without the employee's consent (see §40.327).

(1) You must give this warning to the employee before obtaining any medical information as part of the verification process.

(2) For purposes of this paragraph (d), medical information includes information on medications or other substances affecting the performance of safety-sensitive duties that the employee reports using or medical conditions the employee reports having.

(3) For purposes of this paragraph (d), the persons to whom this information may be provided include the employer, a SAP evaluating the employee as part of the return to duty process (see §40.293(g)), DOT, another Federal safety agency (e.g., the NTSB), or any state safety agency as required by state law.

(e) You must also advise the employee that, after informing any third party about any medication the employee is using pursuant to a legally valid prescription under the Controlled Substances Act, you will allow 5 days for the employee to have the prescribing physician contact you to determine if the medication can be changed to one that does not make the employee medically unqualified or does not pose a significant safety risk. If, as an MRO, you receive such information from the prescribing physician, you must transmit this information to any third party to whom you previously provided information about the safety risks of the employee's other medication.

[65 FR 79526, Dec. 19, 2000, as amended at 66 FR 41952, Aug. 9, 2001]

§ 40.137 On what basis does the MRO verify test results involving marijuana, cocaine, amphetamines, or PCP?

(a) As the MRO, you must verify a confirmed positive test result for marijuana, cocaine, amphetamines, and/or PCP unless the employee presents a legitimate medical explanation for the presence of the drug(s)/metabolite(s) in his or her system.

(b) You must offer the employee an opportunity to present a legitimate medical explanation in all cases.

(c) The employee has the burden of proof that a legitimate medical explanation exists. The employee must present information meeting this burden at the time of the verification interview. As the MRO, you have discretion to extend the time available to the employee for this purpose for up to five days before verifying the test result, if you determine that there is a reasonable basis to believe that the employee will be able to produce relevant evidence concerning a legitimate medical explanation within that time.

(d) If you determine that there is a legitimate medical explanation, you must verify the test result as negative. Otherwise, you must verify the test result as positive.

(e) In determining whether a legitimate medical explanation exists, you may consider the employee's use of a medication from a foreign country. You must exercise your professional judgment consistently with the following principles:

(1) There can be a legitimate medical explanation only with respect to a substance that is obtained legally in a foreign country.

(2) There can be a legitimate medical explanation only with respect to a substance that has a legitimate medical use. Use of a drug of abuse (e.g., heroin, PCP, marijuana) or any other substance (see §40.151(f) and (g)) that cannot be viewed as having a legitimate medical use can never be the basis for a legitimate medical explanation, even if the substance is obtained legally in a foreign country.

(3) Use of the substance can form the basis of a legitimate medical explanation only if it is used consistently with its proper and intended medical purpose.

(4) Even if you find that there is a legitimate medical explanation under this paragraph (e) and verify a test negative, you may have a responsibility to raise fitness-for-duty considerations with the employer (see §40.327).

§ 40.139 On what basis does the MRO verify test results involving opiates?

As the MRO, you must proceed as follows when you receive a laboratory confirmed positive opiate result:

(a) If the laboratory detects the presence of 6-acetylmorphine (6-AM) in the specimen, you must verify the test result positive.

(b) In the absence of 6-AM, if the laboratory detects the presence of either morphine or codeine at 15,000 ng/mL or above, you must verify the test result positive unless the employee presents a legitimate medical explanation for the presence of the drug or drug metabolite in his or her system, as in the case of other drugs (see §40.137). Consumption of food products (e.g., poppy seeds) must not be considered a legitimate medical explanation for the employee having morphine or codeine at these concentrations.

(c) For all other opiate positive results, you must verify a confirmed positive test result for opiates only if you determine that there is clinical evidence, in addition to the urine test, of unauthorized use of any opium, opiate, or opium derivative (i.e., morphine, heroin, or codeine).

(1) As an MRO, it is your responsibility to use your best professional and ethical judgement and discretion to determine whether there is clinical evidence of unauthorized use of opiates. Examples of information that you may consider in making this judgement include, but are not limited to, the following:

(i) Recent needle tracks;

(ii) Behavioral and psychological signs of acute opiate intoxication or withdrawal;

(iii) Clinical history of unauthorized use recent enough to have produced the laboratory test result;

(iv) Use of a medication from a foreign country. See §40.137(e) for guidance on how to make this determination.

(2) In order to establish the clinical evidence referenced in paragraphs (c)(1)(i) and (ii) of this section, personal observation of the employee is essential.

(i) Therefore, you, as the MRO, must conduct, or cause another physician to conduct, a face-to-face examination of the employee.

(ii) No face-to-face examination is needed in establishing the clinical evidence referenced in paragraph (c)(1)(iii) or (iv) of this section.

(3) To be the basis of a verified positive result for opiates, the clinical evidence you find must concern a drug that the laboratory found in the specimen. (For example, if the test confirmed the presence of codeine, and the employee admits to unauthorized use of hydrocodone, you do not have grounds for verifying the test positive. The admission must be for the substance that was found).

(4) As the MRO, you have the burden of establishing that there is clinical evidence of unauthorized use of opiates referenced in this paragraph (c). If you cannot make this determination (e.g., there is not sufficient clinical evidence or history), you must verify the test as negative. The employee does not need to show you that a legitimate medical explanation exists if no clinical evidence is established.

§ 40.141   How does the MRO obtain information for the verification decision?

As the MRO, you must do the following as you make the determinations needed for a verification decision:

(a) You must conduct a medical interview. You must review the employee's medical history and any other relevant biomedical factors presented to you by the employee. You may direct the employee to undergo further medical evaluation by you or another physician.

(b) If the employee asserts that the presence of a drug or drug metabolite in his or her specimen results from taking prescription medication, you must review and take all reasonable and necessary steps to verify the authenticity of all medical records the employee provides. You may contact the employee's physician or other relevant medical personnel for further information.

§ 40.143   [Reserved]

§ 40.145   On what basis does the MRO verify test results involving adulteration or substitution?

(a) As an MRO, when you receive a laboratory report that a specimen is adulterated or substituted, you must treat that report in the same way you treat the laboratory's report of a confirmed positive test for a drug or drug metabolite.

(b) You must follow the same procedures used for verification of a confirmed positive test for a drug or drug metabolite (see §§40.129–40.135, 40.141, 40.151), except as otherwise provided in this section.

(c) In the verification interview, you must explain the laboratory findings to the employee and address technical questions or issues the employee may raise.

(d) You must offer the employee the opportunity to present a legitimate medical explanation for the laboratory findings with respect to presence of the adulterant in, or the creatinine and specific gravity findings for, the specimen.

(e) The employee has the burden of proof that there is a legitimate medical explanation.

(1) To meet this burden in the case of an adulterated specimen, the employee must demonstrate that the adulterant found by the laboratory entered the specimen through physiological means.

(2) To meet this burden in the case of a substituted specimen, the employee must demonstrate that he or she did produce or could have produced urine through physiological means, meeting the creatinine concentration criterion of less than 2 mg/dL and the specific gravity of less than or equal to 1.0010 or greater than or equal to 1.0200 (see §40.93(b)).

(3) The employee must present information meeting this burden at the time of the verification interview. As the MRO, you have discretion to extend the time available to the employee for this purpose for up to five days before verifying the specimen, if you determine that there is a reasonable basis to believe that the employee will be able to produce relevant evidence supporting a legitimate medical explanation within that time.

(f) As the MRO or the employer, you are not responsible for arranging, conducting, or paying for any studies, examinations or analyses to determine whether a legitimate medical explanation exists.

(g) As the MRO, you must exercise your best professional judgment in deciding whether the employee has established a legitimate medical explanation.

(1) If you determine that the employee's explanation does not present a reasonable basis for concluding that there may be a legitimate medical explanation, you must report the test to the DER as a verified refusal to test because of adulteration or substitution, as applicable.

(2) If you believe that the employee's explanation may present a reasonable basis for concluding that there is a legitimate medical explanation, you must direct the employee to obtain, within the five-day period set forth in paragraph (e)(3) of this section, a further medical evaluation. This evaluation must be performed by a licensed physician (the "referral physician"), acceptable to you, with expertise in the medical issues raised by the employee's explanation. (The MRO may perform this evaluation if the MRO has appropriate expertise.)

(i) As the MRO or employer, you are not responsible for finding or paying a referral physician. However, on request of the employee, you must provide reasonable assistance to the employee's efforts to find such a physician. The final choice of the referral physician is the employee's, as long as the physician is acceptable to you.

(ii) As the MRO, you must consult with the referral physician, providing guidance to him or her concerning his or her responsibilities under this section. As part of this consultation, you must provide the following information to the referral physician:

(A) That the employee was required to take a DOT drug test, but the laboratory reported that the specimen was adulterated or substituted, which is treated as a refusal to test;

(B) The consequences of the appropriate DOT agency regulation for refusing to take the required drug test;

(C) That the referral physician must agree to follow the requirements of paragraphs (g)(3) through (g)(4) of this section; and

(D) That the referral physician must provide you with a signed statement of his or her recommendations.

(3) As the referral physician, you must evaluate the employee and consider any evidence the employee presents concerning the employee's medical explanation. You may conduct additional tests to determine whether there is a legitimate medical explanation. Any additional urine tests must be performed in an HHS-certified laboratory.

(4) As the referral physician, you must then make a written recommendation to the MRO about whether the MRO should determine that there is a legitimate medical explanation. As the MRO, you must seriously consider and assess the referral physician's recommendation in deciding whether there is a legitimate medical explanation.

(5) As the MRO, if you determine that there is a legitimate medical explanation, you must cancel the test and inform ODAPC in writing of the determination and the basis for it (e.g., referral physician's findings, evidence produced by the employee).

(6) As the MRO, if you determine that there is not a legitimate medical explanation, you must report the test to the DER as a verified refusal to test because of adulteration or substitution.

(h) The following are examples of types of evidence an employee could present to support an assertion of a legitimate medical explanation for a substituted result.

(1) Medically valid evidence demonstrating that the employee is capable of physiologically producing urine meeting the creatinine and specific gravity criteria of §40.93(b).

(i) To be regarded as medically valid, the evidence must have been gathered using appropriate methodology and controls to ensure its accuracy and reliability.

(ii) Assertion by the employee that his or her personal characteristics (e.g., with respect to race, gender, weight, diet, working conditions) are responsible for the substituted result does not, in itself, constitute a legitimate medical explanation. To make a case that there is a legitimate medical explanation, the employee must present evidence showing that the cited personal characteristics actually result in the physiological production of urine meeting the creatinine and specific gravity criteria of §40.93(b).

(2) Information from a medical evaluation under paragraph (g) of this section that the individual has a medical condition that has been demonstrated to cause the employee to physiologically produce urine meeting the creatinine and specific gravity criteria of §40.93(b).

(i) A finding or diagnosis by the physician that an employee has a medical condition, in itself, does not constitute a legitimate medical explanation.

(ii) To establish there is a legitimate medical explanation, the employee must demonstrate that the cited medical condition actually results in the physiological production of urine meeting the creatinine and specific gravity criteria of §40.93(b).

[65 FR 79526, Dec. 19, 2000, as amended at 68 FR 31626, May 28, 2003; 69 FR 64867, Nov.9, 2004]

§ 40.147   [Reserved]

§ 40.149   May the MRO change a verified drug test result?

(a) As the MRO, you may change a verified test result only in the following situations:

(1) When you have reopened a verification that was done without an interview with an employee (see §40.133(d)).

(2) If you receive information, not available to you at the time of the original verification, demonstrating that the laboratory made an error in identifying (e.g., a paperwork mistake) or testing (e.g., a false positive or negative) the employee's primary or split specimen. For example, suppose the laboratory originally reported a positive test result for Employee X and a negative result for Employee Y. You verified the test results as reported to you. Then the laboratory notifies you that it mixed up the two test results, and X was really negative and Y was really positive. You would change X's test result from positive to negative and contact Y to conduct a verification interview.

(3) If, within 60 days of the original verification decision—

(i) You receive information that could not reasonably have been provided to you at the time of the decision demonstrating that there is a legitimate medical explanation for the presence of drug(s)/metabolite(s) in the employee's specimen; or

(ii) You receive credible new or additional evidence that a legitimate medical explanation for an adulterated or substituted result exists.

Example to Paragraph (a)(3): If the employee's physician provides you a valid prescription that he or she failed to find at the time of the original verification, you may change the test result from positive to negative if you conclude that the prescription provides a legitimate medical explanation for the drug(s)/metabolite(s) in the employee's specimen.

(4) If you receive the information in paragraph (a)(3) of this section after the 60-day period, you must consult with ODAPC prior to changing the result.

(5) When you have made an administrative error and reported an incorrect result.

(b) If you change the result, you must immediately notify the DER in writing, as provided in §§40.163–40.165.

(c) You are the only person permitted to change a verified test result, such as a verified positive test result or a determination that an individual has refused to test because of adulteration or substitution. This is because, as the MRO, you have the sole authority under this part to make medical determinations leading to a verified test (e.g., a determination that there was or was not a legitimate medical explanation for a laboratory test result). For example, an arbitrator is not permitted to overturn the medical judgment of the MRO that the employee failed to present a legitimate medical explanation for a positive, adulterated, or substituted test result of his or her specimen.

[65 FR 79526, Dec. 19, 2000, as amended at 66 FR 41952, Aug. 9, 2001; 73 FR 35971, June 25, 2008]

§ 40.151 What are MROs prohibited from doing as part of the verification process?

As an MRO, you are prohibited from doing the following as part of the verification process:

(a) You must not consider any evidence from tests of urine samples or other body fluids or tissues (e.g., blood or hair samples) that are not collected or tested in accordance with this part. For example, if an employee tells you he went to his own physician, provided a urine specimen, sent it to a laboratory, and received a negative test result or a DNA test result questioning the identity of his DOT specimen, you are required to ignore this test result.

(b) It is not your function to make decisions about factual disputes between the employee and the collector concerning matters occurring at the collection site that are not reflected on the CCF (e.g., concerning allegations that the collector left the area or left open urine containers where other people could access them).

(c) It is not your function to determine whether the employer should have directed that a test occur. For example, if an employee tells you that the employer misidentified her as the subject of a random

test, or directed her to take a reasonable suspicion or post-accident test without proper grounds under a DOT agency drug or alcohol regulation, you must inform the employee that you cannot play a role in deciding these issues.

(d) It is not your function to consider explanations of confirmed positive, adulterated, or substituted test results that would not, even if true, constitute a legitimate medical explanation. For example, an employee may tell you that someone slipped amphetamines into her drink at a party, that she unknowingly ingested a marijuana brownie, or that she traveled in a closed car with several people smoking crack. MROs are unlikely to be able to verify the facts of such passive or unknowing ingestion stories. Even if true, such stories do not present a legitimate medical explanation. Consequently, you must not declare a test as negative based on an explanation of this kind.

(e) You must not verify a test negative based on information that a physician recommended that the employee use a drug listed in Schedule I of the Controlled Substances Act. (e.g., under a state law that purports to authorize such recommendations, such as the "medical marijuana" laws that some states have adopted).

(f) You must not accept an assertion of consumption or other use of a hemp or other non-prescription marijuana-related product as a basis for verifying a marijuana test negative. You also must not accept such an explanation related to consumption of coca teas as a basis for verifying a cocaine test result as negative. Consuming or using such a product is not a legitimate medical explanation.

(g) You must not accept an assertion that there is a legitimate medical explanation for the presence of PCP or 6-AM in a specimen. There are no legitimate medical explanations for the presence of these substances.

(h) You must not accept, as a legitimate medical explanation for an adulterated specimen, an assertion that soap, bleach, or glutaraldehyde entered a specimen through physiological means. There are no physiological means through which these substances can enter a specimen.

(i) You must not accept, as a legitimate medical explanation for a substituted specimen, an assertion that an employee can produce urine with no detectable creatinine. There are no physiological means through which a person can produce a urine specimen having this characteristic.

[65 FR 79526, Dec. 19, 2000, as amended at 66 FR 41952, Aug. 9, 2001]

§ 40.153 How does the MRO notify employees of their right to a test of the split specimen?

(a) As the MRO, when you have verified a drug test as positive for a drug or drug metabolite, or as a refusal to test because of adulteration or substitution, you must notify the employee of his or her right to have the split specimen tested. You must also notify the employee of the procedures for requesting a test of the split specimen.

(b) You must inform the employee that he or she has 72 hours from the time you provide this notification to him or her to request a test of the split specimen.

(c) You must tell the employee how to contact you to make this request. You must provide telephone numbers or other information that will allow the employee to make this request. As the MRO, you must have the ability to receive the employee's calls at all times during the 72 hour period (e.g., by use of an answering machine with a "time stamp" feature when there is no one in your office to answer the phone).

(d) You must tell the employee that if he or she makes this request within 72 hours, the employer must ensure that the test takes place, and that the employee is not required to pay for the test from his or her own funds before the test takes place. You must also tell the employee that the employer may seek reimbursement for the cost of the test (see §40.173).

(e) You must tell the employee that additional tests of the specimen (e.g., DNA tests) are not authorized.

§ 40.155 What does the MRO do when a negative or positive test result is also dilute?

(a) When the laboratory reports that a specimen is dilute, you must, as the MRO, report to the DER that the specimen, in addition to being negative or positive, is dilute.

(b) You must check the "dilute" box (Step 6) on Copy 2 of the CCF.

(c) When you report a dilute specimen to the DER, you must explain to the DER the employer's obligations and choices under §40.197, to include the requirement for an immediate recollection under direct observation if the creatinine concentration of a negative-dilute specimen was greater than or equal to 2mg/dL but less than or equal to 5 mg/dL.

(d) If the employee's recollection under direct observation, in paragraph (c) of this section, results in another negative-dilute, as the MRO, you must:

(1) Review the CCF to ensure that there is documentation that the recollection was directly observed.

(2) If the CCF documentation shows that the recollection was directly observed as required, report this result to the DER as a negative-dilute result.

(3) If CCF documentation indicates that the recollection was not directly observed as required, do not report a result but again explain to the DER that there must be an immediate recollection under direct observation.

[65 FR 79526, Dec. 19, 2000, as amended at 66 FR 41952, Aug. 9, 2001; 68 FR 31626, May 28, 2003; 69 FR 64867, Nov. 9, 2004; 73 FR 35971, June 25, 2008]

§ 40.157 [Reserved]

§ 40.159 What does the MRO do when a drug test result is invalid?

(a) As the MRO, when the laboratory reports that the test result is an invalid result, you must do the following:

(1) Discuss the laboratory results with a certifying scientist to determine if the primary specimen should be tested at another HHS certified laboratory. If the laboratory did not contact you as required by §§ 40.91(e) and 40.96(c), you must contact the laboratory.

(2) If you and the laboratory have determined that no further testing is necessary, contact the employee and inform the employee that the specimen was invalid. In contacting the employee, use the procedures set forth in § 40.131.

(3) After explaining the limits of disclosure (see §§ 40.135(d) and 40.327), you must determine if the employee has a medical explanation for the invalid result. You must inquire about the medications the employee may have taken.

(4) If the employee gives an explanation that is acceptable, you must:

(i) Place a check mark in the "Test Cancelled" box (Step 6) on Copy 2 of the CCF and enter "Invalid Result" and "direct observation collection not required" on the "Remarks" line.

(ii) Report to the DER that the test is cancelled, the reason for cancellation, and that no further action is required unless a negative test result is required (i.e., pre-employment, return-to-duty, or follow-up tests).

(iii) If a negative test result is required and the medical explanation concerns a situation in which the employee has a permanent or long-term medical condition that precludes him or her from providing a valid specimen, as the MRO, you must follow the procedures outlined at § 40.160 for determining if there is clinical evidence that the individual is an illicit drug user.

(5) If the employee is unable to provide an explanation and/or a valid prescription for a medication that interfered with the immunoassay test but denies having adulterated the specimen, you must:

(i) Place a check mark in the "Test Cancelled" box (Step 6) on Copy 2 of the CCF and enter "Invalid Result" and "direct observation collection required" on the "Remarks" line.

(ii) Report to the DER that the test is cancelled, the reason for cancellation, and that a second collection must take place immediately under direct observation.

(iii) Instruct the employer to ensure that the employee has the minimum possible advance notice that he or she must go to the collection site.

(b) You may only report an invalid test result when you are in possession of a legible copy of Copy 1 of the CCF. In addition, you must have Copy 2 of the CCF, a legible copy of it, or any other copy of the CCF containing the employee's signature.

(c) If the employee admits to having adulterated or substituted the specimen, you must, on the same day, write and sign your own statement of what the employee told you. You must then report a refusal to test in accordance with §40.163.

(d) If the employee admits to using a drug, you must, on the same day, write and sign your own statement of what the employee told you. You must then report that admission to the DER for appropriate action under DOT Agency regulations. This test will be reported as cancelled with the reason noted.

(e) If the employee's recollection (required at paragraph (a)(5) of this section) results in another invalid result for the same reason as reported for the first specimen, as the MRO, you must:

(1) Review the CCF to ensure that there is documentation that the recollection was directly observed.

(2) If the CCF review indicates that the recollection was directly observed as required, document that the employee had another specimen with an invalid result for the same reason.

(3) Follow the recording and reporting procedures at (a)(4)(i) and (ii) of this section.

(4) If a negative result is required (i.e., preemployment, return-to-duty, or follow-up tests), follow the procedures at § 40.160 for determining if there is clinical evidence that the individual is an illicit drug user.

(5) If the recollection was not directly observed as required, do not report a result but again explain to the DER that there must be an immediate recollection under direct observation.

(f) If the employee's recollection (required at paragraph (a)(5) of this section) results in another invalid result for a different reason than that reported for the first specimen, as the MRO, you must:

(1) Review the CCF to ensure that there is documentation that the recollection was directly observed.

(2) If the CCF review indicates that the recollection was directly observed as required, document that the employee had another specimen with an invalid result for a different reason.

(3) As the MRO, you should not contact the employee to discuss the result, but rather direct the DER to conduct an immediate recollection under direct observation without prior notification to the employee.

(4) If the CCF documentation indicates that the recollection was not directly observed as required, do not report a result but again explain to the DER that there must be an immediate recollection under direct observation.

(g) If, as the MRO, you receive a laboratory invalid result in conjunction with a positive, adulterated, and/or substituted result and you verify any of those results as being a positive and/or refusal to test, you do not report the invalid result unless the split specimen fails to reconfirm the result(s) of the primary specimen.

[65 FR 79526, Dec. 19, 2000 as amended at 73 FR 35972, June 25, 2008]

§ 40.160   What does the MRO do when a valid test result cannot be produced and a negative result is required?

(a) If a valid test result cannot be produced and a negative result is required, (under § 40.159 (a)(5)(iii) and (e)(4)), as the MRO, you must determine if there is clinical evidence that the individual is currently an illicit drug user. You must make this determination by personally conducting, or causing to be conducted, a medical evaluation. In addition, if appropriate, you may also consult with the employee's physician to gather information you need to reach this determination.

(b) If you do not personally conduct the medical evaluation, as the MRO, you must ensure that one is conducted by a licensed physician acceptable to you.

(c) For purposes of this section, the MRO or the physician conducting the evaluation may conduct an alternative test (e.g., blood) as part of the medically appropriate procedures in determining clinical evidence of drug use.

(d) If the medical evaluation reveals no clinical evidence of drug use, as the MRO, you must report this to the employer as a negative test result with written notations regarding the medical examination. The report must also state why the medical examination was required (i.e., either the basis for the determination that a permanent or long-term medical condition exists or because the recollection under direct observation resulted in another invalid result for the same reason, as appropriate) and for the determination that no signs and symptoms of drug use exist.

(1) Check "Negative" (Step 6) on the CCF.

(2) Sign and date the CCF.

(e) If the medical evaluation reveals clinical evidence of drug use, as the MRO, you must report the result to the employer as a cancelled test with written notations regarding the results of the medical examination. The report must also state why the medical examination was required (i.e., either the basis for the determination that a permanent or long-term medical condition exists or because the recollection under direct observation resulted in another invalid result for the same reason, as appropriate) and state the reason for the determination that signs and symptoms of drug use exist. Because this is a cancelled test, it does not serve the purpose of an actual negative test result (i.e., the employer is not authorized to allow the employee to begin or resume performing safety-sensitive functions, because a negative test result is needed for that purpose).

[73 FR 35972, June 25, 2008]

§ 40.161   What does the MRO do when a drug test specimen is rejected for testing?

As the MRO, when the laboratory reports that the specimen is rejected for testing (e.g., because of a fatal or uncorrected flaw), you must do the following:

(a) Place a check mark in the "Test Cancelled" box (Step 6) on Copy 2 of the CCF and enter the reason on the "Remarks" line.

(b) Report to the DER that the test is cancelled and the reason for cancellation, and that no further action is required unless a negative test is required (e.g., in the case of a pre-employment, return-to-duty, or follow-up test).

(c) You may only report a test cancelled because of a rejected for testing test result when you are in possession of a legible copy of Copy 1 of the CCF. In addition, you must have Copy 2 of the CCF, a legible copy of it, or any other copy of the CCF containing the employee's signature.

§ 40.162   What must MROs do with multiple verified results for the same testing event?

(a) If the testing event is one in which there was one specimen collection with multiple verified non-negative results, as the MRO, you must report them all to the DER. For example, if you verified the specimen as being positive for marijuana and cocaine and as being a refusal to test because the specimen was also adulterated, as the MRO, you should report the positives and the refusal to the DER.

(b) If the testing event was one in which two separate specimen collections (e.g., a specimen out of temperature range and the subsequent observed collection) were sent to the laboratory, as the MRO, you must:

(1) If both specimens were verified negative, report the result as negative.

(2) If either of the specimens was verified negative and the other was verified as one or more non-negative(s), report the non-negative result(s) only. For example, if you verified one specimen as negative and the other as a refusal to test because the second specimen was substituted, as the MRO you should report only the refusal to the DER.

(i) If the first specimen is reported as negative, but the result of the second specimen has not been reported by the laboratory, as the MRO, you should hold—not report—the result of the first specimen until the result of the second specimen is received.

(ii) If the first specimen is reported as non-negative, as the MRO, you should report the result immediately and not wait to receive the result of the second specimen.

(3) If both specimens were verified non-negative, report all of the non-negative results. For example, if you verified one specimen as positive and the other as a refusal to test because the specimen was adulterated, as the MRO, you should report the positive and the refusal results to the DER.

(c) As an exception to paragraphs (a) and (b) of this section, as the MRO, you must follow procedures at § 40.159(f) when any verified non-negative result is also invalid.

[73 FR 35972, June 25, 2008]

§ 40.163   How does the MRO report drug test results?

(a) As the MRO, it is your responsibility to report all drug test results to the employer.

(b) You may use a signed or stamped and dated legible photocopy of Copy 2 of the CCF to report test results.

(c) If you do not report test results using Copy 2 of the CCF for this purpose, you must provide a written report (e.g., a letter) for each test result. This report must, as a minimum, include the following information:

(1) Full name, as indicated on the CCF, of the employee tested;

(2) Specimen ID number from the CCF and the donor SSN or employee ID number;

(3) Reason for the test, if indicated on the CCF (e.g., random, post-accident);

(4) Date of the collection;

(5) Date you received Copy 2 of the CCF;

(6) Result of the test (i.e., positive, negative, dilute, refusal to test, test cancelled) and the date the result was verified by the MRO;

(7) For verified positive tests, the drug(s)/metabolite(s) for which the test was positive;

(8) For cancelled tests, the reason for cancellation; and

(9) For refusals to test, the reason for the refusal determination (e.g., in the case of an adulterated test result, the name of the adulterant).

(d) As an exception to the reporting requirements of paragraph (b) and (c) of this section, the MRO may report negative results using an electronic data file.

(1) If you report negatives using an electronic data file, the report must contain, as a minimum, the information specified in paragraph (c) of this section, as applicable for negative test results.

(2) In addition, the report must contain your name, address, and phone number, the name of any person other than you reporting the results, and the date the electronic results report is released.

(e) You must retain a signed or stamped and dated copy of Copy 2 of the CCF in your records. If you do not use Copy 2 for reporting results, you must maintain a copy of the signed or stamped and dated letter in addition to the signed or stamped and dated Copy 2. If you use the electronic data file to report negatives, you must maintain a retrievable copy of that report in a format suitable for inspection and auditing by a DOT representative.

(f) You must not use Copy 1 of the CCF to report drug test results.

(g) You must not provide quantitative values to the DER or C/TPA for drug or validity test results. However, you must provide the test information in your possession to a SAP who consults with you (see §40.293(g)).

[66 FR 41952, Aug. 9, 2001]

§ 40.165 To whom does the MRO transmit reports of drug test results?

(a) As the MRO, you must report all drug test results to the DER, except in the circumstances provided for in §40.345.

(b) If the employer elects to receive reports of results through a C/TPA, acting as an intermediary as provided in §40.345, you must report the results through the designated C/TPA.

§ 40.167 How are MRO reports of drug results transmitted to the employer?

As the MRO or C/TPA who transmits drug test results to the employer, you must comply with the following requirements:

(a) You must report the results in a confidential manner.

(b) You must transmit to the DER on the same day the MRO verifies the result or the next business day all verified positive test results, results requiring an immediate collection under direct observation, adulterated or substituted specimen results, and other refusals to test.

(1) Direct telephone contact with the DER is the preferred method of immediate reporting. Follow up your phone call with appropriate documentation (see §40.163).

(2) You are responsible for identifying yourself to the DER, and the DER must have a means to confirm your identification.

(3) The MRO's report that you transmit to the employer must contain all of the information required by §40.163.

(c) You must transmit the MRO's report(s) of verified tests to the DER so that the DER receives it within two days of verification by the MRO.

(1) You must fax, courier, mail, or electronically transmit a legible image or copy of either the signed or stamped and dated Copy 2 or the written report (see §40.163(b) and (c)).

(2) Negative results reported electronically (i.e., computer data file) do not require an image of Copy 2 or the written report.

(d) In transmitting test results, you or the C/TPA and the employer must ensure the security of the transmission and limit access to any transmission, storage, or retrieval systems.

(e) MRO reports are not subject to modification or change by anyone other than the MRO, as provided in §40.149(c).

[65 FR 79526, Dec. 19, 2000, as amended at 66 FR 41953, Aug. 9, 2001]

§ 40.169 Where is other information concerning the role of MROs and the verification process found in this regulation?

You can find more information concerning the role of MROs in several sections of this part:

§40.3—Definition.

§§40.47–40.49—Correction of form and kit errors.

§40.67—Role in direct observation and other atypical test situations.

§40.83—Laboratory handling of fatal and correctable flaws.

§40.97—Laboratory handling of test results and quantitative values.

§40.99—Authorization of longer laboratory retention of specimens.

§40.101—Relationship with laboratories; avoidance of conflicts of interest.

§40.105—Notification of discrepancies in blind specimen results.

§40.171—Request for test of split specimen.

§40.187—Action concerning split specimen test results.

§40.193—Role in "shy bladder" situations.

§40.195—Role in cancelling tests.

§§40.199–40.203—Documenting errors in tests.

§40.327—Confidentiality and release of information.

§40.347—Transfer of records.

§40.353—Relationships with service agents.

SUBPART H—SPLIT SPECIMEN TESTS

§ 40.171 How does an employee request a test of a split specimen?

(a) As an employee, when the MRO has notified you that you have a verified positive drug test and/or refusal to test because of adulteration or substitution, you have 72 hours from the time of notification to request a test of the split specimen. The request may be verbal or in writing. If you make this request to the MRO within 72 hours, you trigger the requirements of this section for a test of the split specimen. There is no split specimen testing for an invalid result.

(b)(1) If, as an employee, you have not requested a test of the split specimen within 72 hours, you may present to the MRO information documenting that serious injury, illness, lack of actual notice of the verified test result, inability to contact the MRO (e.g., there was no one in the MRO's office and the answering machine was not working), or other circumstances unavoidably prevented you from making a timely request.

(2) As the MRO, if you conclude from the employee's information that there was a legitimate reason for the employee's failure to contact you within 72 hours, you must direct that the test of the split specimen take place, just as you would when there is a timely request.

(c) When the employee makes a timely request for a test of the split specimen under paragraphs (a) and (b) of this section, you must, as the MRO, immediately provide written notice to the laboratory that tested the primary specimen, directing the laboratory to forward the split specimen to a second HHS-certified laboratory. You must also document the date and time of the employee's request.

[65 FR 79526, Dec. 19, 2000, as amended at 73 FR 35973, June 25, 2008]

§ 40.173 Who is responsible for paying for the test of a split specimen?

(a) As the employer, you are responsible for making sure (e.g., by establishing appropriate accounts with laboratories for testing split specimens) that the MRO, first laboratory, and second laboratory perform the functions noted in §§40.175–40.185 in a timely manner, once the employee has made a timely request for a test of the split specimen.

(b) As the employer, you must not condition your compliance with these requirements on the employee's direct payment to the MRO or laboratory or the employee's agreement to reimburse you for the costs of testing. For example, if you ask the employee to pay for some or all of the cost of testing the split specimen, and the employee is unwilling or unable to do so, you must ensure that the test takes place in a timely manner, even though this means that you pay for it.

(c) As the employer, you may seek payment or reimbursement of all or part of the cost of the split specimen from the employee (e.g., through your written company policy or a collective bargaining agreement). This part takes no position on who ultimately pays the cost of the test, so long as the employer ensures that the testing is conducted as required and the results released appropriately.

§ 40.175 What steps does the first laboratory take with a split specimen?

(a) As the laboratory at which the primary and split specimen first arrive, you must check to see whether the split specimen is available for testing.

(b) If the split specimen is unavailable or appears insufficient, you must then do the following:

(1) Continue the testing process for the primary specimen as you would normally. Report the results for the primary specimen without providing the MRO information regarding the unavailable split specimen.

(2) Upon receiving a letter from the MRO instructing you to forward the split specimen to another laboratory for testing, report to the MRO that the split specimen is unavailable for testing. Provide as much information as you can about the cause of the unavailability.

(c) As the laboratory that tested the primary specimen, you are not authorized to open the split specimen under any circumstances (except when the split specimen is redesignated as provided in §40.83).

(d) When you receive written notice from the MRO instructing you to send the split specimen to another HHS-certified laboratory, you must forward the following items to the second laboratory:

(1) The split specimen in its original specimen bottle, with the seal intact;

(2) A copy of the MRO's written request; and

(3) A copy of Copy 1 of the CCF, which identifies the drug(s)/metabolite(s) or the validity criteria to be tested for.

(e) You must not send to the second laboratory any information about the identity of the employee. Inadvertent disclosure does not, however, cause a fatal flaw.

(f) This subpart does not prescribe who gets to decide which HHS-certified laboratory is used to test the split specimen. That decision is left to the parties involved.

§ 40.177 What does the second laboratory do with the split specimen when it is tested to reconfirm the presence of a drug or drug metabolite?

(a) As the laboratory testing the split specimen, you must test the split specimen for the drug(s)/drug metabolite(s) detected in the primary specimen.

(b) You must conduct this test without regard to the cutoff concentrations of §40.87.

(c) If the test fails to reconfirm the presence of the drug(s)/drug metabolite(s) that were reported positive in the primary specimen, you must conduct validity tests in an attempt to determine the reason for being unable to reconfirm the presence of the drug(s)/metabolite(s). You should conduct the same validity tests as you would conduct on a primary specimen set forth in §40.91.

(d) In addition, if the test fails to reconfirm the presence of the drug(s)/drug metabolite(s) reported in the primary specimen, you may send the specimen or an aliquot of it for testing at another HHS-certified laboratory that has the capability to conduct another reconfirmation test.

[65 FR 79526, Dec. 19, 2000, as amended at 73 FR 35973, June 25, 2008]

§ 40.179 What does the second laboratory do with the split specimen when it is tested to reconfirm an adulterated test result?

(a) As the laboratory testing the split specimen, you must test the split specimen for the adulterant detected in the primary specimen, using the confirmatory test for the adulterant and using criteria in §40.95 and confirmatory cutoff levels required by the HHS Mandatory Guidelines.

(b) In addition, if the test fails to reconfirm the adulterant result reported in the primary specimen, you may send the specimen or an aliquot of it for testing at another HHS-certified laboratory that has the capability to conduct another reconfirmation test.

[65 FR 79526, Dec. 19, 2000, as amended 73 FR 35973, June 25, 2008]

§ 40.181 What does the second laboratory do with the split specimen when it is tested to reconfirm a substituted test result?

As the laboratory testing the split specimen, you must test the split specimen using the confirmatory tests for creatinine and specific gravity, and using criteria set forth in § 40.93(b).

[65 FR 79526, Dec. 19, 2000, as amended 73 FR 35973, June 25, 2008]

§ 40.183 What information do laboratories report to MROs regarding split specimen results?

(a) As the laboratory responsible for testing the split specimen, you must report split specimen test results by checking the "Reconfirmed" box and/or the "Failed to Reconfirm" box (Step 5(b)) on Copy 1 of the CCF, as appropriate, and by providing clarifying remarks using current HHS Mandatory Guidelines requirements.

(b) As the laboratory certifying scientist, enter your name, sign, and date the CCF.

[65 FR 79526, Dec. 19, 2000, as amended 73 FR 35973, June 25, 2008]

§ 40.185 Through what methods and to whom must a laboratory report split specimen results?

(a) As the laboratory testing the split specimen, you must report laboratory results directly, and only, to the MRO at his or her place of business. You must not report results to or through the DER or another service agent (e.g., a C/TPA).

(b) You must fax, courier, mail, or electronically transmit a legible image or copy of the fully-completed Copy 1 of the CCF, which has been signed by the certifying scientist.

(c) You must transmit the laboratory result to the MRO immediately, preferably on the same day or next business day as the result is signed and released.

§ 40.187 What does the MRO do with split specimen laboratory results?

As the MRO, the split specimen laboratory results you receive will fall into five categories. You must take the following action, as appropriate, when a laboratory reports split specimen results to you.

(a) Category 1: The laboratory reconfirmed one or more of the primary specimen results. As the MRO, you must report to the DER and the employee the result(s) that was/were reconfirmed.

(1) In the case of a reconfirmed positive test(s) for drug(s) or drug metabolite(s), the positive is the final result.

(2) In the case of a reconfirmed adulterated or substituted result, the refusal to test is the final result.

(3) In the case of a combination positive and refusal to test results, the final result is both positive and refusal to test.

(b) Category 2: The laboratory failed to reconfirm all of the primary specimen results because, as appropriate, drug(s)/drug metabolite(s) were not detected; adulteration criteria were not met; and/or substitution criteria were not met. As the MRO, you must report to the DER and the employee that the test must be cancelled.

(1) As the MRO, you must inform ODAPC of the failure to reconfirm using the format in Appendix D to this part.

(2) In a case where the split failed to reconfirm because the substitution criteria were not met and the split specimen creatinine concentration was equal to or greater than 2mg/dL but less than or equal to 5mg/dL, as the MRO, you must, in addition to step in (b)(1) of this paragraph, direct the DER to ensure the

immediate collection of another specimen from the employee under direct observation, with no notice given to the employee of this collection requirement until immediately before the collection.

(3) In a case where the split failed to reconfirm and the primary specimen's result was also invalid, direct the DER to ensure the immediate collection of another specimen from the employee under direct observation, with no notice given to the employee of this collection requirement until immediately before the collection.

(c) <u>Category 3</u>: The laboratory failed to reconfirm all of the primary specimen results, and also reported that the split specimen was invalid, adulterated, and/or substituted.

(1) In the case where the laboratory failed to reconfirm all of the primary specimen results and the split was reported as invalid, as the MRO, you must:

(i) Report to the DER and the employee that the test must be cancelled and the reason for the cancellation.

(ii) Direct the DER to ensure the immediate collection of another specimen from the employee under direct observation, with no notice given to the employee of this collection requirement until immediately before the collection.

(iii) Inform ODAPC of the failure to reconfirm using the format in Appendix D to this part.

(2) In the case where the laboratory failed to reconfirm any of the primary specimen results, and the split was reported as adulterated and/or substituted, as the MRO, you must:

(i) Contact the employee and inform the employee that the laboratory has determined that his or her split specimen is adulterated and/or substituted, as appropriate.

(ii) Follow the procedures of § 40.145 to determine if there is a legitimate medical explanation for the laboratory finding of adulteration and/or substitution, as appropriate.

(iii) If you determine that there is a legitimate medical explanation for the adulterated and/or substituted test result, report to the DER and the employee that the test must be cancelled; and inform ODAPC of the failure to reconfirm using the format in Appendix D to this part.

(iv) If you determine that there is not a legitimate medical explanation for the adulterated and/or substituted test result, you must take the following steps:

(A) Report the test to the DER and the employee as a verified refusal to test. Inform the employee that he or she has 72 hours to request a test of the primary specimen to determine if the adulterant found in the split specimen is also present in the primary specimen and/or to determine if the primary specimen meets appropriate substitution criteria.

(B) Except when the request is for a test of the primary specimen and is being made to the laboratory that tested the primary specimen, follow the procedures of §§ 40.153, 40.171, 40.173, 40.179, 40.181, and 40.185, as appropriate.

(C) As the laboratory that tests the primary specimen to reconfirm the presence of the adulterant found in the split specimen and/or to determine that the primary specimen meets appropriate substitution criteria, report your result to the MRO on a photocopy (faxed, mailed, scanned, couriered) of Copy 1 of the CCF.

(D) If the test of the primary specimen reconfirms the adulteration and/or substitution finding of the split specimen, as the MRO you must report the result as a refusal to test as provided in paragraph (a)(2) of this section.

(E) If the test of the primary specimen fails to reconfirm the adulteration and/or substitution finding of the split specimen, as the MRO you must cancel the test, following procedures in paragraph (b) of this section.

(d) <u>Category 4</u>: The laboratory failed to reconfirm one or more but not all of the primary specimen results, and also reported that the split specimen was invalid, adulterated, and/or substituted. As the MRO, in the case where the laboratory reconfirmed one or more of the primary specimen result(s), you must follow procedures in paragraph (a) of this section and:

(1) Report that the split was also reported as being invalid, adulterated, and/or substituted (as appropriate).

(2) Inform the DER to take action only on the reconfirmed result(s).

(e) <u>Category 5</u>: The split specimen was not available for testing or there was no split laboratory available to test the specimen. As the MRO, you must:

(1) Report to the DER and the employee that the test must be cancelled and the reason for the cancellation;

(2) Direct the DER to ensure the immediate recollection of another specimen from the employee under direct observation, with no notice given to the employee of this collection requirement until immediately before the collection; and

(3) Notify ODAPC of the failure to reconfirm using the format in Appendix D to this part.

(f) For all split specimen results, as the MRO you must:

(1) Enter your name, sign, and date (Step 7) of Copy 2 of the CCF.

(2) Send a legible copy of Copy 2 of the CCF (or a signed and dated letter, see § 40.163) to the employer and keep a copy for your records. Transmit the document as provided in § 40.167.

[65 FR 79526, Dec. 19, 2000, as amended at 66 FR 41953, Aug. 9, 2001; 68 FR 31626, May 28, 2003; 73 FR 35973, June 25, 2008]

§ 40.189 Where is other information concerning split specimens found in this regulation?

You can find more information concerning split specimens in several sections of this part:

§40.3—Definition.

§40.65—Quantity of split specimen.

§40.67—Directly observed test when split specimen is unavailable.

§§40.71–40.73—Collection process for split specimens.

§40.83—Laboratory accessioning of split specimens.

§40.99—Laboratory retention of split specimens.

§40.103—Blind split specimens.

§40.153—MRO notice to employees on tests of split specimen.

§§40.193 and 40.201—MRO actions on insufficient or unavailable split specimens.

Appendix D to Part 40—Report format for split specimen failure to reconfirm.

SUBPART I—PROBLEMS IN DRUG TESTS

§ 40.191 What is a refusal to take a DOT drug test, and what are the consequences?

(a) As an employee, you have refused to take a drug test if you:

(1) Fail to appear for any test (except a pre-employment test) within a reasonable time, as determined by the employer, consistent with applicable DOT agency regulations, after being directed to do so by the employer. This includes the failure of an employee (including an owner-operator) to appear for a test when called by a C/TPA (see §40.61(a));

(2) Fail to remain at the testing site until the testing process is complete; Provided, That an employee who leaves the testing site before the testing process commences (see §40.63(c)) for a pre-employment test is not deemed to have refused to test;

(3) Fail to provide a urine specimen for any drug test required by this part or DOT agency regulations; Provided, That an employee who does not provide a urine specimen because he or she has left the testing site before the testing process commences (see §40.63(c)) for a pre-employment test is not deemed to have refused to test;

(4) In the case of a directly observed or monitored collection in a drug test, fail to permit the observation or monitoring of your provision of a specimen (see §§40.67(l) and 40.69(g));

(5) Fail to provide a sufficient amount of urine when directed, and it has been determined, through a required medical evaluation, that there was no adequate medical explanation for the failure (see §40.193(d)(2));

(6) Fail or decline to take an additional drug test the employer or collector has directed you to take (see, for instance, §40.197(b));

(7) Fail to undergo a medical examination or evaluation, as directed by the MRO as part of the verification process, or as directed by the DER under §40.193(d). In the case of a pre-employment drug test, the employee is deemed to have refused to test on this basis only if the pre-employment test is conducted following a contingent offer of employment. If there was no contingent offer of employment, the MRO will cancel the test; or

(8) Fail to cooperate with any part of the testing process (e.g., refuse to empty pockets when directed by the collector, behave in a confrontational way that disrupts the collection process, fail to wash hands after being directed to do so by the collector).

(9) For an observed collection, fail to follow the observer's instructions to raise your clothing above the waist, lower clothing and underpants, and to turn around to permit the observer to determine if you have any type of prosthetic or other device that could be used to interfere with the collection process.

(10) Possess or wear a prosthetic or other device that could be used to interfere with the collection process.

(11) Admit to the collector or MRO that you adulterated or substituted the specimen.

(b) As an employee, if the MRO reports that you have a verified adulterated or substituted test result, you have refused to take a drug test.

(c) As an employee, if you refuse to take a drug test, you incur the consequences specified under DOT agency regulations for a violation of those DOT agency regulations.

(d) As a collector or an MRO, when an employee refuses to participate in the part of the testing process in which you are involved, you must terminate the portion of the testing process in which you are involved, document the refusal on the CCF (including, in the case of the collector, printing the employee's name on Copy 2 of the CCF), immediately notify the DER by any means (e.g., telephone or secure fax machine) that ensures that the refusal notification is immediately received. As a referral physician (e.g., physician evaluating a "shy bladder" condition or a claim of a legitimate medical explanation in a validity testing situation), you must notify the MRO, who in turn will notify the DER.

(1) As the collector, you must note the refusal in the "Remarks" line (Step 2), and sign and date the CCF.

(2) As the MRO, you must note the refusal by checking the "refused to test because" box (Step 6) on Copy 2 of the CCF, and add the reason on the "Remarks" line. You must then sign and date the CCF.

(e) As an employee, when you refuse to take a non-DOT test or to sign a non-DOT form, you have not refused to take a DOT test. There are no consequences under DOT agency regulations for refusing to take a non-DOT test.

[65 FR 79526, Dec. 19, 2000, as amended at 66 FR 41953, Aug. 9, 2001; 68 FR 31626, May 28, 2003; 71 FR 49384, Aug. 23, 2006; 73 FR 35974, June 25, 2008]

§ 40.193 What happens when an employee does not provide a sufficient amount of urine for a drug test?

(a) This section prescribes procedures for situations in which an employee does not provide a sufficient amount of urine to permit a drug test (i.e., 45 mL of urine).

(b) As the collector, you must do the following:

(1) Discard the insufficient specimen, except where the insufficient specimen was out of temperature range or showed evidence of adulteration or tampering (see §40.65(b) and (c)).

(2) Urge the employee to drink up to 40 ounces of fluid, distributed reasonably through a period of up to three hours, or until the individual has provided a sufficient urine specimen, whichever occurs first. It is not a refusal to test if the employee declines to drink. Document on the Remarks line of the CCF (Step 2), and inform the employee of, the time at which the three-hour period begins and ends.

(3) If the employee refuses to make the attempt to provide a new urine specimen or leaves the collection site before the collection process is complete, you must discontinue the collection, note the fact on the "Remarks" line of the CCF (Step 2), and immediately notify the DER. This is a refusal to test.

(4) If the employee has not provided a sufficient specimen within three hours of the first unsuccessful attempt to provide the specimen, you must discontinue the collection, note the fact on the "Remarks" line of the CCF (Step 2), and immediately notify the DER.

(5) Send Copy 2 of the CCF to the MRO and Copy 4 to the DER. You must send or fax these copies to the MRO and DER within 24 hours or the next business day.

(c) As the DER, when the collector informs you that the employee has not provided a sufficient amount of urine (see paragraph (b)(4) of this section), you must, after consulting with the MRO, direct the employee to obtain, within five days, an evaluation from a licensed physician, acceptable to the MRO, who has expertise in the medical issues raised by the employee's failure to provide a sufficient specimen. (The MRO may perform this evaluation if the MRO has appropriate expertise.)

(1) As the MRO, if another physician will perform the evaluation, you must provide the other physician with the following information and instructions:

(i) That the employee was required to take a DOT drug test, but was unable to provide a sufficient amount of urine to complete the test;

(ii) The consequences of the appropriate DOT agency regulation for refusing to take the required drug test;

(iii) That the referral physician must agree to follow the requirements of paragraphs (d) through (g) of this section.

(2) [Reserved]

(d) As the referral physician conducting this evaluation, you must recommend that the MRO make one of the following determinations:

(1) A medical condition has, or with a high degree of probability could have, precluded the employee from providing a sufficient amount of urine. As the MRO, if you accept this recommendation, you must:

(i) Check "Test Cancelled" (Step 6) on the CCF; and

(ii) Sign and date the CCF.

(2) There is not an adequate basis for determining that a medical condition has, or with a high degree of probability could have, precluded the employee from providing a sufficient amount of urine. As the MRO, if you accept this recommendation, you must:

(i) Check "Refusal to test because" (Step 6) on the CCF and enter reason in the remarks line; and

(ii) Sign and date the CCF.

(e) For purposes of this paragraph, a medical condition includes an ascertainable physiological condition (e.g., a urinary system dysfunction) or a medically documented pre-existing psychological disorder, but does not include unsupported assertions of "situational anxiety" or dehydration.

(f) As the referral physician making the evaluation, after completing your evaluation, you must provide a written statement of your recommendations and the basis for them to the MRO. You must not include in this statement detailed information on the employee's medical condition beyond what is necessary to explain your conclusion.

(g) If, as the referral physician making this evaluation in the case of a pre-employment test, you determine that the employee's medical condition is a serious and permanent or long-term disability that is highly likely to prevent the employee from providing a sufficient amount of urine for a very long or indefinite period of time, you must set forth your determination and the reasons for it in your written statement to the MRO. As the MRO, upon receiving such a report, you must follow the requirements of §40.195, where applicable.

(h) As the MRO, you must seriously consider and assess the referral physician's recommendations in making your determination about whether the employee has a medical condition that has, or with a high degree of probability could have, precluded the employee from providing a sufficient amount of urine. You must report your determination to the DER in writing as soon as you make it.

(i) As the employer, when you receive a report from the MRO indicating that a test is cancelled as provided in paragraph (d)(1) of this section, you take no further action with respect to the employee. The employee remains in the random testing pool.

[65 FR 79526, Dec. 19, 2000, as amended at 66 FR 41953, Aug. 9, 2001]

§ 40.195 What happens when an individual is unable to provide a sufficient amount of urine for a pre-employment follow-up or return-to-duty test because of a permanent or long-term medical condition?

(a) This section concerns a situation in which an employee has a medical condition that precludes him or her from providing a sufficient specimen for a pre-employment follow-up or return-to-duty test and the condition involves a permanent or long-term disability. As the MRO in this situation, you must do the following:

(1) You must determine if there is clinical evidence that the individual is an illicit drug user. You must make this determination by personally conducting, or causing to be conducted, a medical evaluation and through consultation with the employee's physician and/or the physician who conducted the evaluation under §40.193(d).

(2) If you do not personally conduct the medical evaluation, you must ensure that one is conducted by a licensed physician acceptable to you.

(3) For purposes of this section, the MRO or the physician conducting the evaluation may conduct an alternative test (e.g., blood) as part of the medically appropriate procedures in determining clinical evidence of drug use.

(b) If the medical evaluation reveals no clinical evidence of drug use, as the MRO, you must report the result to the employer as a negative test with written notations regarding results of both the evaluation conducted under §40.193(d) and any further medical examination. This report must state the basis for the determination that a permanent or long-term medical condition exists, making provision of a sufficient urine specimen impossible, and for the determination that no signs and symptoms of drug use exist.

(1) Check "Negative" (Step 6) on the CCF.

(2) Sign and date the CCF.

(c) If the medical evaluation reveals clinical evidence of drug use, as the MRO, you must report the result to the employer as a cancelled test with written notations regarding results of both the evaluation conducted under §40.193(d) and any further medical examination. This report must state that a permanent or long-term medical condition exists, making provision of a sufficient urine specimen impossible, and state the reason for the determination that signs and symptoms of drug use exist. Because this is a cancelled test, it does not serve the purposes of a negative test (i.e., the employer is not authorized to allow the employee to begin or resume performing safety-sensitive functions, because a negative test is needed for that purpose).

(d) For purposes of this section, permanent or long-term medical conditions are those physiological, anatomic, or psychological abnormalities documented as being present prior to the attempted collection, and considered not amenable to correction or cure for an extended period of time, if ever.

(1) Examples would include destruction (any cause) of the glomerular filtration system leading to renal failure; unrepaired traumatic disruption of the urinary tract; or a severe psychiatric disorder focused on genito-urinary matters.

(2) Acute or temporary medical conditions, such as cystitis, urethritis or prostatitis, though they might interfere with collection for a limited period of time, cannot receive the same exceptional consideration as the permanent or long-term conditions discussed in paragraph (d)(1) of this section.

[65 FR 79526, Dec. 19, 2000, as amended at 66 FR 41953, Aug. 9, 2001]

§ 40.197 What happens when an employer receives a report of a dilute specimen?

(a) As the employer, if the MRO informs you that a positive drug test was dilute, you simply treat the test as a verified positive test. You must not direct the employee to take another test based on the fact that the specimen was dilute.

(b) As an employer, if the MRO informs you that a negative test was dilute, take the following action:

(1) If the MRO directs you to conduct a recollection under direct observation (i.e., because the creatinine concentration of the specimen was equal to or greater than 2mg/dL, but less than or equal to 5 mg/dL (see §40.155(c)), you must do so immediately.

(2) Otherwise (i.e., if the creatinine concentration of the dilute specimen is greater than 5 mg/dL), you may, but are not required to, direct the employee to take another test immediately.

(i) Such recollections must not be collected under direct observation, unless there is another basis for use of direct observation (see §40.67(b) and (c)).

(ii) You must treat all employees the same for this purpose. For example, you must not retest some employees and not others. You may, however, establish different policies for different types of tests (e.g., conduct retests in pre-employment situations, but not in random test situations). You must inform your employees in advance of your decisions on these matters.

(c) The following provisions apply to all tests you direct an employee to take under paragraph (b) of this section:

(1) You must ensure that the employee is given the minimum possible advance notice that he or she must go to the collection site;

(2) You must treat the result of the test you directed the employee to take under paragraph (b) of this section—and not a prior test—as the test result of record, on which you rely for purposes of this part;

(3) If the result of the test you directed the employee to take under paragraph (b)(1) of this section is also negative and dilute, you are not permitted to make the employee take an additional test because the result was dilute.

(4) If the result of the test you directed the employee to take under paragraph (b)(2) of this section is also negative and dilute, you are not permitted to make the employee take an additional test because the result was dilute. Provided, however, that if the MRO directs you to conduct a recollection under direct observation under paragraph (b)(1) of this section, you must immediately do so.

(5) If the employee declines to take a test you directed him or her to take under paragraph (b) of this section, the employee has refused the test for purposes of this part and DOT agency regulations.

[68 FR 31626, May 28, 2003; 69 FR 64867, Nov. 9, 2004; 73 FR 35974, June 25, 2008]

§ 40.199 What problems always cause a drug test to be cancelled?

(a) As the MRO, when the laboratory discovers a "fatal flaw" during its processing of incoming specimens (see §40.83), the laboratory will report to you that the specimen has been "Rejected for Testing" (with the reason stated). You must always cancel such a test.

(b) The following are "fatal flaws":

(1) There is no printed collector's name and no collector's signature;

(2) The specimen ID numbers on the specimen bottle and the CCF do not match;

(3) The specimen bottle seal is broken or shows evidence of tampering (and a split specimen cannot be redesignated, see §40.83(g)); and

(4) Because of leakage or other causes, there is an insufficient amount of urine in the primary specimen bottle for analysis and the specimens cannot be redesignated (see §40.83(g)).

(c) You must report the result as provided in §40.161.

§ 40.201 What problems always cause a drug test to be cancelled and may result in a requirement for another collection?

As the MRO, you must cancel a drug test when a laboratory reports that any of the following problems have occurred. You must inform the DER that the test was cancelled. You must also direct the DER to ensure that an additional collection occurs immediately, if required by the applicable procedures specified in paragraphs (a) through (e) of this section.

(a) The laboratory reports an "Invalid Result." You must follow applicable procedures in §40.159 (recollection under direct observation may be required).

(b) The laboratory reports the result as "Rejected for Testing." You must follow applicable procedures in §40.161 (a recollection may be required).

(c) The laboratory reports that the split specimen failed to reconfirm all of the primary specimen results because the drug(s)/drug metabolite(s) were not detected; adulteration criteria were not met; and/or substitution criteria were not met. You must follow the applicable procedures in § 40.187(b)—no recollection is required in this case, unless the split specimen creatinine concentration for a substituted primary specimen was greater than or equal to 2mg/dL but less than or equal to 5mg/dL, or the primary specimen had an invalid result which was not reported to the DER. Both these cases require recollection under direct observation.

(d) The laboratory reports that the split specimen failed to reconfirm all of the primary specimen results, and that the split specimen was invalid. You must follow the procedures in § 40.187(c)(1)—recollection under direct observation is required in this case.

(e) The laboratory reports that the split specimen failed to reconfirm all of the primary specimen results because the split specimen was not available for testing or there was no split laboratory available to test the specimen. You must follow the applicable procedures in § 40.187(e)—recollection under direct observation is required in this case.

(f) The examining physician has determined that there is an acceptable medical explanation of the employee's failure to provide a sufficient amount of urine. You must follow applicable procedures in §40.193(d)(1) (no recollection is required in this case).

[65 FR 79526, Dec. 19, 2000, as amended at 73 FR 35974, June 25, 2008]

§ 40.203 What problems cause a drug test to be cancelled unless they are corrected?

(a) As the MRO, when a laboratory discovers a "correctable flaw" during its processing of incoming specimens (see §40.83), the laboratory will attempt to correct it. If the laboratory is unsuccessful in this attempt, it will report to you that the specimen has been "Rejected for Testing" (with the reason stated).

(b) The following is a "correctable flaw" that laboratories must attempt to correct: The collector's signature is omitted on the certification statement on the CCF.

(c) As the MRO, when you discover a "correctable flaw" during your review of the CCF, you must cancel the test unless the flaw is corrected.

(d) The following are correctable flaws that you must attempt to correct:

(1) The employee's signature is omitted from the certification statement, unless the employee's failure or refusal to sign is noted on the "Remarks" line of the CCF.

(2) The certifying scientist's signature is omitted on the laboratory copy of the CCF for a positive, adulterated, substituted, or invalid test result.

(3) The collector uses a non-Federal form or an expired Federal form for the test. This flaw may be corrected through the procedure set forth in §40.205(b)(2), provided that the collection testing process has been conducted in accordance with the procedures of this part in an HHS-certified laboratory. During the period August 1–October 31, 2001, you are not required to cancel a test because of the use of an expired Federal form. Beginning November 1, 2001, if the problem is not corrected, you must cancel the test.

[65 FR 79526, Dec. 19, 2000, as amended at 66 FR 41954, Aug. 9, 2001]

§ 40.205 How are drug test problems corrected?

(a) As a collector, you have the responsibility of trying to successfully complete a collection procedure for each employee.

(1) If, during or shortly after the collection process, you become aware of any event that prevents the completion of a valid test or collection (e.g., a procedural or paperwork error), you must try to correct the problem promptly, if doing so is practicable. You may conduct another collection as part of this effort.

(2) If another collection is necessary, you must begin the new collection procedure as soon as possible, using a new CCF and a new collection kit.

(b) If, as a collector, laboratory, MRO, employer, or other person implementing these drug testing regulations, you become aware of a problem that can be corrected (see §40.203), but which has not already been corrected under paragraph (a) of this section, you must take all practicable action to correct the problem so that the test is not cancelled.

(1) If the problem resulted from the omission of required information, you must, as the person responsible for providing that information, supply in writing the missing information and a statement that it is true and accurate. For example, suppose you are a collector, and you forgot to make a notation on the "Remarks" line of the CCF that the employee did not sign the certification. You would, when the problem is called to your attention, supply a signed statement that the employee failed or refused to sign the certification and that your statement is true and accurate. You must supply this information on the same business day on which you are notified of the problem, transmitting it by fax or courier.

(2) If the problem is the use of a non-Federal form or an expired Federal form, you must provide a signed statement (i.e., a memorandum for the record). It must state that the incorrect form contains all the information needed for a valid DOT drug test, and that the incorrect form was used inadvertently or as the only means of conducting a test, in circumstances beyond your control. The statement must also list the steps you have taken to prevent future use of non-Federal forms or expired Federal forms for DOT tests. For this flaw to be corrected, the test of the specimen must have occurred at a HHS-certified laboratory where it was tested consistent with the requirements of this part. You must supply this information on the same business day on which you are notified of the problem, transmitting it by fax or courier.

(3) You must maintain the written documentation of a correction with the CCF.

(4) You must mark the CCF in such a way (e.g., stamp noting correction) as to make it obvious on the face of the CCF that you corrected the flaw.

(c) If the correction does not take place, as the MRO you must cancel the test.

[65 FR 79526, Dec. 19, 2000, as amended at 66 FR 41954, Aug. 9, 2001]

§ 40.207 What is the effect of a cancelled drug test?

(a) A cancelled drug test is neither positive nor negative.

(1) As an employer, you must not attach to a cancelled test the consequences of a positive test or other violation of a DOT drug testing regulation (e.g., removal from a safety-sensitive position).

(2) As an employer, you must not use a cancelled test for the purposes of a negative test to authorize the employee to perform safety-sensitive functions (i.e., in the case of a pre-employment, return-to-duty, or follow-up test).

(3) However, as an employer, you must not direct a recollection for an employee because a test has been cancelled, except in the situations cited in paragraph (a)(2) of this section or other provisions of this part that require another test to be conducted (e.g., §§40.159(a)(5) and 40.187(b)(2), (c)(1), and (e)).

(b) A cancelled test does not count toward compliance with DOT requirements (e.g., being applied toward the number of tests needed to meet the employer's minimum random testing rate).

(c) A cancelled DOT test does not provide a valid basis for an employer to conduct a non-DOT test (i.e., a test under company authority).

[65 FR 79526, Dec. 19, 2000, as amended at 73 FR 35975, June 25, 2008]

§ 40.208 What problem requires corrective action but does not result in the cancellation of a test?

(a) If, as a laboratory, collector, employer, or other person implementing the DOT drug testing program, you become aware that the specimen temperature on the CCF was not checked and the "Remarks" line did not contain an entry regarding the temperature being out of range, you must take corrective action, including securing a memorandum for the record explaining the problem and taking appropriate action to ensure that the problem does not recur.

(b) This error does not result in the cancellation of the test.

(c) As an employer or service agent, this error, even though not sufficient to cancel a drug test result, may subject you to enforcement action under DOT agency regulations or Subpart R of this part.

[66 FR 41954, Aug. 9, 2001]

§ 40.209 What procedural problems do not result in the cancellation of a test and do not require corrective action?

(a) As a collector, laboratory, MRO, employer or other person administering the drug testing process, you must document any errors in the testing process of which you become aware, even if they are not considered problems that will cause a test to be cancelled as listed in this subpart. Decisions about the ultimate impact of these errors will be determined by other administrative or legal proceedings, subject to the limitations of paragraph (b) of this section.

(b) No person concerned with the testing process may declare a test cancelled based on an error that does not have a significant adverse effect on the right of the employee to have a fair and accurate test. Matters that do not result in the cancellation of a test include, but are not limited to, the following:

(1) A minor administrative mistake (e.g., the omission of the employee's middle initial, a transposition of numbers in the employee's social security number);

(2) An error that does not affect employee protections under this part (e.g., the collector's failure to add bluing agent to the toilet bowl, which adversely affects only the ability of the collector to detect tampering with the specimen by the employee);

(3) The collection of a specimen by a collector who is required to have been trained (see §40.33), but who has not met this requirement;

(4) A delay in the collection process (see §40.61(a));

(5) Verification of a test result by an MRO who has the basic credentials to be qualified as an MRO (see §40.121(a) through (b)) but who has not met training and/or documentation requirements (see §40.121(c) through (e));

(6) The failure to directly observe or monitor a collection that the rule requires or permits to be directly observed or monitored, or the unauthorized use of direct observation or monitoring for a collection;

(7) The fact that a test was conducted in a facility that does not meet the requirements of §40.41;

(8) If the specific name of the courier on the CCF is omitted or erroneous;

(9) Personal identifying information is inadvertently contained on the CCF (e.g., the employee signs his or her name on the laboratory copy); or

(10) Claims that the employee was improperly selected for testing.

(c) As an employer or service agent, these types of errors, even though not sufficient to cancel a drug test result, may subject you to enforcement action under DOT agency regulations or action under Subpart R of this part.

[65 FR 79526, Dec. 19, 2000, as amended at 66 FR 41954, Aug. 9, 2001]

SUBPART J—ALCOHOL TESTING PERSONNEL

§ 40.211 Who conducts DOT alcohol tests?

(a) Screening test technicians (STTs) and breath alcohol technicians (BATs) meeting their respective requirements of this subpart are the only people authorized to conduct DOT alcohol tests.

(b) An STT can conduct only alcohol screening tests, but a BAT can conduct alcohol screening and confirmation tests.

(c) As a BAT- or STT-qualified immediate supervisor of a particular employee, you may not act as the STT or BAT when that employee is tested, unless no other STT or BAT is available and DOT agency regulations do not prohibit you from doing so.

§ 40.213 What training requirements must STTs and BATs meet?

To be permitted to act as a BAT or STT in the DOT alcohol testing program, you must meet each of the requirements of this section:

(a) Basic information. You must be knowledgeable about the alcohol testing procedures in this part and the current DOT guidance. These documents and information are available from ODAPC (Department of Transportation, 1200 New Jersey Avenue, SE, Washington DC, 20590, 202–366–3784, or on the ODAPC web site (http://www.dot.gov/ost/dapc).

(b) Qualification training. You must receive qualification training meeting the requirements of this paragraph (b).

(1) Qualification training must be in accordance with the DOT Model BAT or STT Course, as applicable. The DOT Model Courses are available from ODAPC (Department of Transportation, 1200 New Jersey Avenue, SE, Washington DC, 20590, 202–366–3784, or on the ODAPC web site (http://www.dot.gov/ost/dapc). The training can also be provided using a course of instruction equivalent to the DOT Model Courses. On request, ODAPC will review BAT and STT instruction courses for equivalency.

(2) Qualification training must include training to proficiency in using the alcohol testing procedures of this part and in the operation of the particular alcohol testing device(s) (i.e., the ASD(s) or EBT(s)) you will be using.

(3) The training must emphasize that you are responsible for maintaining the integrity of the testing process, ensuring the privacy of employees being tested, and avoiding conduct or statements that could be viewed as offensive or inappropriate.

(4) The instructor must be an individual who has demonstrated necessary knowledge, skills, and abilities by regularly conducting DOT alcohol tests as an STT or BAT, as applicable, for a period of at least a year, who has conducted STT or BAT training, as applicable, under this part for a year, or who has successfully completed a "train the trainer" course.

(c) Initial Proficiency Demonstration. Following your completion of qualification training under paragraph (b) of this section, you must demonstrate proficiency in alcohol testing under this part by completing seven consecutive error-free mock tests (BATs) or five consecutive error-free tests (STTs).

(1) Another person must monitor and evaluate your performance, in person or by a means that provides real-time observation and interaction between the instructor and trainee, and attest in writing that the mock collections are "error-free." This person must be an individual who meets the requirements of paragraph (b)(4) of this section.

(2) These tests must use the alcohol testing devices (e.g., EBT(s) or ASD(s)) that you will use as a BAT or STT.

(3) If you are an STT who will be using an ASD that indicates readings by changes, contrasts, or other readings in color, you must demonstrate as part of the mock test that you are able to discern changes, contrasts, or readings correctly.

(d) Schedule for qualification training and initial proficiency demonstration. The following is the schedule for qualification training and the initial proficiency demonstration you must meet:

(1) If you became a BAT or STT before August 1, 2001, you were required to have met the requirements set forth in paragraphs (b) and (c) of this section, and you do not have to meet them again.

(2) If you become a BAT or STT on or after August 1, 2001, you must meet the requirements of paragraphs (b) and (c) of this section before you begin to perform BAT or STT functions.

(e) Refresher training. No less frequently than every five years from the date on which you satisfactorily complete the requirements of paragraphs (b) and (c) of this section, you must complete refresher training that meets all the requirements of paragraphs (b) and (c) of this section. If you are a BAT or STT who completed qualification training before January 1, 1998, you are not required to complete refresher training until January 1, 2003.

(f) Error Correction Training. If you make a mistake in the alcohol testing process that causes a test to be cancelled (i.e., a fatal or uncorrected flaw), you must undergo error correction training. This training must occur within 30 days of the date you are notified of the error that led to the need for retraining.

(1) Error correction training must be provided and your proficiency documented in writing by a person who meets the requirements of paragraph (b)(4) of this section.

(2) Error correction training is required to cover only the subject matter area(s) in which the error that caused the test to be cancelled occurred.

(3) As part of the error correction training, you must demonstrate your proficiency in the alcohol testing procedures of this part by completing three consecutive error-free mock tests. The mock tests must include one uneventful scenario and two scenarios related to the area(s) in which your error(s) occurred. The person providing the training must monitor and evaluate your performance and attest in writing that the mock tests were error-free.

(g) Documentation. You must maintain documentation showing that you currently meet all requirements of this section. You must provide this documentation on request to DOT agency representatives and to employers and C/TPAs who are negotiating to use your services.

(h) Other persons who may serve as BATs or STTs. (1) Anyone meeting the requirements of this section to be a BAT may act as an STT, provided that the individual has demonstrated initial proficiency in the operation of the ASD that he or she is using, as provided in paragraph (c) of this section.

(2) Law enforcement officers who have been certified by state or local governments to conduct breath alcohol testing are deemed to be qualified as BATs. They are not required to also complete the training requirements of this section in order to act as BATs. In order for a test conducted by such an officer to be accepted under DOT alcohol testing requirements, the officer must have been certified by a state or local government to use the EBT or ASD that was used for the test.

[65 FR 79526, Dec. 19, 2000, as amended at 66 FR 41954, Aug. 9, 2001; 73 FR 33329, June 12, 2008]

§ 40.215 What information about the DER do employers have to provide to BATs and STTs?

As an employer, you must provide to the STTs and BATs the name and telephone number of the appropriate DER (and C/TPA, where applicable) to contact about any problems or issues that may arise during the testing process.

§ 40.217 Where is other information on the role of STTs and BATs found in this regulation?

You can find other information on the role and functions of STTs and BATs in the following sections of this part:

§40.3—Definitions.

§40.223—Responsibility for supervising employees being tested.

§§40.225–40.227—Use of the alcohol testing form.

§§40.241–40.245—Screening test procedures with ASDs and EBTs.

§§40.251–40.255—Confirmation test procedures.

§40.261—Refusals to test.

§§40.263–40.265—Insufficient saliva or breath.

§40.267—Problems requiring cancellation of tests.

§§40.269–40.271—Correcting problems in tests.

SUBPART K—TESTING SITES, FORMS, EQUIPMENT AND SUPPLIES USED IN ALCOHOL TESTING

§ 40.221 Where does an alcohol test take place?

(a) A DOT alcohol test must take place at an alcohol testing site meeting the requirements of this section.

(b) If you are operating an alcohol testing site, you must ensure that it meets the security requirements of §40.223.

(c) If you are operating an alcohol testing site, you must ensure that it provides visual and aural privacy to the employee being tested, sufficient to prevent unauthorized persons from seeing or hearing test results.

(d) If you are operating an alcohol testing site, you must ensure that it has all needed personnel, materials, equipment, and facilities to provide for the collection and analysis of breath and/or saliva samples, and a suitable clean surface for writing.

(e) If an alcohol testing site fully meeting all the visual and aural privacy requirements of paragraph (c) is not readily available, this part allows a reasonable suspicion or post-accident test to be conducted at a site that partially meets these requirements. In this case, the site must afford visual and aural privacy to the employee to the greatest extent practicable.

(f) An alcohol testing site can be in a medical facility, a mobile facility (e.g., a van), a dedicated collection facility, or any other location meeting the requirements of this section.

§ 40.223 What steps must be taken to protect the security of alcohol testing sites?

(a) If you are a BAT, STT, or other person operating an alcohol testing site, you must prevent unauthorized personnel from entering the testing site.

(1) The only people you are to treat as authorized persons are employees being tested, BATs, STTs, and other alcohol testing site workers, DERs, employee representatives authorized by the employer (e.g., on the basis of employer policy or labor-management agreement), and DOT agency representatives.

(2) You must ensure that all persons are under the supervision of a BAT or STT at all times when permitted into the site.

(3) You may remove any person who obstructs, interferes with, or causes unnecessary delay in the testing process.

(b) As the BAT or STT, you must not allow any person other than you, the employee, or a DOT agency representative to actually witness the testing process (see §§40.241–40.255).

(c) If you are operating an alcohol testing site, you must ensure that when an EBT or ASD is not being used for testing, you store it in a secure place.

(d) If you are operating an alcohol testing site, you must ensure that no one other than BATs or other employees of the site have access to the site when an EBT is unsecured.

(e) As a BAT or STT, to avoid distraction that could compromise security, you are limited to conducting an alcohol test for only one employee at a time.

(1) When an EBT screening test on an employee indicates an alcohol concentration of 0.02 or higher, and the same EBT will be used for the confirmation test, you are not allowed to use the EBT for a test on another employee before completing the confirmation test on the first employee.

(2) As a BAT who will conduct both the screening and the confirmation test, you are to complete the entire screening and confirmation process on one employee before starting the screening process on another employee.

(3) You are not allowed to leave the alcohol testing site while the testing process for a given employee is in progress, except to notify a supervisor or contact a DER for assistance in the case an employee or other person who obstructs, interferes with, or unnecessarily delays the testing process.

§ 40.225 What form is used for an alcohol test?

(a) The DOT Alcohol Testing Form (ATF) must be used for every DOT alcohol test beginning February 1, 2002. The ATF must be a three-part carbonless manifold form. The ATF is found in Appendix G to this part. You may view this form on the ODAPC web site (http://www.dot.gov/ost/dapc).

(b) As an employer in the DOT alcohol testing program, you are not permitted to modify or revise the ATF except as follows:

(1) You may include other information needed for billing purposes, outside the boundaries of the form.

(2) You may use a ATF directly generated by an EBT which omits the space for affixing a separate printed result to the ATF, provided the EBT prints the result directly on the ATF.

(3) You may use an ATF that has the employer's name, address, and telephone number preprinted. In addition, a C/TPA's name, address, and telephone number may be included, to assist with negative results.

(4) You may use an ATF in which all pages are printed on white paper. You may modify the ATF by using colored paper, or have clearly discernable borders or designation statements on Copy 2 and Copy 3. When colors are used, they must be green for Copy 2 and blue for Copy 3.

(5) As a BAT or STT, you may add, on the "Remarks" line of the ATF, the name of the DOT agency under whose authority the test occurred.

(6) As a BAT or STT, you may use a ATF that has your name, address, and telephone number preprinted, but under no circumstances can your signature be preprinted.

(c) As an employer, you may use an equivalent foreign-language version of the ATF approved by ODAPC. You may use such a non-English language form only in a situation where both the employee and BAT/STT understand and can use the form in that language.

[65 FR 79526, Dec. 19, 2000, as amended at 66 FR 41954, Aug. 9, 2001]

§ 40.227 May employers use the ATF for non-DOT tests, or non-DOT forms for DOT tests?

(a) No, as an employer, BAT, or STT, you are prohibited from using the ATF for non-DOT alcohol tests. You are also prohibited from using non-DOT forms for DOT alcohol tests. Doing either subjects you to enforcement action under DOT agency regulations.

(b) If the STT or BAT, either by mistake, or as the only means to conduct a test under difficult circumstances (e.g., post-accident test with insufficient time to obtain the ATF), uses a non-DOT form for a DOT test, the use of a non-DOT form does not, in and of itself, require the employer or service agent to cancel the test. However, in order for the test to be considered valid, a signed statement must be obtained from the STT or BAT in accordance with §40.271(b).

§ 40.229 What devices are used to conduct alcohol screening tests?

EBTs and ASDs on the NHTSA conforming products lists (CPL) for evidential and non-evidential devices are the only devices you are allowed to use to conduct alcohol screening tests under this part. You may use an ASD that is on the NHTSA CPL for DOT alcohol tests only if there are instructions for its use in this part. An ASD can be used only for screening tests for alcohol, and may not be used for confirmation tests.

[65 FR 79526, Dec. 19, 2000, as amended at 66 FR 41954, Aug. 9, 2001]

§ 40.231 What devices are used to conduct alcohol confirmation tests?

(a) EBTs on the NHTSA CPL for evidential devices that meet the requirements of paragraph (b) of this section are the only devices you may use to conduct alcohol confirmation tests under this part. Note that, among devices on the CPL for EBTs, only those devices listed without an asterisk (*) are authorized for use in confirmation testing in the DOT alcohol testing program.

(b) To conduct a confirmation test, you must use an EBT that has the following capabilities:

(1) Provides a printed triplicate result (or three consecutive identical copies of a result) of each breath test;

(2) Assigns a unique number to each completed test, which the BAT and employee can read before each test and which is printed on each copy of the result;

(3) Prints, on each copy of the result, the manufacturer's name for the device, its serial number, and the time of the test;

(4) Distinguishes alcohol from acetone at the 0.02 alcohol concentration level;

(5) Tests an air blank; and

(6) Performs an external calibration check.

§ 40.233 What are the requirements for proper use and care of EBTs?

(a) As an EBT manufacturer, you must submit, for NHTSA approval, a quality assurance plan (QAP) for your EBT before NHTSA places the EBT on the CPL.

(1) Your QAP must specify the methods used to perform external calibration checks on the EBT, the tolerances within which the EBT is regarded as being in proper calibration, and the intervals at which these checks must be performed. In designating these intervals, your QAP must take into account factors like frequency of use, environmental conditions (e.g., temperature, humidity, altitude) and type of operation (e.g., stationary or mobile).

(2) Your QAP must also specify the inspection, maintenance, and calibration requirements and intervals for the EBT.

(b) As the manufacturer, you must include, with each EBT, instructions for its use and care consistent with the QAP.

(c) As the user of the EBT (e.g., employer, service agent), you must do the following:

(1) You must follow the manufacturer's instructions (see paragraph (b) of this section), including performance of external calibration checks at the intervals the instructions specify.

(2) In conducting external calibration checks, you must use only calibration devices appearing on NHTSA's CPL for "Calibrating Units for Breath Alcohol Tests."

(3) If an EBT fails an external check of calibration, you must take the EBT out of service. You may not use the EBT again for DOT alcohol testing until it is repaired and passes an external calibration check.

(4) You must maintain records of the inspection, maintenance, and calibration of EBTs as provided in §40.333(a)(2).

(5) You must ensure that inspection, maintenance, and calibration of the EBT are performed by its manufacturer or a maintenance representative certified either by the manufacturer or by a state health agency or other appropriate state agency.

§ 40.235 What are the requirements for proper use and care of ASDs?

(a) As an ASD manufacturer, you must submit, for NHTSA approval, a QAP for your ASD before NHTSA places the ASD on the CPL. Your QAP must specify the methods used for quality control checks, temperatures at which the ASD must be stored and used, the shelf life of the device, and environmental conditions (e.g., temperature, altitude, humidity) that may affect the ASD's performance.

(b) As a manufacturer, you must include with each ASD instructions for its use and care consistent with the QAP. The instructions must include directions on the proper use of the ASD, and, where applicable the time within which the device must be read, and the manner in which the reading is made.

(c) As the user of the ADS (e.g., employer, STT), you must follow the QAP instructions.

(d) You are not permitted to use an ASD that does not pass the specified quality control checks or that has passed its expiration date.

(e) As an employer, with respect to breath ASDs, you must also follow the device use and care requirements of §40.233.

SUBPART L—ALCOHOL SCREENING TESTS

§ 40.241 What are the first steps in any alcohol screening test?

As the BAT or STT you will take the following steps to begin all alcohol screening tests, regardless of the type of testing device you are using:

(a) When a specific time for an employee's test has been scheduled, or the collection site is at the employee's worksite, and the employee does not appear at the collection site at the scheduled time, contact the DER to determine the appropriate interval within which the DER has determined the employee is authorized to arrive. If the employee's arrival is delayed beyond that time, you must notify the DER that the employee has not reported for testing. In a situation where a C/TPA has notified an owner/operator or other individual employee to report for testing and the employee does not appear, the C/TPA must notify the employee that he or she has refused to test.

(b) Ensure that, when the employee enters the alcohol testing site, you begin the alcohol testing process without undue delay. For example, you must not wait because the employee says he or she is not ready or because an authorized employer or employee representative is delayed in arriving.

(1) If the employee is also going to take a DOT drug test, you must, to the greatest extent practicable, ensure that the alcohol test is completed before the urine collection process begins.

(2) If the employee needs medical attention (e.g., an injured employee in an emergency medical facility who is required to have a post-accident test), do not delay this treatment to conduct a test.

(c) Require the employee to provide positive identification. You must see a photo ID issued by the employer (other than in the case of an owner-operator or other self-employer individual) or a Federal, state, or local government (e.g., a driver's license). You may not accept faxes or photocopies of identification. Positive identification by an employer representative (not a co-worker or another employee being tested) is also acceptable. If the employee cannot produce positive identification, you must contact a DER to verify the identity of the employee.

(d) If the employee asks, provide your identification to the employee. Your identification must include your name and your employer's name but is not required to include your picture, address, or telephone number.

(e) Explain the testing procedure to the employee, including showing the employee the instructions on the back of the ATF.

(f) Complete Step 1 of the ATF.

(g) Direct the employee to complete Step 2 on the ATF and sign the certification. If the employee refuses to sign this certification, you must document this refusal on the "Remarks" line of the ATF and immediately notify the DER. This is a refusal to test.

§ 40.243 What is the procedure for an alcohol screening test using an EBT or non-evidential breath ASD?

As the BAT or STT, you must take the following steps:

(a) Select, or allow the employee to select, an individually wrapped or sealed mouthpiece from the testing materials.

(b) Open the individually wrapped or sealed mouthpiece in view of the employee and insert it into the device in accordance with the manufacturer's instructions.

(c) Instruct the employee to blow steadily and forcefully into the mouthpiece for at least six seconds or until the device indicates that an adequate amount of breath has been obtained.

(d) Show the employee the displayed test result.

(e) If the device is one that prints the test number, testing device name and serial number, time, and result directly onto the ATF, you must check to ensure that the information has been printed correctly onto the ATF.

(f) If the device is one that prints the test number, testing device name and serial number, time and result, but on a separate printout rather than directly onto the ATF, you must affix the printout of the information to the designated space on the ATF with tamper-evident tape or use a self-adhesive label that is tamper-evident.

(g) If the device is one that does not print the test number, testing device name and serial number, time,

and result, or it is a device not being used with a printer, you must record this information in Step 3 of the ATF.

§ 40.245 What is the procedure for an alcohol screening test using a saliva ASD or a breath tube ASD?

(a) As the STT or BAT, you must take the following steps when using the saliva ASD:

(1) Check the expiration date on the device or on the package containing the device and show it to the employee. You may not use the device after its expiration date.

(2) Open an individually wrapped or sealed package containing the device in the presence of the employee.

(3) Offer the employee the opportunity to use the device. If the employee uses it, you must instruct the employee to insert it into his or her mouth and use it in a manner described by the device's manufacturer.

(4) If the employee chooses not to use the device, or in all cases in which a new test is necessary because the device did not activate (see paragraph (a)(7) of this section), you must insert the device into the employee's mouth and gather saliva in the manner described by the device's manufacturer. You must wear single-use examination or similar gloves while doing so and change them following each test.

(5) When the device is removed from the employee's mouth, you must follow the manufacturer's instructions regarding necessary next steps in ensuring that the device has activated.

(6)(i) If you were unable to successfully follow the procedures of paragraphs (a)(3) through (a)(5) of this section (e.g., the device breaks, you drop the device on the floor), you must discard the device and conduct a new test using a new device.

(ii) The new device you use must be one that has been under your control or that of the employee before the test.

(iii) You must note on the "Remarks" line of the ATF the reason for the new test. (Note: You may continue using the same ATF with which you began the test.)

(iv) You must offer the employee the choice of using the device or having you use it unless the employee, in the opinion of the STT or BAT, was responsible (e.g., the employee dropped the device) for the new test needing to be conducted.

(v) If you are unable to successfully follow the procedures of paragraphs (a)(3) through (a)(5) of this section on the new test, you must end the collection and put an explanation on the "Remarks" line of the ATF.

(vi) You must then direct the employee to take a new test immediately, using an EBT for the screening test.

(7) If you are able to successfully follow the procedures of paragraphs (a)(3)–(a)(5) of this section, but the device does not activate, you must discard the device and conduct a new test, in the same manner as provided in paragraph (a)(6) of this section. In this case, you must place the device into the employee's mouth to collect saliva for the new test.

(8) You must read the result displayed on the device no sooner than the device's manufacturer instructs. In all cases the result displayed must be read within 15 minutes of the test. You must then show the device and it's reading to the employee and enter the result on the ATF.

(9) You must never re-use devices, swabs, gloves or other materials used in saliva testing.

(10) You must note the fact that you used a saliva ASD in Step 3 of the ATF.

(b) As the STT or BAT, you must take the following steps when using the breath tube ASD:

(1) Check the expiration date on the detector device and the electronic analyzer or on the package containing the device and the analyzer and show it to the employee. You must not use the device or the analyzer after their expiration date. You must not use an analyzer which is not specifically pre-calibrated for the device being used in the collection.

(2) Remove the device from the package and secure an inflation bag onto the appropriate end of the device, as directed by the manufacturer on the device's instructions.

(3) Break the tube's ampoule in the presence of the employee.

(4) Offer the employee the opportunity to use the device. If the employee chooses to use (e.g. hold) the device, instruct the employee to blow forcefully and steadily into the blowing end of device until the inflation bag fills with air (approximately 12 seconds).

(5) If the employee chooses not to hold the device, you must hold it and provide the use instructions in paragraph (b)(4) of this section.

(6) When the employee completes the breath process, take the device from the employee (or if you were holding it, remove it from the employee's mouth), remove the inflation bag, and prepare the device to be read by the analyzer in accordance with the manufacturer's directions.

(7)(i) If you were unable to successfully follow the procedures of paragraphs (b)(4) through (b)(6) of this section (e.g., the device breaks apart, the employee did not fill the inflation bag), you must discard the device and conduct a new test using a new one.

(ii) The new device you use must be one that has been under your control or that of the employer before the test.

(iii) You must note on the "Remarks" line of the ATF the reason for the new test. (Note: You may continue using the same ATF with which you began the test.)

(iv) You must offer the employee the choice of holding the device or having you hold it unless the employee, in the your opinion, was responsible (e.g., the employee failed to fill the inflation bag) for the new test needing to be conducted.

(v) If you are unable to successfully follow the procedures of paragraphs (b)(4) through (b)(6) of this section on the new test, you must end the collection and put an explanation on the "Remarks" line of the ATF.

(vi) You must then direct the employee to take a new test immediately, using another type of ASD (e.g., saliva device) or an EBT.

(8) If you were able to successfully follow the procedures of paragraphs (b)(4) through (b)(6) of this section and after having waited the required amount of time directed by the manufacturer for the detector device to incubate, you must place the device in the analyzer in accordance with the manufacturer's directions. The result must be read from the analyzer no earlier then the required incubation time of the device. In all cases, the result must be read within 15 minutes of the test.

(9) You must follow the manufacturer's instructions for determining the result of the test. You must show the analyzer result to the employee and record the result on Step 3 of the ATF.

(10) You must never re-use detector devices or any gloves used in breath tube testing. The inflation bag must be voided of air following removal from a device. Inflation bags and electronic analyzers may be re-used but only in accordance with the manufacturer's directions.

(11) You must note the fact that you used a breath tube device in Step 3 of the ATF.

[67 FR 61522, Oct. 1, 2002, as amended at 72 FR 1299, Jan. 11, 2007]

§ 40.247 What procedures does the BAT or STT follow after a screening test result?

(a) If the test result is an alcohol concentration of less than 0.02, as the BAT or STT, you must do the following:

(1) Sign and date Step 3 of the ATF; and

(2) Transmit the result to the DER in a confidential manner, as provided in §40.255.

(b) If the test result is an alcohol concentration of 0.02 or higher, as the BAT or STT, you must direct the employee to take a confirmation test.

(1) If you are the BAT who will conduct the confirmation test, you must then conduct the test using the procedures beginning at §40.251.

(2) If you are not the BAT who will conduct the confirmation test, direct the employee to take a con-

firmation test, sign and date Step 3 of the ATF, and give the employee Copy 2 of the ATF.

(3) If the confirmation test will be performed at a different site from the screening test, you must take the following additional steps:

(i) Advise the employee not to eat, drink, put anything (e.g., cigarette, chewing gum) into his or her mouth, or belch;

(ii) Tell the employee the reason for the waiting period required by §40.251(a) (i.e., to prevent an accumulation of mouth alcohol from leading to an artificially high reading);

(iii) Explain that following your instructions concerning the waiting period is to the employee's benefit;

(iv) Explain that the confirmation test will be conducted at the end of the waiting period, even if the instructions have not been followed;

(v) Note on the "Remarks" line of the ATF that the waiting period instructions were provided;

(vi) Instruct the person accompanying the employee to carry a copy of the ATF to the BAT who will perform the confirmation test; and

(vii) Ensure that you or another BAT, STT, or employer representative observe the employee as he or she is transported to the confirmation testing site. You must direct the employee not to attempt to drive a motor vehicle to the confirmation testing site.

(c) If the screening test is invalid, you must, as the BAT or STT, tell the employee the test is cancelled and note the problem on the "Remarks" line of the ATF. If practicable, repeat the testing process (see §40. 271).

SUBPART M—ALCOHOL CONFIRMATION TESTS

§ 40.251 What are the first steps in an alcohol confirmation test?

As the BAT for an alcohol confirmation test, you must follow these steps to begin the confirmation test process:

(a) You must carry out a requirement for a waiting period before the confirmation test, by taking the following steps:

(1) You must ensure that the waiting period lasts at least 15 minutes, starting with the completion of the screening test. After the waiting period has elapsed, you should begin the confirmation test as soon as possible, but not more than 30 minutes after the completion of the screening test.

(i) If the confirmation test is taking place at a different location from the screening test (see §40.247(b)(3)) the time of transit between sites counts toward the waiting period if the STT or BAT who conducted the screening test provided the waiting period instructions.

(ii) If you cannot verify, through review of the ATF, that waiting period instructions were provided, then you must carry out the waiting period requirement.

(iii) You or another BAT or STT, or an employer representative, must observe the employee during the waiting period.

(2) Concerning the waiting period, you must tell the employee:

(i) Not to eat, drink, put anything (e.g., cigarette, chewing gum) into his or her mouth, or belch;

(ii) The reason for the waiting period (i.e., to prevent an accumulation of mouth alcohol from leading to an artificially high reading);

(iii) That following your instructions concerning the waiting period is to the employee's benefit; and

(iv) That the confirmation test will be conducted at the end of the waiting period, even if the instructions have not been followed.

(3) If you become aware that the employee has not followed the instructions, you must note this on the "Remarks" line of the ATF.

(b) If you did not conduct the screening test for the employee, you must require positive identification of the employee, explain the confirmation procedures, and use a new ATF. You must note on the "Remarks" line of the ATF that a different BAT or STT conducted the screening test.

(c) Complete Step 1 of the ATF.

(d) Direct the employee to complete Step 2 on the ATF and sign the certification. If the employee refuses to sign this certification, you must document this refusal on the "Remarks" line of the ATF and immediately notify the DER. This is a refusal to test.

(e) Even if more than 30 minutes have passed since the screening test result was obtained, you must begin the confirmation test procedures in §40.253, not another screening test.

(f) You must note on the "Remarks" line of the ATF the time that elapsed between the two events, and if the confirmation test could not begin within 30 minutes of the screening test, the reason why.

(g) Beginning the confirmation test procedures after the 30 minutes have elapsed does not invalidate the screening or confirmation tests, but it may constitute a regulatory violation subject to DOT agency sanction.

§ 40.253 What are the procedures for conducting an alcohol confirmation test?

As the BAT conducting an alcohol confirmation test, you must follow these steps in order to complete the confirmation test process:

(a) In the presence of the employee, you must conduct an air blank on the EBT you are using before beginning the confirmation test and show the reading to the employee.

(1) If the reading is 0.00, the test may proceed. If the reading is greater than 0.00, you must conduct another air blank.

(2) If the reading on the second air blank is 0.00, the test may proceed. If the reading is greater than 0.00, you must take the EBT out of service.

(3) If you take an EBT out of service for this reason, no one may use it for testing until the EBT is found to be within tolerance limits on an external check of calibration.

(4) You must proceed with the test of the employee using another EBT, if one is available.

(b) You must open a new individually wrapped or sealed mouthpiece in view of the employee and insert it into the device in accordance with the manufacturer's instructions.

(c) You must ensure that you and the employee read the unique test number displayed on the EBT.

(d) You must instruct the employee to blow steadily and forcefully into the mouthpiece for at least six seconds or until the device indicates that an adequate amount of breath has been obtained.

(e) You must show the employee the result displayed on the EBT.

(f) You must show the employee the result and unique test number that the EBT prints out either directly onto the ATF or onto a separate printout.

(g) If the EBT provides a separate printout of the result, you must attach the printout to the designated space on the ATF with tamper-evident tape, or use a self-adhesive label that is tamper-evident.

[65 FR 79526, Dec. 19, 2000, as amended at 66 FR 41954, Aug. 9, 2001]

§ 40.255 What happens next after the alcohol confirmation test result?

(a) After the EBT has printed the result of an alcohol confirmation test, you must, as the BAT, take the following additional steps:

(1) Sign and date Step 3 of the ATF.

(2) If the alcohol confirmation test result is lower than 0.02, nothing further is required of the employee. As the BAT, you must sign and date Step 3 of the ATF.

(3) If the alcohol confirmation test result is 0.02 or higher, direct the employee to sign and date Step 4 of the ATF. If the employee does not do so, you must note this on the "Remarks" line of the ATF. However, this is not considered a refusal to test.

(4) If the test is invalid, tell the employee the test is cancelled and note the problem on the "Remarks"

line of the ATF. If practicable, conduct a re-test (see §40.271).

(5) Immediately transmit the result directly to the DER in a confidential manner.

(i) You may transmit the results using Copy 1 of the ATF, in person, by telephone, or by electronic means. In any case, you must immediately notify the DER of any result of 0.02 or greater by any means (e.g., telephone or secure fax machine) that ensures the result is immediately received by the DER. You must not transmit these results through C/TPAs or other service agents.

(ii) If you do not make the initial transmission in writing, you must follow up the initial transmission with Copy 1 of the ATF.

(b) As an employer, you must take the following steps with respect to the receipt and storage of alcohol test result information:

(1) If you receive any test results that are not in writing (e.g., by telephone or electronic means), you must establish a mechanism to establish the identity of the BAT sending you the results.

(2) You must store all test result information in a way that protects confidentiality.

SUBPART N—PROBLEMS IN ALCOHOL TESTING

§ 40.261 What is a refusal to take an alcohol test, and what are the consequences?

(a) As an employee, you are considered to have refused to take an alcohol test if you:

(1) Fail to appear for any test (except a pre-employment test) within a reasonable time, as determined by the employer, consistent with applicable DOT agency regulations, after being directed to do so by the employer. This includes the failure of an employee (including an owner-operator) to appear for a test when called by a C/TPA (see §40.241(a));

(2) Fail to remain at the testing site until the testing process is complete; Provided, That an employee who leaves the testing site before the testing process commences (see §40.243(a)) for a pre-employment test is not deemed to have refused to test;

(3) Fail to provide an adequate amount of saliva or breath for any alcohol test required by this part or DOT agency regulations; Provided, That an employee who does not provide an adequate amount of breath or saliva because he or she has left the testing site before the testing process commences (see §40.243(a)) for a pre-employment test is not deemed to have refused to test;

(4) Fail to provide a sufficient breath specimen, and the physician has determined, through a required medical evaluation, that there was no adequate medical explanation for the failure (see §40.265(c));

(5) Fail to undergo a medical examination or evaluation, as directed by the employer as part of the insufficient breath procedures outlined at §40.265(c);

(6) Fail to sign the certification at Step 2 of the ATF (see §§40.241(g) and 40.251(d)); or

(7) Fail to cooperate with any part of the testing process.

(b) As an employee, if you refuse to take an alcohol test, you incur the same consequences specified under DOT agency regulations for a violation of those DOT agency regulations.

(c) As a BAT or an STT, or as the physician evaluating a "shy lung" situation, when an employee refuses to test as provided in paragraph (a) of this section, you must terminate the portion of the testing process in which you are involved, document the refusal on the ATF (or in a separate document which you cause to be attached to the form), immediately notify the DER by any means (e.g., telephone or secure fax machine) that ensures the refusal notification is immediately received. You must make this notification directly to the DER (not using a C/TPA as an intermediary).

(d) As an employee, when you refuse to take a non-DOT test or to sign a non-DOT form, you have not refused to take a DOT test. There are no consequences under DOT agency regulations for such a refusal.

[65 FR 79526, Dec. 19, 2000, as amended at 66 FR 41954, Aug. 9, 2001]

§ 40.263 What happens when an employee is unable to provide a sufficient amount of saliva for an alcohol screening test?

(a) As the STT, you must take the following steps if an employee is unable to provide sufficient saliva to complete a test on a saliva screening device (e.g., the employee does not provide sufficient saliva to activate the device).

(1) You must conduct a new screening test using a new screening device.

(2) If the employee refuses to make the attempt to complete the new test, you must discontinue testing, note the fact on the "Remarks" line of the ATF, and immediately notify the DER. This is a refusal to test.

(3) If the employee has not provided a sufficient amount of saliva to complete the new test, you must note the fact on the "Remarks" line of the ATF and immediately notify the DER.

(b) As the DER, when the STT informs you that the employee has not provided a sufficient amount of saliva (see paragraph (a)(3) of this section), you must immediately arrange to administer an alcohol test to the employee using an EBT or other breath testing device.

§ 40.265 What happens when an employee is unable to provide a sufficient amount of breath for an alcohol test?

(a) If an employee does not provide a sufficient amount of breath to permit a valid breath test, you must take the steps listed in this section.

(b) As the BAT or STT, you must instruct the employee to attempt again to provide a sufficient amount of breath and about the proper way to do so.

(1) If the employee refuses to make the attempt, you must discontinue the test, note the fact on the "Remarks" line of the ATF, and immediately notify the DER. This is a refusal to test.

(2) If the employee again attempts and fails to provide a sufficient amount of breath, you may provide another opportunity to the employee to do so if you believe that there is a strong likelihood that it could result in providing a sufficient amount of breath.

(3) When the employee's attempts under paragraph (b)(2) of this section have failed to produce a sufficient amount of breath, you must note the fact on the "Remarks" line of the ATF and immediately notify the DER.

(4) If you are using an EBT that has the capability of operating manually, you may attempt to conduct the test in manual mode.

(5) If you are qualified to use a saliva ASD and you are in the screening test stage, you may change to a saliva ASD only to complete the screening test.

(c) As the employer, when the BAT or STT informs you that the employee has not provided a sufficient amount of breath, you must direct the employee to obtain, within five days, an evaluation from a licensed physician who is acceptable to you and who has expertise in the medical issues raised by the employee's failure to provide a sufficient specimen.

(1) You are required to provide the physician who will conduct the evaluation with the following information and instructions:

(i) That the employee was required to take a DOT breath alcohol test, but was unable to provide a sufficient amount of breath to complete the test;

(ii) The consequences of the appropriate DOT agency regulation for refusing to take the required alcohol test;

(iii) That the physician must provide you with a signed statement of his or her conclusions; and

(iv) That the physician, in his or her reasonable medical judgment, must base those conclusions on one of the following determinations:

(A) A medical condition has, or with a high degree of probability could have, precluded the employee from providing a sufficient amount of breath. The physician must not include in the signed statement detailed information on the employee's medical condition. In this case, the test is cancelled.

(B) There is not an adequate basis for determining that a medical condition has, or with a high degree of probability could have, precluded the employee from providing a sufficient amount of breath. This constitutes a refusal to test.

(C) For purposes of paragraphs (c)(1)(iv)(A) and (B) of this section, a medical condition includes an ascertainable physiological condition (e.g., a respiratory system dysfunction) or a medically documented pre-existing psychological disorder, but does not include unsupported assertions of "situational anxiety" or hyperventilation.

(2) As the physician making the evaluation, after making your determination, you must provide a written statement of your conclusions and the basis for them to the DER directly (and not through a C/TPA acting as an intermediary). You must not include in this statement detailed information on the employee's medical condition beyond what is necessary to explain your conclusion.

(3) Upon receipt of the report from the examining physician, as the DER you must immediately inform the employee and take appropriate action based upon your DOT agency regulations.

§ 40.267   What problems always cause an alcohol test to be cancelled?

As an employer, a BAT, or an STT, you must cancel an alcohol test if any of the following problems occur. These are "fatal flaws." You must inform the DER that the test was cancelled and must be treated as if the test never occurred. These problems are:

(a) In the case of a screening test conducted on a saliva ASD or a breath tube ASD:

(1) The STT or BAT reads the result either sooner than or later than the time allotted by the manufacturer and this Part (see §40.245(a)(8) for the saliva ASD and §40.245(b)(8) for the breath tube ASD).

(2) The saliva ASD does not activate (see §40.245(a)(7); or

(3) The device is used for a test after the expiration date printed on the device or on its package (see §40.245(a)(1) for the saliva ASD and §40.245(b)(1) for the breath tube ASD).

(4) The breath tube ASD is tested with an analyzer which has not been pre-calibrated for that device's specific lot (see §40.245(b)(1)).

(b) In the case of a screening or confirmation test conducted on an EBT, the sequential test number or alcohol concentration displayed on the EBT is not the same as the sequential test number or alcohol concentration on the printed result (see §40.253(c), (e) and (f)).

(c) In the case of a confirmation test:

(1) The BAT conducts the confirmation test before the end of the minimum 15-minute waiting period (see §40.251(a)(1));

(2) The BAT does not conduct an air blank before the confirmation test (see §40.253(a));

(3) There is not a 0.00 result on the air blank conducted before the confirmation test (see §40.253(a)(1) and (2));

(4) The EBT does not print the result (see §40.253(f)); or

(5) The next external calibration check of the EBT produces a result that differs by more than the tolerance stated in the QAP from the known value of the test standard. In this case, every result of 0.02 or above obtained on the EBT since the last valid external calibration check is cancelled (see §40.233(a)(1) and (c)(3)).

[65 FR 79526, Dec. 19, 2000, as amended at 67 FR 61522, Oct. 1, 2002; 71 FR 49384. Aug. 23, 2006; 72 FR 1299, Jan. 11, 2007]

§ 40.269   What problems cause an alcohol test to be cancelled unless they are corrected?

As a BAT or STT, or employer, you must cancel an alcohol test if any of the following problems occur, unless they are corrected. These are "correctable flaws." These problems are:

(a) The BAT or STT does not sign the ATF (see §§40.247(a)(1) and 40.255(a)(1)).

(b) The BAT or STT fails to note on the "Remarks" line of the ATF that the employee has not signed the ATF after the result is obtained (see §40.255(a)(3)).

(c) The BAT or STT uses a non-DOT form for the test (see §40.225(a)).

[65 FR 79526, Dec. 19, 2000, amended at 71 FR 49384, Aug. 23, 2006]

§ 40.271   How are alcohol testing problems corrected?

(a) As a BAT or STT, you have the responsibility of trying to complete successfully an alcohol test for each employee.

(1) If, during or shortly after the testing process, you become aware of any event that will cause the test to be cancelled (see §40.267), you must try to correct the problem promptly, if practicable. You may repeat the testing process as part of this effort.

(2) If repeating the testing process is necessary, you must begin a new test as soon as possible. You must use a new ATF, a new sequential test number, and, if needed, a new ASD and/or a new EBT. It is permissible to use additional technical capabilities of the EBT

(e.g., manual operation) if you have been trained to do so in accordance with §40.213(c).

(3) If repeating the testing process is necessary, you are not limited in the number of attempts to complete the test, provided that the employee is making a good faith effort to comply with the testing process.

(4) If another testing device is not available for the new test at the testing site, you must immediately notify the DER and advise the DER that the test could not be completed. As the DER who receives this information, you must make all reasonable efforts to ensure that the test is conducted at another testing site as soon as possible.

(b) If, as an STT, BAT, employer or other service agent administering the testing process, you become aware of a "correctable flaw" (see §40.269) that has not already been corrected, you must take all practicable action to correct the problem so that the test is not cancelled.

(1) If the problem resulted from the omission of required information, you must, as the person responsible for providing that information, supply in writing the missing information and a signed statement that it is true and accurate. For example, suppose you are a BAT and you forgot to make a notation on the "Remarks" line of the ATF that the employee did not sign the certification. You would, when the problem is called to your attention, supply a signed statement that the employee failed or refused to sign the certification after the result was obtained, and that your signed statement is true and accurate.

(2) If the problem is the use of a non-DOT form, you must, as the person responsible for the use of the incorrect form, certify in writing that the incorrect form contains all the information needed for a valid DOT alcohol test. You must also provide a signed statement that the incorrect form was used inadvertently or as the only means of conducting a test, in circumstances beyond your control, and the steps you have taken to prevent future use of non-DOT forms for DOT tests. You must supply this information on the same business day on which you are notified of the problem, transmitting it by fax or courier.

(c) If you cannot correct the problem, you must cancel the test.

§ 40.273 What is the effect of a cancelled alcohol test?

(a) A cancelled alcohol test is neither positive nor negative.

(1) As an employer, you must not attach to a cancelled test the consequences of a test result that is 0.02 or greater (e.g., removal from a safety-sensitive position).

(2) As an employer, you must not use a cancelled test in a situation where an employee needs a test result that is below 0.02 (e.g., in the case of a return-to-duty or follow-up test to authorize the employee to perform safety-sensitive functions).

(3) As an employer, you must not direct a recollection for an employee because a test has been cancelled, except in the situations cited in paragraph (a)(2) of this section or other provisions of this part.

(b) A cancelled test does not count toward compliance with DOT requirements, such as a minimum random testing rate.

(c) When a test must be cancelled, if you are the BAT, STT, or other person who determines that the cancellation is necessary, you must inform the affected DER within 48 hours of the cancellation.

(d) A cancelled DOT test does not provide a valid basis for an employer to conduct a non-DOT test (i.e., a test under company authority).

§ 40.275 What is the effect of procedural problems that are not sufficient to cancel an alcohol test?

(a) As an STT, BAT, employer, or a service agent administering the testing process, you must document any errors in the testing process of which you become aware, even if they are not "fatal flaws" or "correctable flaws" listed in this subpart. Decisions about the ultimate impact of these errors will be determined by administrative or legal proceedings, subject to the limitation of paragraph (b) of this section.

(b) No person concerned with the testing process may declare a test cancelled based on a mistake in the process that does not have a significant adverse effect on the right of the employee to a fair and accurate test. For example, it is inconsistent with this part to cancel a test based on a minor administrative mistake (e.g., the omission of the employee's middle initial) or an error that does not affect employee protections under this part. Nor does the failure of an employee to sign in Step 4 of the ATF result in the cancellation of the test. Nor is a test to be cancelled on the basis of a claim by an employee that he or she was improperly selected for testing.

(c) As an employer, these errors, even though not sufficient to cancel an alcohol test result, may subject you to enforcement action under DOT agency regulations.

§ 40.277 Are alcohol tests other than saliva or breath permitted under these regulations?

No, other types of alcohol tests (e.g., blood and urine) are not authorized for testing done under this part. Only saliva or breath for screening tests and breath for confirmation tests using approved devices are permitted.

SUBPART O—SUBSTANCE ABUSE PROFESSIONALS AND THE RETURN-TO-DUTY PROCESS

§ 40.281   Who is qualified to act as a SAP?

To be permitted to act as a SAP in the DOT drug and alcohol testing program, you must meet each of the requirements of this section:

(a) Credentials. You must have one of the following credentials:

(1) You are a licensed physician (Doctor of Medicine or Osteopathy);

(2) You are a licensed or certified social worker;

(3) You are a licensed or certified psychologist;

(4) You are a licensed or certified employee assistance professional;

(5) You are a state-licensed or certified marriage and family therapist; or

(6) You are a drug and alcohol counselor certified by the National Association of Alcoholism and Drug Abuse Counselors Certification Commission (NAADAC); or by the International Certification Reciprocity Consortium/Alcohol and Other Drug Abuse (ICRC); or by the National Board for Certified Counselors, Inc. and Affiliates/Master Addictions Counselor (NBCC).

(b) Basic knowledge. You must be knowledgeable in the following areas:

(1) You must be knowledgeable about and have clinical experience in the diagnosis and treatment of alcohol and controlled substances-related disorders.

(2) You must be knowledgeable about the SAP function as it relates to employer interests in safety-sensitive duties.

(3) You must be knowledgeable about this part, the DOT agency regulations applicable to the employers for whom you evaluate employees, and the DOT SAP Guidelines, and you keep current on any changes to these materials. These documents are available from ODAPC (Department of Transportation, 1200 New Jersey Avenue, SE, Washington DC, 20590, 202–366–3784, or on the ODAPC web site (http://www.dot.gov/ost/dapc).

(c) Qualification training. You must receive qualification training meeting the requirements of this paragraph (c).

(1) Qualification training must provide instruction on the following subjects:

(i) Background, rationale, and coverage of the Department's drug and alcohol testing program;

(ii) 49 CFR Part 40 and DOT agency drug and alcohol testing rules;

(iii) Key DOT drug testing requirements, including collections, laboratory testing, MRO review, and problems in drug testing;

(iv) Key DOT alcohol testing requirements, including the testing process, the role of BATs and STTs, and problems in alcohol tests;

(v) SAP qualifications and prohibitions;

(vi) The role of the SAP in the return-to-duty process, including the initial employee evaluation, referrals for education and/or treatment, the follow-up evaluation, continuing treatment recommendations, and the follow-up testing plan;

(vii) SAP consultation and communication with employers, MROs, and treatment providers;

(viii) Reporting and recordkeeping requirements;

(ix) Issues that SAPs confront in carrying out their duties under the program.

(2) Following your completion of qualification training under paragraph (c)(1) of this section, you must satisfactorily complete an examination administered by a nationally-recognized professional or training organization. The examination must comprehensively cover all the elements of qualification training listed in paragraph (c)(1) of this section.

(3) The following is the schedule for qualification training you must meet:

(i) If you became a SAP before August 1, 2001, you must meet the qualification training requirement no later than December 31, 2003.

(ii) If you become a SAP between August 1, 2001, and December 31, 2003, you must meet the qualification training requirement no later than December 31, 2003.

(iii) If you become a SAP on or after January 1, 2004, you must meet the qualification training requirement before you begin to perform SAP functions.

(d) Continuing education. During each three-year period from the date on which you satisfactorily complete the examination under paragraph (c)(2) of this section, you must complete continuing education consisting of at least 12 professional development hours (e.g., CEUs) relevant to performing SAP functions.

(1) This continuing education must include material concerning new technologies, interpretations, recent guidance, rule changes, and other information about developments in SAP practice, pertaining to the DOT program, since the time you met the qualification training requirements of this section.

(2) Your continuing education activities must include documentable assessment tools to assist you in determining whether you have adequately learned the material.

(e) Documentation. You must maintain documentation showing that you currently meet all requirements of this section. You must provide this documentation on request to DOT agency representatives and to employers and C/TPAs who are using or contemplating using your services.

[65 FR 79526, Dec. 19, 2000, as amended at 69 FR 3022, Jan. 22, 2004; 71 FR 49384, Aug. 23, 2006; 71 FR 55347, Sept. 22, 2006; 73 FR 33329, June 12, 2008]

§ 40.283 How does a certification organization obtain recognition for its members as SAPs?

(a) If you represent a certification organization that wants DOT to authorize its certified drug and alcohol counselors to be added to §40.281(a)(6), you may submit a written petition to DOT requesting a review of your petition for inclusion.

(b) You must obtain the National Commission for Certifying Agencies (NCCA) accreditation before DOT will act on your petition.

(c) You must also meet the minimum requirements of Appendix E to this part before DOT will act on your petition.

[65 FR 79526, Dec. 19, 2000, as amended at 71 FR 49384, Aug. 23, 2006]

§ 40.285 When is a SAP evaluation required?

(a) As an employee, when you have violated DOT drug and alcohol regulations, you cannot again perform any DOT safety-sensitive duties for any employer until and unless you complete the SAP evaluation, referral, and education/treatment process set forth in this subpart and in applicable DOT agency regulations. The first step in this process is a SAP evaluation.

(b) For purposes of this subpart, a verified positive DOT drug test result, a DOT alcohol test with a result indicating an alcohol concentration of 0.04 or greater, a refusal to test (including by adulterating or substituting a urine specimen) or any other violation of the prohibition on the use of alcohol or drugs under a DOT agency regulation constitutes a DOT drug and alcohol regulation violation.

§ 40.287 What information is an employer required to provide concerning SAP services to an employee who has a DOT drug and alcohol regulation violation?

As an employer, you must provide to each employee (including an applicant or new employee) who violates a DOT drug and alcohol regulation a listing of SAPs readily available to the employee and acceptable to you, with names, addresses, and telephone numbers. You cannot charge the employee any fee for compiling or providing this list. You may provide this list yourself or through a C/TPA or other service agent.

§ 40.289 Are employers required to provide SAP and treatment services to employees?

(a) As an employer, you are not required to provide a SAP evaluation or any subsequent recommended education or treatment for an employee who has violated a DOT drug and alcohol regulation.

(b) However, if you offer that employee an opportunity to return to a DOT safety-sensitive duty following a violation, you must, before the employee again performs that duty, ensure that the employee receives an evaluation by a SAP meeting the requirements of §40.281 and that the employee successfully complies with the SAP's evaluation recommendations.

(c) Payment for SAP evaluations and services is left for employers and employees to decide and may be governed by existing management-labor agreements and health care benefits.

§ 40.291 What is the role of the SAP in the evaluation, referral, and treatment process of an employee who has violated DOT agency drug and alcohol testing regulations?

(a) As a SAP, you are charged with:

(1) Making a face-to-face clinical assessment and evaluation to determine what assistance is needed by the employee to resolve problems associated with alcohol and/or drug use;

(2) Referring the employee to an appropriate education and/or treatment program;

(3) Conducting a face-to-face follow-up evaluation to determine if the employee has actively participated in the education and/or treatment program and has demonstrated successful compliance with the initial assessment and evaluation recommendations;

(4) Providing the DER with a follow-up drug and/or alcohol testing plan for the employee; and

(5) Providing the employee and employer with recommendations for continuing education and/or treatment.

(b) As a SAP, you are not an advocate for the employer or employee. Your function is to protect the public interest in safety by professionally evaluating the employee and recommending appropriate education/treatment, follow-up tests, and aftercare.

§ 40.293 What is the SAP's function in conducting the initial evaluation of an employee?

As a SAP, for every employee who comes to you following a DOT drug and alcohol regulation violation, you must accomplish the following:

(a) Provide a comprehensive face-to-face assessment and clinical evaluation.

(b) Recommend a course of education and/or treatment with which the employee must demonstrate successful compliance prior to returning to DOT safety-sensitive duty.

(1) You must make such a recommendation for every individual who has violated a DOT drug and alcohol regulation.

(2) You must make a recommendation for education and/or treatment that will, to the greatest extent possible, protect public safety in the event that the employee returns to the performance of safety-sensitive functions.

(c) Appropriate education may include, but is not limited to, self-help groups (e.g., Alcoholics Anonymous) and community lectures, where attendance can be independently verified, and bona fide drug and alcohol education courses.

(d) Appropriate treatment may include, but is not limited to, in-patient hospitalization, partial in-patient treatment, out-patient counseling programs, and aftercare.

(e) You must provide a written report directly to the DER highlighting your specific recommendations for assistance (see §40.311(c)).

(f) For purposes of your role in the evaluation process, you must assume that a verified positive test result has conclusively established that the employee committed a DOT drug and alcohol regulation violation. You must not take into consideration in any way, as a factor in determining what your recommendation will be, any of the following:

(1) A claim by the employee that the test was unjustified or inaccurate;

(2) Statements by the employee that attempt to mitigate the seriousness of a violation of a DOT drug or alcohol regulation (e.g., related to assertions of use of hemp oil, "medical marijuana" use, "contact positives," poppy seed ingestion, job stress); or

(3) Personal opinions you may have about the justification or rationale for drug and alcohol testing.

(g) In the course of gathering information for purposes of your evaluation in the case of a drug-related violation, you may consult with the MRO. As the MRO, you are required to cooperate with the SAP and provide available information the SAP requests. It is not necessary to obtain the consent of the employee to provide this information.

§ 40.295 May employees or employers seek a second SAP evaluation if they disagree with the first SAP's recommendations?

(a) As an employee with a DOT drug and alcohol regulation violation, when you have been evaluated by a SAP, you must not seek a second SAP's evaluation in order to obtain another recommendation.

(b) As an employer, you must not seek a second SAP's evaluation if the employee has already been evaluated by a qualified SAP. If the employee, contrary to paragraph (a) of this section, has obtained a second SAP evaluation, as an employer you may not rely on it for any purpose under this part.

§ 40.297 Does anyone have the authority to change a SAP's initial evaluation?

(a) Except as provided in paragraph (b) of this section, no one (e.g., an employer, employee, a managed-care provider, any service agent) may change in any way the SAP's evaluation or recommendations for assistance. For example, a third party is not permitted to make more or less stringent a SAP's recommendation by changing the SAP's evaluation or seeking another SAP's evaluation.

(b) The SAP who made the initial evaluation may modify his or her initial evaluation and recommendations based on new or additional information (e.g., from an education or treatment program).

§ 40.299 What is the SAP's role and what are the limits on a SAP's discretion in referring employees for education and treatment?

(a) As a SAP, upon your determination of the best recommendation for assistance, you will serve as a referral source to assist the employee's entry into a education and/or treatment program.

(b) To prevent the appearance of a conflict of interest, you must not refer an employee requiring assistance to your private practice or to a person or organization from which you receive payment or to a person or organization in which you have a financial interest. You are precluded from making referrals to entities with which you are financially associated.

(c) There are four exceptions to the prohibitions contained in paragraph (b) of this section. You may refer an employee to any of the following providers of assistance, regardless of your relationship with them:

(1) A public agency (e.g., treatment facility) operated by a state, county, or municipality;

(2) The employer or a person or organization under contract to the employer to provide alcohol or drug treatment and/or education services (e.g., the employer's contracted treatment provider);

(3) The sole source of therapeutically appropriate treatment under the employee's health insurance program (e.g., the single substance abuse in-patient treatment program made available by the employee's insurance coverage plan); or

(4) The sole source of therapeutically appropriate treatment reasonably available to the employee (e.g., the only treatment facility or education program reasonably located within the general commuting area).

§ 40.301 What is the SAP's function in the follow-up evaluation of an employee?

(a) As a SAP, after you have prescribed assistance under §40.293, you must re-evaluate the employee to determine if the employee has successfully carried out your education and/or treatment recommendations.

(1) This is your way to gauge for the employer the employee's ability to demonstrate successful compliance with the education and/or treatment plan.

(2) Your evaluation may serve as one of the reasons the employer decides to return the employee to safety-sensitive duty.

(b) As the SAP making the follow-up evaluation determination, you must:

(1) Confer with or obtain appropriate documentation from the appropriate education and/or treatment program professionals where the employee was referred; and

(2) Conduct a face-to-face clinical interview with the employee to determine if the employee demonstrates successful compliance with your initial evaluation recommendations.

(c) (1) If the employee has demonstrated successful compliance, you must provide a written report directly to the DER highlighting your clinical determination that the employee has done so with your initial evaluation recommendation (see §40.311(d)).

(2) You may determine that an employee has successfully demonstrated compliance even though the employee has not yet completed the full regimen of education and/or treatment you recommended or needs additional assistance. For example, if the employee has successfully completed the 30-day inpatient program you prescribed, you may make a "successful compliance" determination even though you conclude that the employee has not yet completed the out-patient counseling you recommended or should continue in an aftercare program.

(d)(1) As the SAP, if you believe, as a result of the follow-up evaluation, that the employee has not demonstrated successful compliance with your recommendations, you must provide written notice directly to the DER (see §40.311(e)).

(2) As an employer who receives the SAP's written notice that the employee has not successfully complied with the SAP's recommendations, you must not return the employee to the performance of safety-sensitive duties.

(3) As the SAP, you may conduct additional follow-up evaluation(s) if the employer determines that doing so is consistent with the employee's progress as you have reported it and with the employer's policy and/or labor-management agreements.

(4) As the employer, following a SAP report that the employee has not demonstrated successful compliance, you may take personnel action consistent with your policy and/or labor-management agreements.

§ 40.303 What happens if the SAP believes the employee needs additional treatment, aftercare, or support group services even after the employee returns to safety-sensitive duties?

(a) As a SAP, if you believe that ongoing services (in addition to follow-up tests) are needed to assist an employee to maintain sobriety or abstinence from drug use after the employee resumes the performance of safety-sensitive duties, you must provide recommendations for these services in your follow-up evaluation report (see §40.311(d)(10)).

(b) As an employer receiving a recommendation for these services from a SAP, you may, as part of a return-to-duty agreement with the employee, require the employee to participate in the recommended services. You may monitor and document the employee's participation in the recommended services. You may also make use of SAP and employee assistance program (EAP) services in assisting and monitoring employees' compliance with SAP recommendations. Nothing in this section permits an employer to fail to carry out its obligations with respect to follow-up testing (see §40.309).

(c) As an employee, you are obligated to comply with the SAP's recommendations for these services. If you fail or refuse to do so, you may be subject to disciplinary action by your employer.

§ 40.305 How does the return-to-duty process conclude?

(a) As the employer, if you decide that you want to permit the employee to return to the performance of safety-sensitive functions, you must ensure that the employee takes a return-to-duty test. This test cannot occur until after the SAP has determined that the employee has successfully complied with prescribed education and/or treatment. The employee must have a negative drug test result and/or an alcohol test with an alcohol concentration of less than 0.02 before resuming performance of safety-sensitive duties.

(b) As an employer, you must not return an employee to safety-sensitive duties until the employee meets the conditions of paragraph (a) of this section. However, you are not required to return an employee to safety-sensitive duties because the employee has met these conditions. That is a personnel decision that you have the discretion to make, subject to collective bargaining agreements or other legal requirements.

(c) As a SAP or MRO, you must not make a "fitness for duty" determination as part of this re-evaluation unless required to do so under an applicable DOT agency regulation. It is the employer, rather than you, who must decide whether to put the employee back to work in a safety-sensitive position.

§ 40.307 What is the SAP's function in pre-scribing the employee's follow-up tests?

(a) As a SAP, for each employee who has committed a DOT drug or alcohol regulation violation, and who seeks to resume the performance of safety-sensitive functions, you must establish a written follow-up testing plan. You do not establish this plan until after you determine that the employee has successfully complied with your recommendations for education and/or treatment.

(b) You must present a copy of this plan directly to the DER (see §40.311(d)(9)).

(c) You are the sole determiner of the number and frequency of follow-up tests and whether these tests will be for drugs, alcohol, or both, unless otherwise directed by the appropriate DOT agency regulation. For example, if the employee had a positive drug test, but your evaluation or the treatment program professionals determined that the employee had an alcohol problem as well, you should require that the employee have follow-up tests for both drugs and alcohol.

(d) However, you must, at a minimum, direct that the employee be subject to six unannounced follow-up tests in the first 12 months of safety-sensitive duty following the employee's return to safety-sensitive functions.

(1) You may require a greater number of follow-up tests during the first 12-month period of safety-sensitive duty (e.g., you may require one test a month during the 12-month period; you may require two tests per month during the first 6-month period and one test per month during the final 6-month period).

(2) You may also require follow-up tests during the 48 months of safety-sensitive duty following this first 12-month period.

(3) You are not to establish the actual dates for the follow-up tests you prescribe. The decision on specific dates to test is the employer's.

(4) As the employer, you must not impose additional testing requirements (e.g., under company authority) on the employee that go beyond the SAP's follow-up testing plan.

(e) The requirements of the SAP's follow-up testing plan "follow the employee" to subsequent employers or through breaks in service.

Example 1 to Paragraph (e): The employee returns to duty with Employer A. Two months afterward, after completing the first two of six follow-up tests required by the SAP's plan, the employee quits his job with Employer A and begins to work in a similar position for Employer B. The employee remains obligated to complete the four additional tests during the next 10 months of safety-sensitive duty, and Employer B is responsible for ensuring that the employee does so. Employer B learns of this obligation through the inquiry it makes under §40.25.

Example 2 to Paragraph (e): The employee returns to duty with Employer A. Three months later, after the employee completes the first two of six follow-up tests required by the SAP's plan, Employer A lays the employee off for economic or seasonal employment reasons. Four months later, Employer A recalls the employee. Employer A must ensure that the employee completes the remaining four follow-up tests during the next nine months.

(f) As the SAP, you may modify the determinations you have made concerning follow-up tests. For example, even if you recommended follow-up testing beyond the first 12-months, you can terminate the testing requirement at any time after the first year of testing. You must not, however, modify the requirement that the employee take at least six follow-up tests within the first 12 months after returning to the performance of safety-sensitive functions.

§ 40.309 What are the employer's responsibilities with respect to the SAP's directions for follow-up tests?

(a) As the employer, you must carry out the SAP's follow-up testing requirements. You may not allow the employee to continue to perform safety-sensitive functions unless follow-up testing is conducted as directed by the SAP.

(b) You should schedule follow-up tests on dates of your own choosing, but you must ensure that the tests are unannounced with no discernable pattern as to their timing, and that the employee is given no advance notice.

(c) You cannot substitute any other tests (e.g., those carried out under the random testing program) conducted on the employee for this follow-up testing requirement.

(d) You cannot count a follow-up test that has been cancelled as a completed test. A cancelled follow-up test must be recollected.

§ 40.311 What are the requirements concerning SAP reports?

(a) As the SAP conducting the required evaluations, you must send the written reports required by this section in writing directly to the DER and not to a third party or entity for forwarding to the DER (except as provided in §40.355(e)). You may, however, forward the document simultaneously to the DER and to a C/TPA.

(b) As an employer, you must ensure that you receive SAP written reports directly from the SAP performing the evaluation and that no third party or entity changed the SAP's report in any way.

(c) The SAP's written report, following an initial evaluation that determines what level of assistance is needed to address the employee's drug and/or alcohol problems, must be on the SAP's own letterhead (and not the letterhead of another service agent) signed and dated by the SAP, and must contain the following delineated items:

(1) Employee's name and SSN;

(2) Employer's name and address;

(3) Reason for the assessment (specific violation of DOT regulations and violation date);

(4) Date(s) of the assessment;

(5) SAP's education and/or treatment recommendation; and

(6) SAP's telephone number.

(d) The SAP's written report concerning a follow-up evaluation that determines the employee has demonstrated successful compliance must be on the SAP's own letterhead (and not the letterhead of another service agent), signed by the SAP and dated, and must contain the following items:

(1) Employee's name and SSN;

(2) Employer's name and address;

(3) Reason for the initial assessment (specific violation of DOT regulations and violation date);

(4) Date(s) of the initial assessment and synopsis of the treatment plan;

(5) Name of practice(s) or service(s) providing the recommended education and/or treatment;

(6) Inclusive dates of employee's program participation;

(7) Clinical characterization of employee's program participation;

(8) SAP's clinical determination as to whether the employee has demonstrated successful compliance;

(9) Follow-up testing plan;

(10) Employee's continuing care needs with specific treatment, aftercare, and/or support group services recommendations; and

(11) SAP's telephone number.

(e) The SAP's written report concerning a follow-up evaluation that determines the employee has not demonstrated successful compliance must be on the SAP's own letterhead (and not the letterhead of another service agent), signed by the SAP and dated, and must contain the following items:

(1) Employee's name and SSN;

(2) Employer's name and address;

(3) Reason for the initial assessment (specific DOT violation and date);

(4) Date(s) of initial assessment and synopsis of treatment plan;

(5) Name of practice(s) or service(s) providing the recommended education and/or treatment;

(6) Inclusive dates of employee's program participation;

(7) Clinical characterization of employee's program participation;

(8) Date(s) of the first follow-up evaluation;

(9) Date(s) of any further follow-up evaluation the SAP has scheduled;

(10) SAP's clinical reasons for determining that the employee has not demonstrated successful compliance; and

(11) SAP's telephone number.

(f) As a SAP, you must also provide these written reports directly to the employee if the employee has no current employer and to the gaining DOT regulated employer in the event the employee obtains another transportation industry safety-sensitive position.

(g) As a SAP, you are to maintain copies of your reports to employers for 5 years, and your employee clinical records in accordance with Federal, state, and local laws regarding record maintenance, confidentiality, and release of information. You must make these records available, on request, to DOT agency representatives (e.g., inspectors conducting an audit or safety investigation) and representatives of the NTSB in an accident investigation.

(h) As an employer, you must maintain your reports from SAPs for 5 years from the date you received them.

§ 40.313 Where is other information on SAP functions and the return-to-duty process found in this regulation?

You can find other information on the role and functions of SAPs in the following sections of this part:

§40.3—Definition.

§40.347—Service agent assistance with SAP-required follow-up testing.

§40.355—Transmission of SAP reports.

§40.329(c)—Making SAP reports available to employees on request.

Appendix E to Part 40—SAP Equivalency Requirements for Certification Organizations.

SUBPART P—CONFIDENTIALITY AND RELEASE OF INFORMATION

§ 40.321 What is the general confidentiality rule for drug and alcohol test information?

Except as otherwise provided in this subpart, as a service agent or employer participating in the DOT drug or alcohol testing process, you are prohibited from releasing individual test results or medical information about an employee to third parties without the employee's specific written consent.

(a) A "third party" is any person or organization to whom other subparts of this regulation do not explicitly authorize or require the transmission of information in the course of the drug or alcohol testing process.

(b) "Specific written consent" means a statement signed by the employee that he or she agrees to the release of a particular piece of information to a particular, explicitly identified, person or organization at a particular time. "Blanket releases," in which an employee agrees to a release of a category of information (e.g., all test results) or to release information to a category of parties (e.g., other employers who are members of a C/TPA, companies to which the employee may apply for employment), are prohibited under this part.

§ 40.323 May program participants release drug or alcohol test information in connection with legal proceedings?

(a) As an employer, you may release information pertaining to an employee's drug or alcohol test without the employee's consent in certain legal proceedings.

(1) These proceedings include a lawsuit (e.g., a wrongful discharge action), grievance (e.g., an arbitration concerning disciplinary action taken by the employer), or administrative proceeding (e.g., an unemployment compensation hearing) brought by, or on behalf of, an employee and resulting from a positive DOT drug or alcohol test or a refusal to test (including, but not limited to, adulterated or substituted test results).

(2) These proceedings also include a criminal or civil action resulting from an employee's performance of safety-sensitive duties, in which a court of competent jurisdiction determines that the drug or alcohol test information sought is relevant to the case and issues an order directing the employer to produce the information. For example, in personal injury litigation following a truck or bus collision, the court could determine that a post-accident drug test result of an employee is relevant to determining whether the driver or the driver's employer was negligent. The employer is authorized to respond to the court's order to produce the records.

(b) In such a proceeding, you may release the information to the decisionmaker in the proceeding (e.g., the court in a lawsuit). You may release the information only with a binding stipulation that the decisionmaker to whom it is released will make it available only to parties to the proceeding.

(c) If you are a service agent, and the employer requests its employee's drug or alcohol testing information from you to use in a legal proceeding as authorized in paragraph (a) of this section (e.g., the laboratory's data package), you must provide the requested information to the employer.

(d) As an employer or service agent, you must immediately notify the employee in writing of any information you release under this section.

§ 40.325 [Reserved]

§ 40.327 When must the MRO report medical information gathered in the verification process?

(a) As the MRO, you must, except as provided in paragraph (c) of this section, report drug test results and medical information you learned as part of the verification process to third parties without the employee's consent if you determine, in your reasonable medical judgment, that:

(1) The information is likely to result in the employee being determined to be medically unqualified under an applicable DOT agency regulation; or

(2) The information indicates that continued performance by the employee of his or her safety-sensitive function is likely to pose a significant safety risk.

(b) The third parties to whom you are authorized to provide information by this section include the employer, a physician or other health care provider responsible for determining the medical qualifications of the employee under an applicable DOT agency safety regulation, a SAP evaluating the employee as part of the return to duty process (see §40.293(g)), a DOT agency, or the National Transportation Safety Board in the course of an accident investigation.

(c) If the law of a foreign country (e.g., Canada) prohibits you from providing medical information to the employer, you may comply with that prohibition.

§ 40.329 What information must laboratories, MROs, and other service agents release to employees?

(a) As an MRO or service agent you must provide, within 10 business days of receiving a written request from an employee, copies of any records pertaining to the employee's use of alcohol and/or drugs, including records of the employee's DOT-mandated drug and/or alcohol tests. You may charge no more than the cost of preparation and reproduction for copies of these records.

(b) As a laboratory, you must provide, within 10 business days of receiving a written request from an employee, and made through the MRO, the records relating to the results of the employee's drug test (i.e., laboratory report and data package). You may charge no more than the cost of preparation and reproduction for copies of these records.

(c) As a SAP, you must make available to an employee, on request, a copy of all SAP reports (see §40.311). However, you must redact follow-up testing information from the report before providing it to the employee.

[65 FR 79526, Dec. 19, 2000, as amended at 66 FR 41954, Aug. 9, 2001]

§ 40.331 To what additional parties must employers and service agents release information?

As an employer or service agent you must release information under the following circumstances:

(a) If you receive a specific, written consent from an employee authorizing the release of information about that employee's drug or alcohol tests to an identified person, you must provide the information to the identified person. For example, as an employer, when you receive a written request from a former employee to provide information to a subsequent employer, you must do so. In providing the information, you must comply with the terms of the employee's consent.

(b) If you are an employer, you must, upon request of DOT agency representatives, provide the following:

(1) Access to your facilities used for this part and DOT agency drug and alcohol program functions.

(2) All written, printed, and computer-based drug and alcohol program records and reports (including copies of name-specific records or reports), files, materials, data, documents/documentation, agreements, contracts, policies, and statements that are required by this part and DOT agency regulations. You must provide this information at your principal place of business in the time required by the DOT agency.

(3) All items in paragraph (b)(2) of this section must be easily accessible, legible, and provided in an organized manner. If electronic records do not meet these standards, they must be converted to printed documentation that meets these standards.

(c) If you are a service agent, you must, upon request of DOT agency representatives, provide the following:

(1) Access to your facilities used for this part and DOT agency drug and alcohol program functions.

(2) All written, printed, and computer-based drug and alcohol program records and reports (including copies of name-specific records or reports), files, materials, data, documents/documentation, agreements, contracts, policies, and statements that are required by this part and DOT agency regulations. You must provide this information at your principal place of business in the time required by the DOT agency.

(3) All items in paragraph (c)(2) of this section must be easily accessible, legible, and provided in an organized manner. If electronic records do not meet these standards, they must be converted to printed documentation that meets these standards.

(d) If requested by the National Transportation Safety Board as part of an accident investigation, you must provide information concerning post-accident tests administered after the accident.

(e) If requested by a Federal, state or local safety agency with regulatory authority over you or the employee, you must provide drug and alcohol test records concerning the employee.

(f) Except as otherwise provided in this part, as a laboratory you must not release or provide a specimen or a part of a specimen to a requesting party, without first obtaining written consent from ODAPC. If a party seeks a court order directing you to release a specimen or part of a specimen contrary to any provision of this part, you must take necessary legal steps to contest the issuance of the order (e.g., seek to quash a subpoena, citing the requirements of §40.13). This part does not require you to disobey a court order, however.

(g) Notwithstanding any other provision of this Part, as an employer of Commercial Motor Vehicle (CMV) drivers holding commercial driving licenses (CDLs) or as a third party administrator for owner-operator CMV drivers with CDLs, you are authorized to comply with State laws requiring you to provide to State CDL licensing authorities information about all violations of DOT drug and alcohol testing rules (including positive tests and refusals) by any CMV driver holding a CDL.

[65 FR 79526, Dec. 19, 2000, as amended at 66 FR 41955, Aug. 9, 2001; 73 FR 33737, June 13, 2008]

§ 40.333 What records must employers keep?

(a) As an employer, you must keep the following records for the following periods of time:

(1) You must keep the following records for five years:

(i) Records of alcohol test results indicating an alcohol concentration of 0.02 or greater;

(ii) Records of verified positive drug test results;

(iii) Documentation of refusals to take required alcohol and/or drug tests (including substituted or adulterated drug test results);

(iv) SAP reports; and

(v) All follow-up tests and schedules for follow-up tests.

(2) You must keep records for three years of information obtained from previous employers under §40.25 concerning drug and alcohol test results of employees.

(3) You must keep records of the inspection, maintenance, and calibration of EBTs, for two years.

(4) You must keep records of negative and cancelled drug test results and alcohol test results with a concentration of less than 0.02 for one year.

(b) You do not have to keep records related to a program requirement that does not apply to you (e.g., a maritime employer who does not have a DOT-mandated random alcohol testing program need not maintain random alcohol testing records).

(c) You must maintain the records in a location with controlled access.

(d) A service agent may maintain these records for you. However, you must ensure that you can produce these records at your principal place of business in the time required by the DOT agency. For example, as a motor carrier, when an FMCSA inspector requests your records, you must ensure that you can provide them within two business days.

(e) If you store records electronically, where permitted by this part, you must ensure that the records are easily accessible, legible, and formatted and stored in an organized manner. If electronic records do not meet these criteria, you must convert them to printed documentation in a rapid and readily auditable manner, at the request of DOT agency personnel.

[65 FR 79526, Dec. 19, 2000, as amended at 66 FR 41955, Aug. 9, 2001]

SUBPART Q—ROLES AND RESPONSIBILITIES OF SERVICE AGENTS

§ 40.341 Must service agents comply with DOT drug and alcohol testing requirements?

(a) As a service agent, the services you provide to transportation employers must meet the requirements of this part and the DOT agency drug and alcohol testing regulations.

(b) If you do not comply, DOT may take action under the Public Interest Exclusions procedures of this part (see Subpart R of this part) or applicable provisions of other DOT agency regulations.

§ 40.343 What tasks may a service agent perform for an employer?

As a service agent, you may perform for employers the tasks needed to comply with DOT agency drug and alcohol testing regulations, subject to the requirements and limitations of this part.

§ 40.345 In what circumstances may a C/TPA act as an intermediary in the transmission of drug and alcohol testing information to employers?

(a) As a C/TPA or other service agent, you may act as an intermediary in the transmission of drug and alcohol testing information in the circumstances specified in this section only if the employer chooses to have you do so. Each employer makes the decision about whether to receive some or all of this informa-

tion from you, acting as an intermediary, rather than directly from the service agent who originates the information (e.g., an MRO or BAT).

(b) The specific provisions of this part concerning which you may act as an intermediary are listed in Appendix F to this part. These are the only situations in which you may act as an intermediary. You are prohibited from doing so in all other situations.

(c) In every case, you must ensure that, in transmitting information to employers, you meet all requirements (e.g., concerning confidentiality and timing) that would apply if the service agent originating the information (e.g., an MRO or collector) sent the information directly to the employer. For example, if you transmit drug testing results from MROs to DERs, you must transmit each drug test result to the DER in compliance with the MRO requirements set forth in §40.167.

§ 40.347 What functions may C/TPAs perform with respect to administering testing?

As a C/TPA, except as otherwise specified in this part, you may perform the following functions for employers concerning random selection and other selections for testing.

(a) You may operate random testing programs for employers and may assist (i.e., through contracting with laboratories or collection sites, conducting collections) employers with other types of testing (e.g., pre-employment, post-accident, reasonable suspicion, return-to-duty, and follow-up).

(b) You may combine employees from more than one employer or one transportation industry in a random pool if permitted by all the DOT agency drug and alcohol testing regulations involved.

(1) If you combine employees from more than one transportation industry, you must ensure that the random testing rate is at least equal to the highest rate required by each DOT agency.

(2) Employees not covered by DOT agency regulations may not be part of the same random pool with DOT covered employees.

(c) You may assist employers in ensuring that follow-up testing is conducted in accordance with the plan established by the SAP. However, neither you nor the employer are permitted to randomly select employees from a "follow-up pool" for follow-up testing.

§ 40.349 What records may a service agent receive and maintain?

(a) Except where otherwise specified in this part, as a service agent you may receive and maintain all records concerning DOT drug and alcohol testing programs, including positive, negative, and refusal to test individual test results. You do not need the employee's consent to receive and maintain these records.

(b) You may maintain all information needed for operating a drug/alcohol program (e.g., CCFs, ATFs, names of employees in random pools, random selection lists, copies of notices to employers of selected employees) on behalf of an employer.

(c) If a service agent originating drug or alcohol testing information, such as an MRO or BAT, sends the information directly to the DER, he or she may also provide the information simultaneously to you, as a C/TPA or other service agent who maintains this information for the employer.

(d) If you are serving as an intermediary in transmitting information that is required to be provided to the employer, you must ensure that it reaches the employer in the same time periods required elsewhere in this part.

(e) You must ensure that you can make available to the employer within two business days any information the employer is asked to produce by a DOT agency representative.

(f) On request of an employer, you must, at any time on the request of an employer, transfer immediately all records pertaining to the employer and its employees to the employer or to any other service agent the employer designates. You must carry out this transfer as soon as the employer requests it. You are not required to obtain employee consent for this transfer. You must not charge more than your reasonable administrative costs for conducting this transfer. You may not charge a fee for the release of these records.

(g) If you are planning to go out of business or your organization will be bought by or merged with another organization, you must immediately notify all employers and offer to transfer all records pertaining to the employer and its employees to the employer or to any other service agent the employer designates. You must carry out this transfer as soon as the employer requests it. You are not required to obtain employee consent for this transfer. You must not charge more than your reasonable administrative costs for conducting this transfer. You may not charge a fee for the release of these records.

[65 FR 79526, Dec. 19, 2000, as amended at 66 FR 41955, Aug. 9, 2001]

§ 40.351 What confidentiality requirements apply to service agents?

Except where otherwise specified in this part, as a service agent the following confidentiality requirements apply to you:

(a) When you receive or maintain confidential information about employees (e.g., individual test results), you must follow the same confidentiality regulations as the employer with respect to the use and release of this information.

(b) You must follow all confidentiality and records retention requirements applicable to employers.

(c) You may not provide individual test results or other confidential information to another employer without a specific, written consent from the employee. For example, suppose you are a C/TPA that has employers X and Y as clients. Employee Jones works for X, and you maintain Jones' drug and alcohol test for X. Jones wants to change jobs and work for Y. You may not inform Y of the result of a test conducted for X without having a specific, written consent from Jones. Likewise, you may not provide this information to employer Z, who is not a C/TPA member, without this consent.

(d) You must not use blanket consent forms authorizing the release of employee testing information.

(e) You must establish adequate confidentiality and security measures to ensure that confidential employee records are not available to unauthorized persons. This includes protecting the physical security of records, access controls, and computer security measures to safeguard confidential data in electronic data bases.

§ 40.353 What principles govern the interaction between MROs and other service agents?

As a service agent other than an MRO (e.g., a C/TPA), the following principles govern your interaction with MROs:

(a) You may provide MRO services to employers, directly or through contract, if you meet all applicable provisions of this part.

(b) If you employ or contract for an MRO, the MRO must perform duties independently and confidentially. When you have a relationship with an MRO, you must structure the relationship to ensure that this independence and confidentiality are not compromised. Specific means (including both physical and operational measures, as appropriate) to separate MRO functions and other service agent functions are essential.

(c) Only your staff who are actually under the day-to-day supervision and control of an MRO with respect to MRO functions may perform these functions. This does not mean that those staff may not perform other functions at other times. However, the designation of your staff to perform MRO functions under MRO supervision must be limited and not used as a subterfuge to circumvent confidentiality and other requirements of this part and DOT agency regulations. You must ensure that MRO staff operate under controls sufficient to ensure that the independence and confidentiality of the MRO process are not compromised.

(d) Like other MROs, an MRO you employ or contract with must personally conduct verification interviews with employees and must personally make all verification decisions. Consequently, your staff cannot perform these functions.

§ 40.355 What limitations apply to the activities of service agents?

As a service agent, you are subject to the following limitations concerning your activities in the DOT drug and alcohol testing program.

(a) You must not require an employee to sign a consent, release, waiver of liability, or indemnification agreement with respect to any part of the drug or alcohol testing process covered by this part (including, but not limited to, collections, laboratory testing, MRO, and SAP services). No one may do so on behalf of a service agent.

(b) You must not act as an intermediary in the transmission of drug test results from the laboratory to the MRO. That is, the laboratory may not send results to you, with you in turn sending them to the MRO for verification. For example, a practice in which the laboratory transmits results to your computer system, and you then assign the results to a particular MRO, is not permitted.

(c) You must not transmit drug test results directly from the laboratory to the employer (by electronic or other means) or to a service agent who forwards them to the employer. All confirmed laboratory results must be processed by the MRO before they are released to any other party.

(d) You must not act as an intermediary in the transmission of alcohol test results of 0.02 or higher from the STT or BAT to the DER.

(e) Except as provided in paragraph (f) of this section, you must not act as an intermediary in the transmission of individual SAP reports to the actual employer. That is, the SAP may not send such reports to you, with you in turn sending them to the actual employer. However, you may maintain individual SAP summary reports and follow-up testing plans after they are sent to the DER, and the SAP may transmit such reports to you simultaneously with sending them to the DER.

(f) As an exception to paragraph (e) of this section, you may act as an intermediary in the transmission of SAP report from the SAP to an owner-operator or other self-employed individual.

(g) Except as provided in paragraph (h) of this section, you must not make decisions to test an employee based upon reasonable suspicion, post-accident, return-to-duty, and follow-up determination criteria. These are duties the actual employer cannot delegate to a C/TPA. You may, however, provide advice and information to employers regarding these testing issues and how the employer should schedule required testing.

(h) As an exception to paragraph (g) of this section, you may make decisions to test an employee based upon reasonable suspicion, post-accident, return-to-duty, and follow-up determination criteria with respect to an owner-operator or other self-employed individual.

(i) Except as provided in paragraph (j) of this section, you must not make a determination that an employee has refused a drug or alcohol test. This is a non-delegable duty of the actual employer. You may, however, provide advice and information to employers regarding refusal-to-test issues.

(j) As an exception to paragraph (i) of this section, you may make a determination that an employee has refused a drug or alcohol test, if:

(1) You schedule a required test for an owner-operator or other self-employed individual, and the individual fails to appear for the test without a legitimate reason; or

(2) As an MRO, you determine that an individual has refused to test on the basis of adulteration or substitution.

(k) You must not act as a DER. For example, while you may be responsible for transmitting information to the employer about test results, you must not act on behalf of the employer in actions to remove employees from safety-sensitive duties.

(l) In transmitting documents to laboratories, you must ensure that you send to the laboratory that conducts testing only the laboratory copy of the CCF. You must not transmit other copies of the CCF or any ATFs to the laboratory.

(m) You must not impose conditions or requirements on employers that DOT regulations do not authorize. For example, as a C/TPA serving employers in the pipeline or motor carrier industry, you must not require employers to have provisions in their DOT plans that PHMSA or FMCSA regulations do not require.

(n) You must not intentionally delay the transmission of drug or alcohol testing-related documents concerning actions you have performed, because of a payment dispute or other reasons.

Example 1 to Paragraph (n): A laboratory that has tested a specimen must not delay transmitting the documentation of the test result to an MRO because of a billing or payment dispute with the MRO or a C/TPA.

Example 2 to Paragraph (n): An MRO or SAP who has interviewed an employee must not delay sending a verified test result or SAP report to the employer because of such a dispute with the employer or employee.

Example 3 to Paragraph (n): A collector who has performed a urine specimen collection must not delay sending the drug specimen and CCF to the laboratory because of a payment or other dispute with the laboratory or a C/TPA.

Example 4 to Paragraph (n): A BAT who has conducted an alcohol test must not delay sending test result information to an employer or C/TPA because of a payment or other dispute with the employer or C/TPA.

(o) While you must follow the DOT agency regulations, the actual employer remains accountable to DOT for compliance, and your failure to implement any aspect of the program as required in this part and other applicable DOT agency regulations makes the employer subject to enforcement action by the Department.

[65 FR 79526, Dec. 19, 2000, as amended at 66 FR 41955, Aug. 9, 2001]

SUBPART R—PUBLIC INTEREST EXCLUSIONS

§ 40.361 What is the purpose of a public interest exclusion (PIE)?

(a) To protect the public interest, including protecting transportation employers and employees from serious noncompliance with DOT drug and alcohol testing rules, the Department's policy is to ensure that employers conduct business only with responsible service agents.

(b) The Department therefore uses PIEs to exclude from participation in DOT's drug and alcohol testing program any service agent who, by serious noncompliance with this part or other DOT agency drug and alcohol testing regulations, has shown that it is not currently acting in a responsible manner.

(c) A PIE is a serious action that the Department takes only to protect the public interest. We intend to use PIEs only to remedy situations of serious noncompliance. PIEs are not used for the purpose of punishment.

(d) Nothing in this subpart precludes a DOT agency or the Inspector General from taking other action authorized by its regulations with respect to service agents or employers that violate its regulations.

§ 40.363 On what basis may the Department issue a PIE?

(a) If you are a service agent, the Department may issue a PIE concerning you if we determine that you have failed or refused to provide drug or alcohol testing services consistent with the requirements of this part or a DOT agency drug and alcohol regulation.

(b) The Department also may issue a PIE if you have failed to cooperate with DOT agency representatives concerning inspections, complaint investigations, compliance and enforcement reviews, or requests for documents and other information about compliance with this part or DOT agency drug and alcohol regulations.

§ 40.365 What is the Department's policy concerning starting a PIE proceeding?

(a) It is the Department's policy to start a PIE proceeding only in cases of serious, uncorrected noncompliance with the provisions of this part, affecting such matters as safety, the outcomes of test results, privacy and confidentiality, due process and fairness for employees, the honesty and integrity of the testing program, and cooperation with or provision of information to DOT agency representatives.

(b) The following are examples of the kinds of serious noncompliance that, as a matter of policy, the Department views as appropriate grounds for starting a PIE proceeding. These examples are not intended to be an exhaustive or exclusive list of the grounds for starting a PIE proceeding. We intend them to illustrate the level of seriousness that the Department believes supports starting a PIE proceeding. The examples follow:

(1) For an MRO, verifying tests positive without interviewing the employees as required by this part or providing MRO services without meeting the qualifications for an MRO required by this part;

(2) For a laboratory, refusing to provide information to the Department, an employer, or an employee as required by this part; failing or refusing to conduct a validity testing program when required by this part; or a pattern or practice of testing errors that result in the cancellation of tests. (As a general matter of policy, the Department does not intend to initiate a PIE proceeding concerning a laboratory with respect to matters on which HHS initiates certification actions under its laboratory guidelines.);

(3) For a collector, a pattern or practice of directly observing collections when doing so is unauthorized, or failing or refusing to directly observe collections when doing so is mandatory;

(4) For collectors, BATs, or STTs, a pattern or practice of using forms, testing equipment, or collection kits that do not meet the standards in this part;

(5) For a collector, BAT, or STT, a pattern or practice of "fatal flaws" or other significant uncorrected errors in the collection process;

(6) For a laboratory, MRO or C/TPA, failing or refusing to report tests results as required by this part or DOT agency regulations;

(7) For a laboratory, falsifying, concealing, or destroying documentation concerning any part of the drug testing process, including, but not limited to, documents in a "litigation package";

(8) For SAPs, providing SAP services while not meeting SAP qualifications required by this part or performing evaluations without face-to-face interviews;

(9) For any service agent, maintaining a relationship with another party that constitutes a conflict of interest under this part (e.g., a laboratory that derives a financial benefit from having an employer use a specific MRO);

(10) For any service agent, representing falsely that the service agent or its activities is approved or certified by the Department or a DOT agency;

(11) For any service agent, disclosing an employee's test result information to any party this part or a DOT agency regulation does not authorize, including by obtaining a "blanket" consent from employees or by creating a data base from which employers or others can retrieve an employee's DOT test results without the specific consent of the employee;

(12) For any service agent, interfering or attempting to interfere with the ability of an MRO to communicate with the Department, or retaliating against an MRO for communicating with the Department;

(13) For any service agent, directing or recommending that an employer fail or refuse to implement any provision of this part; or

(14) With respect to noncompliance with a DOT agency regulation, conduct that affects important provisions of Department-wide concern (e.g., failure to properly conduct the selection process for random testing).

§ 40.367 Who initiates a PIE proceeding?

The following DOT officials may initiate a PIE proceeding:

(a) The drug and alcohol program manager of a DOT agency;

(b) An official of ODAPC, other than the Director; or

(c) The designee of any of these officials.

§ 40.369 What is the discretion of an initiating official in starting a PIE proceeding?

(a) Initiating officials have broad discretion in deciding whether to start a PIE proceeding.

(b) In exercising this discretion, the initiating official must consider the Department's policy regarding the seriousness of the service agent's conduct (see §40.365) and all information he or she has obtained to this point concerning the facts of the case. The initiating official may also consider the availability of the resources needed to pursue a PIE proceeding.

(c) A decision not to initiate a PIE proceeding does not necessarily mean that the Department regards a service agent as being in compliance or that the Department may not use other applicable remedies in a situation of noncompliance.

§ 40.371 On what information does an initiating official rely in deciding whether to start a PIE proceeding?

(a) An initiating official may rely on credible information from any source as the basis for starting a PIE proceeding.

(b) Before sending a correction notice (see §40.373), the initiating official informally contacts the service agent to determine if there is any information that may affect the initiating official's determination about whether it is necessary to send a correction notice. The initiating official may take any information resulting from this contact into account in determining whether to proceed under this subpart.

§ 40.373 Before starting a PIE proceeding, does the initiating official give the service agent an opportunity to correct problems?

(a) If you are a service agent, the initiating official must send you a correction notice before starting a PIE proceeding.

(b) The correction notice identifies the specific areas in which you must come into compliance in order to avoid being subject to a PIE proceeding.

(c) If you make and document changes needed to come into compliance in the areas listed in the correction notice to the satisfaction of the initiating official within 60 days of the date you receive the notice, the initiating official does not start a PIE proceeding. The initiating official may conduct appropriate fact finding to verify that you have made and maintained satisfactory corrections. When he or she is satisfied that you are in compliance, the initiating official sends you a notice that the matter is concluded.

§ 40.375 How does the initiating official start a PIE proceeding?

(a) As a service agent, if your compliance matter is not correctable (see §40.373(a)), or if have not resolved compliance matters as provided in §40.373(c), the initiating official starts a PIE proceeding by sending you a notice of proposed exclusion (NOPE). The NOPE contains the initiating official's recommendations concerning the issuance of a PIE, but it is not a decision by the Department to issue a PIE.

(b) The NOPE includes the following information:

(1) A statement that the initiating official is recommending that the Department issue a PIE concerning you;

(2) The factual basis for the initiating official's belief that you are not providing drug and/or alcohol testing services to DOT-regulated employers consistent with the requirements of this part or are in serious noncompliance with a DOT agency drug and alcohol regulation;

(3) The factual basis for the initiating official's belief that your noncompliance has not been or cannot be corrected;

(4) The initiating official's recommendation for the scope of the PIE;

(5) The initiating official's recommendation for the duration of the PIE; and

(6) A statement that you may contest the issuance of the proposed PIE, as provided in §40.379.

(c) The initiating official sends a copy of the NOPE to the ODAPC Director at the same time he or she sends the NOPE to you.

§ 40.377 Who decides whether to issue a PIE?

(a) The ODAPC Director, or his or her designee, decides whether to issue a PIE. If a designee is acting as the decisionmaker, all references in this subpart to the Director refer to the designee.

(b) To ensure his or her impartiality, the Director plays no role in the initiating official's determination about whether to start a PIE proceeding.

(c) There is a "firewall" between the initiating official and the Director. This means that the initiating official and the Director are prohibited from having any discussion, contact, or exchange of information with one another about the matter, except for documents and discussions that are part of the record of the proceeding.

§ 40.379 How do you contest the issuance of a PIE?

(a) If you receive a NOPE, you may contest the issuance of the PIE.

(b) If you want to contest the proposed PIE, you must provide the Director information and argument in opposition to the proposed PIE in writing, in person, and/or through a representative. To contest the proposed PIE, you must take one or more of the steps listed in this paragraph (b) within 30 days after you receive the NOPE.

(1) You may request that the Director dismiss the proposed PIE without further proceedings, on the basis that it does not concern serious noncompliance with this part or DOT agency regulations, consistent with the Department's policy as stated in §40.365.

(2) You may present written information and arguments, consistent with the provisions of §40.381, contesting the proposed PIE.

(3) You may arrange with the Director for an informal meeting to present your information and arguments.

(c) If you do not take any of the actions listed in paragraph (b) of this section within 30 days after you receive the NOPE, the matter proceeds as an uncontested case. In this event, the Director makes his or her decision based on the record provided by the initiating official (i.e., the NOPE and any supporting information or testimony) and any additional information the Director obtains.

§ 40.381 What information do you present to contest the proposed issuance of a PIE?

(a) As a service agent who wants to contest a proposed PIE, you must present at least the following information to the Director:

(1) Specific facts that contradict the statements contained in the NOPE (see §40.375(b)(2) and (3)). A general denial is insufficient to raise a genuine dispute over facts material to the issuance of a PIE;

(2) Identification of any existing, proposed or prior PIE; and

(3) Identification of your affiliates, if any.

(b) You may provide any information and arguments you wish concerning the proposed issuance, scope and duration of the PIE (see §40.375(b)(4) and (5)).

(c) You may provide any additional relevant information or arguments concerning any of the issues in the matter.

§ 40.383 What procedures apply if you contest the issuance of a PIE?

(a) DOT conducts PIE proceedings in a fair and informal manner. The Director may use flexible procedures to allow you to present matters in opposition. The Director is not required to follow formal rules of evidence or procedure in creating the record of the proceeding.

(b) The Director will consider any information or argument he or she determines to be relevant to the decision on the matter.

(c) You may submit any documentary evidence you want the Director to consider. In addition, if you have arranged an informal meeting with the Director, you may present witnesses and confront any person the initiating official presents as a witness against you.

(d) In cases where there are material factual issues in dispute, the Director or his or her designee may conduct additional fact-finding.

(e) If you have arranged a meeting with the Director, the Director will make a transcribed record of the meeting available to you on your request. You must pay the cost of transcribing and copying the meeting record.

§ 40.385 Who bears the burden of proof in a PIE proceeding?

(a) As the proponent of issuing a PIE, the initiating official bears the burden of proof.

(b) This burden is to demonstrate, by a preponderance of the evidence, that the service agent was in serious noncompliance with the requirements of this part for drug and/or alcohol testing-related services or with the requirements of another DOT agency drug and alcohol testing regulation.

§ 40.387 What matters does the Director decide concerning a proposed PIE?

(a) Following the service agent's response (see §40.379(b)) or, if no response is received, after 30 days have passed from the date on which the service agent received the NOPE, the Director may take one of the following steps:

(1) In response to a request from the service agent (see §40.379(b)(1)) or on his or her own motion, the Director may dismiss a PIE proceeding if he or she determines that it does not concern serious noncompliance with this part or DOT agency regulations, consistent with the Department's policy as stated in §40.365.

(i) If the Director dismisses a proposed PIE under this paragraph (a), the action is closed with respect to the noncompliance alleged in the NOPE.

(ii) The Department may initiate a new PIE proceeding against you on the basis of different or subsequent conduct that is in noncompliance with this part or other DOT drug and alcohol testing rules.

(2) If the Director determines that the initiating official's submission does not have complete information needed for a decision, the Director may remand the matter to the initiating official. The initiating official may resubmit the matter to the Director when the needed information is complete. If the basis for the proposed PIE has changed, the initiating official must send an amended NOPE to the service agent.

(b) The Director makes determinations concerning the following matters in any PIE proceeding that he or she decides on the merits:

(1) Any material facts that are in dispute;

(2) Whether the facts support issuing a PIE;

(3) The scope of any PIE that is issued; and

(4) The duration of any PIE that is issued.

§ 40.389 What factors may the Director consider?

This section lists examples of the kind of mitigating and aggravating factors that the Director may consider in determining whether to issue a PIE concerning you, as well as the scope and duration of a PIE. This list is not exhaustive or exclusive. The Director may consider other factors if appropriate in the circumstances of a particular case. The list of examples follows:

(a) The actual or potential harm that results or may result from your noncompliance;

(b) The frequency of incidents and/or duration of the noncompliance;

(c) Whether there is a pattern or prior history of noncompliance;

(d) Whether the noncompliance was pervasive within your organization, including such factors as the following:

(1) Whether and to what extent your organization planned, initiated, or carried out the noncompliance;

(2) The positions held by individuals involved in the noncompliance, and whether your principals tolerated their noncompliance; and

(3) Whether you had effective standards of conduct and control systems (both with respect to your own organization and any contractors or affiliates) at the time the noncompliance occurred;

(e) Whether you have demonstrated an appropriate compliance disposition, including such factors as the following:

(1) Whether you have accepted responsibility for the noncompliance and recognize the seriousness of the conduct that led to the cause for issuance of the PIE;

(2) Whether you have cooperated fully with the Department during the investigation. The Director may consider when the cooperation began and whether you disclosed all pertinent information known to you;

(3) Whether you have fully investigated the circumstances of the noncompliance forming the basis for the PIE and, if so, have made the result of the investigation available to the Director;

(4) Whether you have taken appropriate disciplinary action against the individuals responsible for the activity that constitutes the grounds for issuance of the PIE; and

(5) Whether your organization has taken appropriate corrective actions or remedial measures, including implementing actions to prevent recurrence;

(f) With respect to noncompliance with a DOT agency regulation, the degree to which the noncompliance affects matters common to the DOT drug and alcohol testing program;

(g) Other factors appropriate to the circumstances of the case.

§ 40.391 What is the scope of a PIE?

(a) The scope of a PIE is the Department's determination about the divisions, organizational elements, types of services, affiliates, and/or individuals (including direct employees of a service agent and its contractors) to which a PIE applies.

(b) If, as a service agent, the Department issues a PIE concerning you, the PIE applies to all your divisions, organizational elements, and types of services that are involved with or affected by the noncompliance that forms the factual basis for issuing the PIE.

(c) In the NOPE (see §40.375(b)(4)), the initiating official sets forth his or her recommendation for the scope of the PIE. The proposed scope of the PIE is one of the elements of the proceeding that the service agent may contest (see §40.381(b)) and about which the Director makes a decision (see §40.387(b)(3)).

(d) In recommending and deciding the scope of the PIE, the initiating official and Director, respectively, must take into account the provisions of paragraphs (e) through (j) of this section.

(e) The pervasiveness of the noncompliance within a service agent's organization (see §40.389(d)) is an important consideration in determining the scope of a PIE. The appropriate scope of a PIE grows broader as the pervasiveness of the noncompliance increases.

(f) The application of a PIE is not limited to the specific location or employer at which the conduct that forms the factual basis for issuing the PIE was discovered.

(g) A PIE applies to your affiliates, if the affiliate is involved with or affected by the conduct that forms the factual basis for issuing the PIE.

(h) A PIE applies to individuals who are officers, employees, directors, shareholders, partners, or other individuals associated with your organization in the following circumstances:

(1) Conduct forming any part of the factual basis of the PIE occurred in connection with the individual's performance of duties by or on behalf of your organization; or

(2) The individual knew of, had reason to know of, approved, or acquiesced in such conduct. The individual's acceptance of benefits derived from such conduct is evidence of such knowledge, acquiescence, or approval.

(i) If a contractor to your organization is solely responsible for the conduct that forms the factual basis for a PIE, the PIE does not apply to the service agent itself unless the service agent knew or should have known about the conduct and did not take action to correct it.

(j) PIEs do not apply to drug and alcohol testing that DOT does not regulate.

(k) The following examples illustrate how the Department intends the provisions of this section to work:

Example 1 to §40.391. Service Agent P provides a variety of drug testing services. P's SAP services are involved in a serious violation of this Part 40. However, P's other services fully comply with this part, and P's overall management did not plan or concur in the noncompliance, which in fact was contrary to P's articulated standards. Because the noncompliance was isolated in one area of the organization's activities, and did not pervade the entire organization, the scope of the PIE could be limited to SAP services.

Example 2 to §40.391. Service Agent Q provides a similar variety of services. The conduct forming the factual basis for a PIE concerns collections for a transit authority. As in Example 1, the noncompliance is not pervasive throughout Q's organization. The PIE would apply to collections at all locations served by Q, not just the particular transit authority or not just in the state in which the transit authority is located.

Example 3 to §40.391. Service Agent R provides a similar array of services. One or more of the following problems exists: R's activities in several areas—collections, MROs, SAPs, protecting the confidentiality of information—are involved in serious noncompliance;

DOT determines that R's management knew or should have known about serious noncompliance in one or more areas, but management did not take timely corrective action; or, in response to an inquiry from DOT personnel, R's management refuses to provide information about its operations. In each of these three cases, the scope of the PIE would include all aspects of R's services.

Example 4 to §40.391. Service Agent W provides only one kind of service (e.g., laboratory or MRO services). The Department issues a PIE concerning these services. Because W only provides this one kind of service, the PIE necessarily applies to all its operations.

Example 5 to §40.391. Service Agent X, by exercising reasonably prudent oversight of its collection contractor, should have known that the contractor was making numerous "fatal flaws" in tests. Alternatively, X received a correction notice pointing out these problems in its contractor's collections. In neither case did X take action to correct the problem. X, as well as the contractor, would be subject to a PIE with respect to collections.

Example 6 to §40.391. Service Agent Y could not reasonably have known that one of its MROs was regularly failing to interview employees before verifying tests positive. When it received a correction notice, Y immediately dismissed the erring MRO. In this case, the MRO would be subject to a PIE but Y would not.

Example 7 to §40.391. The Department issues a PIE with respect to Service Agent Z. Z provides services for DOT-regulated transportation employers, a Federal agency under the HHS-regulated Federal employee testing program, and various private businesses and public agencies that DOT does not regulate. The PIE applies only to the DOT-regulated transportation employers with respect to their DOT-mandated testing, not to the Federal agency or the other public agencies and private businesses. The PIE does not prevent the non-DOT regulated entities from continuing to use Z's services.

§ 40.393 How long does a PIE stay in effect?

(a) In the NOPE (see §40.375(b)(5)), the initiating official proposes the duration of the PIE. The duration of the PIE is one of the elements of the proceeding that the service agent may contest (see §40.381(b)) and about which the Director makes a decision (see §40.387(b)(4)).

(b) In deciding upon the duration of the PIE, the Director considers the seriousness of the conduct on which the PIE is based and the continued need to protect employers and employees from the service agent's noncompliance. The Director considers factors such as those listed in §40.389 in making this decision.

(c) The duration of a PIE will be between one and five years, unless the Director reduces its duration under §40.407.

§ 40.395 Can you settle a PIE proceeding?

Any time before the Director's decision, you and the initiating official can, with the Director's concurrence, settle a PIE proceeding.

§ 40.397 When does the Director make a PIE decision?

Director makes his or her decision within 60 days of the date when the record of a PIE proceeding is complete (including any meeting with the Director and any additional fact-finding that is necessary). The Director may extend this period for good cause for additional periods of up to 30 days.

§ 40.399 How does the Department notify service agents of its decision?

You are a service agent involved in a PIE proceeding, the Director provides you written notice as soon as he or she makes a PIE decision. The notice includes the following elements:

(a) If the decision is not to issue a PIE, a statement of the reasons for the decision, including findings of fact with respect to any material factual issues that were in dispute.

(b) If the decision is to issue a PIE—

(1) A reference to the NOPE;

(2) A statement of the reasons for the decision, including findings of fact with respect to any material factual issues that were in dispute;

(3) A statement of the scope of the PIE; and

(4) A statement of the duration of the PIE.

§ 40.401 How does the Department notify employers and the public about a PIE?

(a) The Department maintains a document called the "List of Excluded Drug and Alcohol Service Agents." This document may be found on the Department's web site (http://www.dot.gov/ost/dapc). You may also request a copy of the document from ODAPC.

(b) When the Director issues a PIE, he or she adds to the List the name and address of the service agent, and any other persons or organizations, to whom the PIE applies and information about the scope and duration of the PIE.

(c) When a service agent ceases to be subject to a PIE, the Director removes this information from the List.

(d) The Department also publishes a Federal Register notice to inform the public on any occasion on which a service agent is added to or taken off the List.

§ 40.403 Must a service agent notify its clients when the Department issues a PIE?

(a) As a service agent, if the Department issues a PIE concerning you, you must notify each of your DOT-regulated employer clients, in writing, about the issuance, scope, duration, and effect of the PIE. You may meet this requirement by sending a copy of the Director's PIE decision or by a separate notice. You must send this notice to each client within three business days of receiving from the Department the notice provided for in §40.399(b).

(b) As part of the notice you send under paragraph (a) of this section, you must offer to transfer immediately all records pertaining to the employer and its employees to the employer or to any other service agent the employer designates. You must carry out this transfer as soon as the employer requests it.

[65 FR 79526, Dec. 19, 2000, as amended at 66 FR 41955, Aug. 9, 2001]

§ 40.405 May the Federal courts review PIE decisions?

Director's decision is a final administrative action of the Department. Like all final administrative actions of Federal agencies, the Director's decision is subject to judicial review under the Administrative Procedure Act (5 U.S.C. 551 et seq).

§ 40.407 May a service agent ask to have a PIE reduced or terminated?

(a) Yes, as a service agent concerning whom the Department has issued a PIE, you may request that the Director terminate a PIE or reduce its duration and/or scope. This process is limited to the issues of duration and scope. It is not an appeal or reconsideration of the decision to issue the PIE.

(b) Your request must be in writing and supported with documentation.

(c) You must wait at least nine months from the date on which the Director issued the PIE to make this request.

(d) The initiating official who was the proponent of the PIE may provide information and arguments concerning your request to the Director.

(e) If the Director verifies that the sources of your noncompliance have been eliminated and that all drug or alcohol testing-related services you would provide to DOT-regulated employers will be consistent with the requirements of this part, the Director may issue a notice terminating or reducing the PIE.

§ 40.409 What does the issuance of a PIE mean to transportation employers?

(a) As an employer, you are deemed to have notice of the issuance of a PIE when it appears on the List mentioned in §40.401(a) or the notice of the PIE appears in the Federal Register as provided in §40.401(d). You should check this List to ensure that any service agents you are using or planning to use are not subject to a PIE.

(b) As an employer who is using a service agent concerning whom a PIE is issued, you must s using the services of the service agent no later than 90 days after the Department has published the decision in the Federal Register or posted it on its web site. You may apply to the ODAPC Director for an extension of 30 days if you demonstrate that you cannot find a substitute service agent within 90 days.

(c) Except during the period provided in paragraph (b) of this section, you must not, as an employer, use the services of a service agent that are covered by a PIE that the Director has issued under this subpart. If you do so, you are in violation of the Department's regulations and subject to applicable DOT agency sanctions (e.g., civil penalties, withholding of Federal financial assistance).

(d) You also must not obtain drug or alcohol testing services through a contractor or affiliate of the service agent to whom the PIE applies.

Example to Paragraph (d): Service Agent R was subject to a PIE with respect to SAP services. As an employer, not only must you not use R's own SAP services, but you also must not use SAP services you arrange through R, such as services provided by a subcontractor or affiliate of R or a person or organization that receives financial gain from its relationship with R.

(e) This section's prohibition on using the services of a service agent concerning which the Director has issued a PIE applies to employers in all industries subject to DOT drug and alcohol testing regulations.

Example to Paragraph (e): The initiating official for a PIE was the FAA drug and alcohol program manager, and the conduct forming the basis of the PIE pertained to the aviation industry. As a motor carrier, transit authority, pipeline, railroad, or maritime employer, you are also prohibited from using the services of the service agent involved in connection with the DOT drug and alcohol testing program.

(f) The issuance of a PIE does not result in the cancellation of drug or alcohol tests conducted using the service agent involved before the issuance of the Director's decision or up to 90 days following its publication in the Federal Register or posting on the Department's web site, unless otherwise specified in the Director's PIE decision or the Director grants an extension as provided in paragraph (b) of this section.

Example to Paragraph (f): The Department issues a PIE concerning Service Agent N on September 1. All tests conducted using N's services before September 1, and through November 30, are valid for all purposes under DOT drug and alcohol testing regulations, assuming they meet all other regulatory requirements.

§ 40.411 What is the role of the DOT Inspector General's office?

(a) Any person may bring concerns about waste, fraud, or abuse on the part of a service agent to the attention of the DOT Office of Inspector General.

(b) In appropriate cases, the Office of Inspector General may pursue criminal or civil remedies against a service agent.

(c) The Office of Inspector General may provide factual information to other DOT officials for use in a PIE proceeding.

§ 40.413 How are notices sent to service agents?

(a) If you are a service agent, DOT sends notices to you, including correction notices, notices of proposed exclusion, decision notices, and other notices, in any of the ways mentioned in paragraph (b) or (c) of this section.

(b) DOT may send a notice to you, your identified counsel, your agent for service of process, or any of your partners, officers, directors, owners, or joint venturers to the last known street address, fax number, or e-mail address. DOT deems the notice to have been received by you if sent to any of these persons.

(c) DOT considers notices to be received by you—

(1) When delivered, if DOT mails the notice to the last known street address, or five days after we send it if the letter is undeliverable;

(2) When sent, if DOT sends the notice by fax or five days after we send it if the fax is undeliverable; or

(3) When delivered, if DOT sends the notice by e-mail or five days after DOT sends it if the e-mail is undeliverable.

APPENDIX A TO PART 40—DOT STANDARDS FOR URINE COLLECTION KITS

The Collection Kit Contents

1. Collection Container

a. Single-use container, made of plastic, large enough to easily catch and hold at least 55 mL of urine voided from the body.

b. Must have graduated volume markings clearly noting levels of 45 mL and above.

c. Must have a temperature strip providing graduated temperature readings 32–38°C/90–100°F, that is affixed or can be affixed at a proper level on the outside of the collection container. Other methodologies (e.g., temperature device built into the wall of the container) are acceptable provided the temperature measurement is accurate and such that there is no potential for contamination of the specimen.

d. Must be individually wrapped in a sealed plastic bag or shrink wrapping; or must have a peelable, sealed lid or other easily visible tamper-evident system.

e. May be made available separately at collection sites to address shy bladder situations when several voids may be required to complete the testing process.

2. Plastic Specimen Bottles

a. Each bottle must be large enough to hold at least 35 mL; or alternatively, they may be two distinct sizes of specimen bottles provided that the bottle designed to hold the primary specimen holds at least 35 mL of urine and the bottle designed to hold the split specimen holds at least 20 mL.

b. Must have screw-on or snap-on caps that prevent seepage of the urine from the bottles during shipment.

c. Must have markings clearly indicating the appropriate levels (30 mL for the primary specimen and 15 mL for the split) of urine that must be poured into the bottles.

d. Must be designed so that the required tamper-evident bottle seals made available on the CCF fit with no damage to the seal when the employee initials it nor with the chance that the seal overlap would conceal printed information.

e. Must be wrapped (with caps) together in a sealed plastic bag or shrink wrapping separate from the collection container; or must be wrapped (with cap) individually in sealed plastic bags or shrink wrapping; or must have peelable, sealed lid or other easily visible tamper-evident system.

f. Plastic material must be leach resistant.

3. Leak-Resistant Plastic Bag

a. Must have two sealable compartments or pouches which are leak-resistant; one large enough to hold two specimen bottles and the other large enough to hold the CCF paperwork.

b. The sealing methodology must be such that once the compartments are sealed, any tampering or attempts to open either compartment will be evident.

4. Absorbent material

Each kit must contain enough absorbent material to absorb the entire contents of both specimen bottles. Absorbent material must be designed to fit inside the leak-resistant plastic bag pouch into which the specimen bottles are placed.

5. Shipping Container

a. Must be designed to adequately protect the specimen bottles from shipment damage in the transport of specimens from the collection site to the laboratory (e.g., standard courier box, small cardboard box, plastic container).

b. May be made available separately at collection sites rather than being part of an actual kit sent to collection sites.

c. A shipping container is not necessary if a laboratory courier hand-delivers the specimen bottles in the plastic leak-proof bags from the collection site to the laboratory.

APPENDIX B TO PART 40—DOT DRUG TESTING SEMI-ANNUAL LABORATORY REPORT TO EMPLOYERS

The following items are required on each report:

Reporting Period: (inclusive dates)

Laboratory Identification: (name and address)

Employer Identification: (name; may include Billing Code or ID code)

C/TPA Identification: (where applicable; name and address)

1. Specimen Results Reported (total number)

By Type of Test

    (a) Pre-employment (number)

    (b) Post-Accident (number)

    (c) Random (number)

    (d) Reasonable Suspicion/Cause (number)

    (e) Return-to-Duty (number)

    (f) Follow-up (number)

    (g) Type of Test Not Noted on CCF (number)

2. Specimens Reported

    (a) Negative (number)

    (b) Negative and Dilute (number)

3. Specimens Reported as Rejected for Testing (total number)

By Reason

    (a) Fatal flaw (number)

    (b) Uncorrected Flaw (number)

4. Specimens Reported as Positive (total number)

By Drug

    (a) Marijuana Metabolite (number)

    (b) Cocaine Metabolite (number)

    (c) Opiates (number)

        (1) Codeine (number)

        (2) Morphine (number)

        (3) 6-AM (number)

    (d) Phencyclidine (number)

    (e) Amphetamines (number)

        (1) Amphetamine (number)

        (2) Methamphetamine (number)

5. Adulterated (number)

6. Substituted (number)

7. Invalid Result (number)

[65 FR 79526, Dec. 19, 2000, as amended 73 FR 35975, June 25, 2008]

APPENDIX C TO PART 40—DOT DRUG TESTING SEMI-ANNUAL LABORATORY REPORT TO DOT

Mail, fax, or email to:

U.S. Department of Transportation

Office of Drug and Alcohol Policy and Compliance

W62-300

1200 New Jersey Avenue, S.E.

Washington, DC 20590

Fax: (202) 366-3897

Email: ODAPCWebMail@dot.gov

The following items are required on each report:

Reporting Period: (inclusive dates)

Laboratory Identification: (name and address)

1. DOT Specimen Results Reported (number)

2. Negative Results Reported (number)

3. Rejected for Testing Reported (number)

 By Reason (number)

4. Positive Results Reported (number)

 By Drug (number)

5. Adulterated Results Reported (number)

 By Reason (number)

6. Substituted Results Reported (number)

7. Invalid Results Reported (number)

 By Reason (number)

[73 FR 35975, June 25, 2008]

APPENDIX D TO PART 40—REPORT FORMAT: SPLIT SPECIMEN FAILURE TO RECONFIRM

Mail, fax, or submit electronically to:

U.S. Department of Transportation

Office of Drug and Alcohol Policy and Compliance

W62-300

1200 New Jersey Avenue, S.E.

Washington, DC 20590

Fax: (202) 366-3897

Submit Electronically: http://www.dot.gov/ost/dapc/mro_split.html

The following items are required on each report:

1. MRO name, address, phone number, and fax number.

2. Collection site name, address, and phone number.

3. Date of collection.

4. Specimen I.D. number.

5. Laboratory accession number.

6. Primary specimen laboratory name, address, and phone number.

7. Date result reported or certified by primary laboratory.

8. Split specimen laboratory name, address, and phone number.

9. Date split specimen result reported or certified by split specimen laboratory.

10. Primary specimen results (e.g., name of drug, adulterant) in the primary specimen.

11. Reason for split specimen failure-to-reconfirm result (e.g., drug or adulterant not present, specimen invalid, split not collected, insufficient volume).

12. Actions taken by the MRO (e.g., notified employer of failure to reconfirm and requirement for recollection).

13. Additional information explaining the reason for cancellation.

14. Name of individual submitting the report (if not the MRO).

[65 FR 79526, Dec. 19, 2000, as amended 73 FR 35975, June 25, 2008]

APPENDIX E TO PART 40—SAP EQUIVALENCY REQUIREMENTS FOR CERTIFICATION ORGANIZATIONS

1. Experience: Minimum requirements are for three years of full-time supervised experience or 6,000 hours of supervised experience as an alcoholism and/or drug abuse counselor. The supervision must be provided by a licensed or certified practitioner. Supervised experience is important if the individual is to be considered a professional in the field of alcohol and drug abuse evaluation and counseling.

2. Education: There exists a requirement of 270 contact hours of education and training in alcoholism and/or drug abuse or related training. These hours can take the form of formal education, in-service training, and professional development courses. Part of any professional counselor's development is participation in formal and non-formal education opportunities within the field.

3. Continuing Education: The certified counselor must receive at least 40–60 hours of continuing education units (CEU) during each two year period. These CEUs are important to the counselor's keeping abreast of changes and improvements in the field.

4. Testing: A passing score on a national test is a requirement. The test must accurately measure the application of the knowledge, skills, and abilities possessed by the counselor. The test establishes a national standard that must be met to practice.

5. Testing Validity: The certification examination must be reviewed by an independent authority for validity (examination reliability and relationship to the knowledge, skills, and abilities required by the counseling field). The reliability of the exam is paramount if counselor attributes are to be accurately measured. The examination passing score point must be placed at an appropriate minimal level score as gauged by statistically reliable methodology.

6. Measurable Knowledge Base: The certification process must be based upon measurable knowledge possessed by the applicant and verified through collateral data and testing. That level of knowledge must be of sufficient quantity to ensure a high quality of SAP evaluation and referral services.

7. Measurable Skills Base: The certification process must be based upon measurable skills possessed by the applicant and verified through collateral data and testing. That level of skills must be of sufficient quality to ensure a high quality of SAP evaluation and referral services.

8. Quality Assurance Plan: The certification agency must ensure that a means exists to determine that applicant records are verified as being true by the certification staff. This is an important check to ensure that true information is being accepted by the certifying agency.

9. Code of Ethics: Certified counselors must pledge to adhere to an ethical standard for practice. It must be understood that code violations could result in de-certification. These standards are vital in maintaining the integrity of practitioners. High ethical standards are required to ensure quality of client care and confidentiality of client information as well as to guard against inappropriate referral practices.

10. Re-certification Program: Certification is not just a one-time event. It is a continuing privilege with continuing requirements. Among these are continuing education, continuing state certification, and concomitant adherence to the code of ethics. Re-certification serves as a protector of client interests by removing poor performers from the certified practice.

11. Fifty State Coverage: Certification must be available to qualified counselors in all 50 states and, therefore, the test must be available to qualified applicants in all 50 states. Because many companies are multi-state operators, consistency in SAP evaluation quality and opportunities is paramount. The test need not be given in all 50 states but should be accessible to candidates from all states.

12. National Commission for Certifying Agencies (NCCA) Accreditation: Having NCCA accreditation is a means of demonstrating to the Department of Transportation that your certification has been reviewed by a panel of impartial experts that have determined that your examination(s) has met stringent and appropriate testing standards.

APPENDIX F TO PART 40—DRUG AND ALCOHOL TESTING INFORMATION THAT C/TPAS MAY TRANSMIT TO EMPLOYERS

1. If you are a C/TPA, you may, acting as an intermediary, transmit the information in the following sections of this part to the DER for an employer, if the employer chooses to have you do so. These are the only items that you are permitted to transmit to the employer as an intermediary. The use of C/TPA intermediaries is prohibited in all other cases, such as transmission of laboratory drug test results to MROs, the transmission of medical information from MROs to employers, the transmission of SAP reports to employers, the transmission of positive alcohol test results, and the transmission of medical information from MROs to employers.

2. In every case, you must ensure that, in transmitting the information, you meet all requirements (e.g., concerning confidentiality and timing) that would apply if the party originating the information (e.g., an MRO or collector) sent the information directly to the employer. For example, if you transmit MROs' drug testing results to DERs, you must transmit each drug test result to the DER in compliance with the requirements for MROs set forth in §40.167.

Drug Testing Information

§40.25: Previous two years' test results

§40.35: Notice to collectors of contact information for DER

§40.61(a): Notification to DER that an employee is a "no show" for a drug test

§40.63(e): Notification to DER of a collection under direct observation

§40.65(b)(6) and (7) and (c)(2) and (3): Notification to DER of a refusal to provide a specimen or an insufficient specimen

§40.73(a)(9): Transmission of CCF copies to DER (However, MRO copy of CCF must be sent by collector directly to the MRO, not through the C/TPA.)

§40.111(a): Transmission of laboratory statistical report to employer

§40.127(f): Report of test results to DER

§§40.127(g), 40.129(d), 40.159(a)(4)(ii); 40.161(b): Reports to DER that test is cancelled

§40.129 (d): Report of test results to DER

§40.129(g)(1): Report to DER of confirmed positive test in stand-down situation

§§40.149(b): Report to DER of changed test result

§40.155(a): Report to DER of dilute specimen

§40.167(b) and (c): Reports of test results to DER

§40.187(a) through (e): Reports to DER concerning the reconfirmation of tests

§40.191(d): Notice to DER concerning refusals to test

§40.193(b)(3): Notification to DER of refusal in shy bladder situation

§40.193(b)(4): Notification to DER of insufficient specimen

§40.193(b)(5): Transmission of CCF copies to DER (not to MRO)

§40.199: Report to DER of cancelled test and direction to DER for additional collection

§40.201: Report to DER of cancelled test

Alcohol Testing Information

§40.215: Notice to BATs and STTs of contact information for DER

§40.241(b)(1): Notification to DER that an employee is a "no show" for an alcohol test

§40.247(a)(2): Transmission of alcohol screening test results only when the test result is less than 0.02

§40.255(a)(4): Transmission of alcohol confirmation test results only when the test result is less than 0.02

§40.263(a)(3) and 263(b)(3): Notification of insufficient saliva and failure to provide sufficient amount of breath

[65 FR 79526, Dec. 19, 2000, as amended at 66 FR 41955, Aug. 9, 2001; 73 FR 35975, June 25, 2008]

APPENDIX G TO PART 40—ALCOHOL TESTING FORM

The following form is the alcohol testing form required for use in the DOT alcohol testing program beginning August 1, 2001. Employers are authorized to use this form effective February 25, 2010.

U.S. Department of Transportation (DOT)
Alcohol Testing Form
(The instructions for completing this form are on the back of Copy 3)

Step 1: TO BE COMPLETED BY ALCOHOL TECHNICIAN

A: Employee Name _____

(Print)   (First, M.I., Last)

B: SSN or Employee ID No. _____

C: Employer Name _____
    Street
    City, Sate, Zip _____

    DER Name and _____
    Telephone No.   ( )
                        DER Name   DER Phone Number

D: Reason for Test: Random   Reasonable Susp   Post-Accident   Return to Duty   Follow-up   Pre-employment

STEP 2: TO BE COMPLETED BY EMPLOYEE

I certify that I am about to submit to alcohol testing required by US Department of Transportation regulations and that the identifying information provided on the form is true and correct.

_____   ___/___/___
Signature of Employee   Date Month Day Year

STEP 3: TO BE COMPLETED BY ALCOHOL TECHNICIAN

(If the technician conducting the screening test is not the same technician who will be conducting the confirmation test, each technician must complete their own form.) I certify that I have conducted alcohol testing on the above named individual in accordance with the procedures established in the US Department of Transportation regulation, 49 CFR Part 40, that I am qualified to operate the testing device(s) identified, and that the results are as recorded.

TECHNICIAN: BAT   STT   DEVICE: SALIVA   BREATH*   15-Minute Wait: Yes   No

SCREENING TEST: *(For BREATH DEVICE* write in the space below only if the testing device is not designed to print.)*

Test #   Testing Device Name   Device Serial # *OR* Lot # & Exp Date   Activation Time   Reading Time   Result

CONFIRMATION TEST: *Results MUST be affixed to each copy of this form or printed directly onto the form.*

REMARKS:
_____
_____
_____

_____   _____
Alcohol Technician's Company   Company Street Address

_____   _____ ( )
(PRINT) Alcohol Technician's Name (First, M.I., Last)   Company City, State, Zip   Phone Number

_____   ___/___/___
Signature of Alcohol Technician   Date Month Day Year

STEP 4: TO BE COMPLETED BY EMPLOYEE IF TEST RESULT IS 0.02 OR HIGHER

I certify that I have submitted to the alcohol test, the results of which are accurately recorded on this form. I understand that I must not drive, perform safety-sensitive duties, or operate heavy equipment because the results are 0.02 or greater.

_____   ___/___/___
Signature of Employee   Date Month Day Year

Form DOT F 1380 (Rev. 5/2008)   OMB No. 2105-0529

COPY 1 – ORIGINAL – FORWARD TO THE EMPLOYER

U.S. Department of Transportation (DOT)
Alcohol Testing Form
(The instructions for completing this form are on the back of Copy 3)

Step 1: TO BE COMPLETED BY ALCOHOL TECHNICIAN

A: Employee Name _____
(Print)   (First, M.I., Last)

B: SSN or Employee ID No. _____

C: Employer Name _____
Street _____
City, State, Zip _____

DER Name and _____
Telephone No. ( )
DER Name   DER Phone Number

D: Reason for Test: ☐ Random   Reasonable Susp ☐ Post-Accident ☐ Return to Duty ☐ Follow-up ☐ Pre-employment

STEP 2: TO BE COMPLETED BY EMPLOYEE

I certify that I am about to submit to alcohol testing required by US Department of Transportation regulations and that the identifying information provided on the form is true and correct.

_____   __/__/__
Signature of Employee   Date Month Day Year

STEP 3: TO BE COMPLETED BY ALCOHOL TECHNICIAN

(If the technician conducting the screening test is not the same technician who will be conducting the confirmation test, each technician must complete their own form.) I certify that I have conducted alcohol testing on the above named individual in accordance with the procedures established in the US Department of Transportation regulation, 49 CFR Part 40, that I am qualified to operate the testing device(s) identified, and that the results are as recorded.

TECHNICIAN: ☐ BAT ☐ STT   DEVICE: ☐ SALIVA ☐ BREATH* 15-Minute Wait: ☐ Yes ☐ No

SCREENING TEST: *(For BREATH DEVICE* write in the space below only if the testing device is not designed to print.)*

_____ _____ _____ _____ _____ _____
Test # Testing Device Name Device Serial # OR Lot # & Exp Date Activation Time Reading Time Result

CONFIRMATION TEST: Results *MUST* be affixed to each copy of this form or printed directly onto the form.

REMARKS:
_____
_____
_____

_____   _____
Alcohol Technician's Company   Company Street Address
                                                  ( )
_____   _____
(PRINT) Alcohol Technician's Name (First, M.I., Last) Company City, State, Zip   Phone Number

_____   __/__/__
Signature of Alcohol Technician   Date Month Day Year

STEP 4: TO BE COMPLETED BY EMPLOYEE IF TEST RESULT IS 0.02 OR HIGHER

I certify that I have submitted to the alcohol test, the results of which are accurately recorded on this form. I understand that I must not drive, perform safety-sensitive duties, or operate heavy equipment because the results are 0.02 or greater.

_____   __/__/__
Signature of Employee   Date Month Day Year

Form DOT F 1380 (Rev. 5/2008)   OMB No. 2105-0529

COPY 2 – EMPLOYEE RETAINS

U.S. Department of Transportation (DOT)
Alcohol Testing Form
(The instructions for completing this form are on the back of Copy 3)

Step 1: TO BE COMPLETED BY ALCOHOL TECHNICIAN

A: Employee Name _____

       (Print)   (First, M.I., Last)

B: SSN or Employee ID No. _____

C: Employer Name _____
   Street _____
   City, State, Zip _____

DER Name and _____
Telephone No.   (   )

          DER Name   DER Phone Number

D: Reason for Test: ☐ Random ☐ Reasonable Susp ☐ Post-Accident ☐ Return to Duty ☐ Follow-up ☐ Pre-employment

STEP 2: TO BE COMPLETED BY EMPLOYEE

I certify that I am about to submit to alcohol testing required by US Department of Transportation regulations and that the identifying information provided on the form is true and correct.

_____   _____/_____/_____

Signature of Employee   Date   Month   Day   Year

STEP 3: TO BE COMPLETED BY ALCOHOL TECHNICIAN

(If the technician conducting the screening test is not the same technician who will be conducting the confirmation test, each technician must complete their own form.) I certify that I have conducted alcohol testing on the above named individual in accordance with the procedures established in the US Department of Transportation regulation, 49 CFR Part 40, that I am qualified to operate the testing device(s) identified, and that the results are as recorded.

TECHNICIAN: ☐ BAT ☐ STT   DEVICE: ☐ SALIVA ☐ BREATH*   15-Minute Wait: ☐ Yes ☐ No

SCREENING TEST: *(For BREATH DEVICE* write in the space below only if the testing device is not designed to print.)*

Test #   Testing Device Name   Device Serial # *OR* Lot # & Exp Date   Activation Time   Reading Time   Result

CONFIRMATION TEST: *Results MUST be affixed to each copy of this form or printed directly onto the form.*

REMARKS: _____
_____
_____

Alcohol Technician's Company _____   Company Street Address _____

(PRINT) Alcohol Technician's Name (First, M.I., Last)   Company City, State, Zip   ( )   Phone Number

Signature of Alcohol Technician _____   _____/_____/_____
                          Date   Month   Day   Year

STEP 4: TO BE COMPLETED BY EMPLOYEE IF TEST RESULT IS 0.02 OR HIGHER

I certify that I have submitted to the alcohol test, the results of which are accurately recorded on this form. I understand that I must not drive, perform safety-sensitive duties, or operate heavy equipment because the results are 0.02 or greater.

_____   _____/_____/_____

Signature of Employee   Date   Month   Day   Year

Form DOT F 1380 (Rev. 5/2008)   OMB No. 2105-0529

COPY 3 – ALCOHOL TECHNICIAN RETAINS

BACK OF PAGES 1 and 2

INSTRUCTIONS FOR COMPLETING THE U.S. DEPARTMENT OF TRANSPORTATION ALCOHOL TESTING FORM

NOTE: Use a ballpoint pen, press hard, and check all copies for legibility.

STEP 1   The Breath Alcohol Technician (BAT) or Screening Test Technician (STT) completes the information required in this step. Be sure to print the employee's name and check the box identifying the reason for the test.

NOTE: If the employee refuses to provide SSN or I.D. number, be sure to indicate this in the remarks section in STEP 3. Proceed with STEP 2.

STEP 2   Instruct the employee to read, sign, and date the employee certification statement in STEP 2.

NOTE: If the employee refuses to sign the certification statement, do not proceed with the alcohol test. Contact the designated employer representative.

STEP 3   The BAT or STT completes the information required in this step and checks the type of device (saliva or breath) being used. After conducting the alcohol screening test, do the following (as appropriate):

Enter the information for the screening test (test number, testing device name, testing device serial number or lot number and expiration date, time of test with any device-dependent activation times, and the results), on the front of the AFT. For a breath testing device capable of printing, the information may be part of the printed record.

NOTE: Be sure to enter the result of the test exactly as it is indicated on the breath testing device, e.g., 0.00, 0.02, 0.04, etc.

Affix the printed information to the front of the form in the space provided, or to the back of the form, in a tamper-evident manner (e.g., tape) such that it does not obscure the original printed information, or the device may print the results directly on the ATF. If the results of the screening test are less than 0.02, print, sign your name, and enter today's date in the space provided. The test process is complete.

If the results of the screening test are 0.02 or greater, a confirmation test must be administered in accordance with DOT regulations. An EVIDENTIAL BREATH TESTING device that is capable of printing confirmation test information must be used in conducting this test.

Ensure that a waiting period of at least 15 minutes occurs before the confirmation test begins. Check the box indicating that the waiting period lasted at least 15 minutes.

After conducting the alcohol confirmation test, affix the printed information to the front of the form in the space provided, or to the back of the form, in a tamper-evident manner (e.g., tape) such that it does not obscure the original information, or the device may print the results directly on the ATF. Print, sign your name, and enter the date in the space provided. Go to STEP 4.

STEP 4   If the employee has a breath alcohol confirmation test result of 0.02 or higher, instruct the employee to read, sign, and date the employee certification statement in STEP 4.

NOTE: If the employee refuses to sign the certification statement in STEP 4, be sure to indicate this in the remarks line in STEP 3.

Immediately notify the DER if the employee has a breath alcohol confirmation test result of 0.02 or higher.

Forward Copy 1 to the employer. Give Copy 2 to the employee. Retain Copy 3 for BAT/STT records.

BACK OF PAGE 3

APPENDIX H TO PART 40—DOT DRUG AND ALCOHOL TESTING MANAGEMENT INFORMATION SYSTEM (MIS) DATA COLLECTION FORM

The following form and instructions must be used when an employer is required to report MIS data to a DOT agency.

U.S. DEPARTMENT OF TRANSPORTATION DRUG AND ALCOHOL TESTING MIS DATA COLLECTION FORM INSTRUCTION SHEET

This Management Information System (MIS) form is made-up of four sections: employer information; covered employees (i.e., employees performing DOT regulated safety-sensitive duties) information; drug testing data; and alcohol testing data. The employer information needs only to be provided once per submission. However, you must submit a separate page of data for each employee category for which you report testing data. If you are preparing reports for more than one DOT agency then you must submit DOT agency-specific forms.

Please type or print entries legibly in black ink.

TIP ~ Read the entire instructions before starting. Please note that USCG-regulated employers do not report alcohol test results on the MIS form.

Calendar Year Covered by this Report: Enter the appropriate year.

Section I. Employer

1. Enter your company's name, to include when applicable, your "doing business as" name; current address, city, state, and zip code; and an e-mail address, if available.

2. Enter the printed name, signature, and complete telephone number of the company official certifying the accuracy of the report and the date that person certified the report as complete.

3. If someone other than the certifying official completed the MIS form, enter that person's name and phone number on the appropriate lines provided.

4. If a Consortium/Third Party Administrator (C/TPA) performs administrative services for your drug and alcohol program operation, enter its name and phone number on the appropriate lines provided.

5. DOT Agency Information: Check the box next to the DOT agency for which you are completing this MIS form. Again, if you are submitting to multiple DOT agencies, you must use separate forms for each DOT agency.

a. If you are completing the form for FMCSA, enter your FMCSA DOT Number, as appropriate. In addition, you must indicate whether you are an owner-operator (i.e., an employer who employs only himself or herself as a driver) and whether you are exempt from providing MIS data. Exemptions are noted in the FMCSA regulation at 382.103(d).

b. If you are completing the form for FAA, enter your FAA Certificate Number and FAA Antidrug Plan / Registration Number, when applicable.

c. If you are completing the form for PHMSA, check the additional box(s) indicating your type of operation.

d. If you are completing the form for FRA, enter the number of observed/documented Part 219 "Rule G" Observations for covered employees.

e. If you are submitting the form for USCG, enter the vessel ID number. If there is more than one number, enter the numbers separately.

Section II. Covered Employees

1. In Box II-A, enter the total number of covered employees (i.e., employees performing DOT regulated safety-sensitive duties) who work for your company. Then enter, in Box II-B, the total number of employee categories that number represents. If you have employees, some of whom perform duties under one DOT agency and others of whom perform duties under another DOT agency, enter only the number of those employees performing duties under the DOT agency for whom you are submitting the form. If you have covered employees who perform multi-DOT agency functions (e.g., an employee drives a commercial motor vehicle and performs pipeline maintenance duties for you), count the employee only on the MIS report for the DOT agency regulating more than 50 percent of the employee's safety sensitive function.

[Example: If you are submitting the information for the FRA and you have 2000 covered employees performing duties in all FRA-covered service categories—you would enter "2000" in the first box (II-A) and "5" in the second box (II-B), because FRA has five safety-sensitive employee categories and you have employees in all of these groups. If you have 1000 employees performing safety-sensitive duties in three FRA-covered service categories (e.g., engine service, train service, and dispatcher/operation), you would enter "1000" in the first box (II-A) and "3" in the second box (II-B).]

TIP ~ To calculate the total number of covered employees, add the total number of covered employees eligible for testing during each random testing selection period for the year and divide that total by the number of random testing periods. (However, no company will need to factor the average number of employees more often than once per month). For instance, a company conducting random testing quarterly needs to add the total of covered employees they had in the random pool when each selection was made; then divide this number by 4 to obtain the yearly average number of covered employees. It is extremely important that you place all eligible employees into these random pools. [As an example, if Company A had 1500 employees in the first quarter

U.S. DEPARTMENT OF TRANSPORTATION DRUG AND ALCOHOL TESTING MIS DATA COLLECTION FORM

Calendar Year Covered by this Report: _____   OMB No. 2105-0529

I. Employer:

Company Name:_____

Doing Business As (DBA) Name (if applicable):_____

Address:_____ E-mail: _____

Name of Certifying Official: _____ Signature: _____

Telephone: (____)_____ Date Certified: _____

Prepared by (if different): _____ Telephone: (____)_____

C/TPA Name and Telephone (if applicable): _____ (____)_____

Check the DOT agency for which you are reporting MIS data; and complete the information on that same line as appropriate:

___ FMCSA – Motor Carrier: DOT #: _____ Owner-operator: (circle one) YES or NO Exempt (Circle One) YES or NO

___ FAA – Aviation: Certificate # (if applicable): _____ Plan / Registration # (if applicable):_____

___ PHMSA – Pipeline: (Check) Gas Gathering__ Gas Transmission__ Gas Distribution__ Transport Hazardous Liquids__ Transport Carbon Dioxide__

___ FRA – Railroad: Total Number of observed/documented Part 219 "Rule G" Observations for covered employees: _____

___ USCG – Maritime: Vessel ID # (USCG- or State-Issued): _____ (If more than one vessel, list separately.)

___ FTA – Transit

II. Covered Employees: (A) Enter Total Number Safety-Sensitive Employees In All Employee Categories:

(B) Enter Total Number of Employee Categories:

(C)

Employee Category Employees	Total Number of in this	If you have multiple employee categories, complete Sections I and II (A) & (B). Take that filled-in form and make one copy for each employee category and complete Sections II (C), III, and IV for each separate employee category.

III. Drug Testing Data:

Type of Test	1 Total Number Of Test Results [Should equal the sum of Columns 2, 3, 9, 10,	2 Verified Negative Results	3 Verified Positive Results – For One Or More Drugs	4 Positive For Marijuana	5 Positive For Cocaine	6 Positive For PCP	7 Positive For Opiates	8 Positive For Amphetamines	Refusal Results 9 Adulterated	10 Substituted	11 "Shy Bladder" ~ With No Medical Explanation	12 Other Refusals To Submit To Testing	13 Cancelled Results
Pre-Employment													
Random													
Post-Accident													
Reasonable Susp./Cause													
Return-to-Duty													
Follow-Up													
TOTAL													

IV. Alcohol Testing Data:

Type of Test	1 Total Number Of Screening Test Results [Should equal the sum of Columns 2, 3, 7, and 8]	2 Screening Tests With Results Below 0.02	3 Screening Tests With Results 0.02 Or Greater	4 Number Of Confirmation Tests Results	5 Confirmation Tests With Results 0.02 Through 0.039	6 Confirmation Tests With Results 0.04 Or Greater	Refusal Results 7 "Shy Lung" ~ With No Medical Explanation	8 Other Refusals To Submit To Testing	9 Cancelled Results
Pre-Employment									
Random									
Post-Accident									
Reasonable Susp./Cause									
Return-to-Duty									
Follow-Up									
TOTAL									

random pool, 2250 in the second quarter, 2750 in the third quarter; and 1500 in the fourth quarter; 1500 + 2250 + 2750 + 1500 = 8000; 8000/4 = 2000; the total number of covered employees for the year would be reported as, "2000".

If you conduct random selections more often than once per month (e.g., you select daily, weekly, bi-weekly), you do not need to compute this total number of covered employees rate more than on a once per month basis. Therefore, employers need not compute the covered employees rate more than 12 times per year.]

2. If you are reporting multiple employee categories, enter the specific employee category in box II-C; and provide the number of employees performing safety-sensitive duties in that specific category.

[Example: You are submitting data to the FTA and you have 2000 covered employees. You have 1750 personnel performing revenue vehicle operation and the remaining 250 are performing revenue vehicle and equipment maintenance. When you provide vehicle operation information, you would enter "Revenue Vehicle Operation" in the first II-C box and "1750" in the second II-C box. When you provide data on the maintenance personnel, you would enter "Revenue Vehicle and Equipment Maintenance" in the first II-C box and "250" in the second II-C box.]

TIP ~ A separate form for each employee category must be submitted. You may do this by filling out a single MIS form through Section II-B and then make one copy for each additional employee category you are reporting. [For instance, if you are submitting the MIS form for the FMCSA, you need only submit one form for all FMCSA covered employees working for you—your only category of employees is "driver." If you are reporting testing data to the FAA and you employ only flight crewmembers, flight attendants, and aircraft maintenance workers, you need to complete one form each for category—three forms in all. If you are reporting to FAA and have all FAA categories of covered employees, you must submit eight forms.]

Here is a full listing of covered-employee categories:

FMCSA (one category): Driver

FAA (eight categories): Flight Crewmember; Flight Attendant; Flight Instructor; Aircraft Dispatcher; Aircraft Maintenance; Ground Security Coordinator; Aviation Screener; Air Traffic Controller

PHMSA (one category): Operation/Maintenance/Emergency Response

FRA (five categories): Engine Service; Train Service; Dispatcher/Operation; Signal Service; Other [Includes yardmasters, hostlers (non-engineer craft), bridge tenders; switch tenders, and other miscellaneous employees performing 49 CFR 228.5 (c) defined covered service.]

USCG (one category): Crewmember

FTA (five categories): Revenue Vehicle Operation; Revenue Vehicle and Equipment Maintenance; Revenue Vehicle Control/Dispatch; CDL/Non-Revenue Vehicle; Armed Security Personnel

Section III. Drug Testing Data

This section summarizes the drug testing results for all covered employees (to include applicants). The table in this section requires drug test data by test type and by result. The categories of test types are: Pre-Employment; Random; Post-Accident; Reasonable Suspicion/Reasonable Cause; Return-to-Duty, and Follow-Up.

The categories of type of results are: Total Number of Test Results [excluding cancelled tests and blind specimens]; Verified Negative; Verified Positive; Positive for Marijuana; Positive for Cocaine; Positive for PCP; Positive for Opiates; Positive for Amphetamines; Refusals due to Adulterated, Substituted, "Shy Bladder" with No Medical Explanation, and Other Refusals to Submit to Testing; and Cancelled Results.

TIP ~ Do not enter data on blind specimens submitted to laboratories. Be sure to enter all pre-employment testing data regardless of whether an applicant was hired or not. You do not need to separate reasonable suspicion and reasonable cause drug testing data on the MIS form. [Therefore, if you conducted only reasonable suspicion drug testing (i.e., FMCSA and FTA), enter that data; if you conducted only reasonable cause drug testing (i.e., FAA, PHMSA, and USCG); or if you conducted both under FRA drug testing rules, simply enter the data with no differentiation.] For USCG, enter any "Serious Marine Incident" testing in the Post-Accident row. For FRA, do not enter post accident data (the FRA does not collect this data on the MIS form). Finally, you may leave blank any row or column in which there were no results, or you may enter "0" (zero) instead. Please note that cancelled tests are not included in the "total number of test results" column.

■ **Section III, Column 1. Total Number of Test Results** ~ This column requires a count of the total number of test results in each testing category during the entire reporting year. Count the number of test results as the number of testing events resulting in negative, positive, and refusal results. Do not count cancelled tests and blind specimens in this total.

[Example: A company that conducted fifty pre-employment tests would enter "50" on the Pre-Employment row. If it conducted one hundred random tests, "100" would be entered on the Random row. If that company did no post-accident, reasonable suspicion, reasonable cause, return-to-duty, or follow-up tests, those categories will be left blank or zeros entered.]

■ **Section III, Column 2. Verified Negative Results** ~ This column requires a count of the number of tests in each testing category that the Medical Review Officer (MRO) reported as negative. Do not count a negative-dilute result if, subsequently, the employee underwent a second collection; the second test is the test of record.

[Example: If forty-seven of the company's fifty pre-employment tests were reported negative, "47" would be entered in Column 2 on the Pre-Employment row. If ninety of the company's one hundred random test results were reported negative, "90" would be entered in Column 2 on the Random row. Because the company did no other testing, those other categories would be left blank or zeros entered.]

■ **Section III, Column 3. Verified Positive Results ~ For One Or More Drugs** ~ This column requires a count of the number of tests in each testing category that the MRO reported as positive for one or more drugs. When the MRO reports a test positive for two drugs, it would count as one positive test.

[Example: If one of the fifty pre-employment tests was positive for two drugs, "1" would be entered in Column 3 on the Pre-Employment row. If four of the company's one hundred random test results were reported positive (three for one drug and one for two drugs), "4" would be entered in Column 3 on the Random row.]

■ **Section III, Columns 4 through 8. Positive** (for specific drugs) ~ These columns require entry of the by-drug data for which specimens were reported positive by the MRO.

[Example: The pre-employment positive test reported by the MRO was positive for marijuana, "1" would be entered in Column 4 on the Pre-Employment row. If three of the four positive results for random testing were reported by the MRO to be positive for marijuana, "3" would be entered in Column 4 on the Random row. If one of the four positive results for random testing was reported positive for both PCP and opiates, "1" would be entered in Column 6 on the Random row and "1" would be entered in Column 7 of the Random row.]

TIP ~ Column 1 should equal the sum of Columns 2, 3, 9, 10, 11, and 12. Remember you have not counted specimen results that were ultimately cancelled or were from blind specimens. So, Column 1 = Column 2 + Column 3 + Column 9 + Column 10 + Column 11 + Column 12. Certainly, double check your records to determine if your actual results count is reflective of all negative, positive, and refusal counts.

An MRO may report that a specimen is positive for more than one drug. When that happens, to use the company example above (i.e., one random test was positive for both PCP and opiates), the positive results should be recorded in the appropriate columns—PCP and opiates in this case. There is no expectation for Columns 4 through 8 numbers to add up to the numbers in Column 3 when you report multiple positives.

■ **Section III, Columns 9 through 12. Refusal Results** ~ The refusal section is divided into four refusal groups—they are: Adulterated; Substituted; "Shy Bladder" ~ With No Medical Explanation; and Other Refusals To Submit to Testing. The MRO reports two of these refusal types—adulterated and substituted specimen results—because of laboratory test findings.

When an individual does not provide enough urine at the collection site, the MRO conducts or causes to have conducted a medical evaluation to determine if there exists a medical reason for the person's inability to provide the appropriate amount of urine. If there is no medical reason to support the inability, the MRO reports the result to the employer as a refusal to test: Refusals of this type are reported in the "Shy Bladder" ~ With No Medical Explanation category.

Finally, additional reasons exist for a test to be considered a refusal. Some examples are: the employee fails to report to the collection site as directed by the employer; the employee leaves the collection site without permission; the employee fails to empty his or her pockets at the collection site; the employee refuses to have a required shy bladder evaluation. Again, these are only four examples: there are more.

■ **Section III, Column 9. Adulterated** ~ This column requires the count of the number of tests reported by the MRO as refusals because the specimens were adulterated.

[Example: If one of the fifty pre-employment tests was adulterated, "1" would be entered in Column 9 of the Pre-Employment row.]

■ **Section III, Column 10. Substituted** ~ This column requires the count of the number of tests reported by the MRO as refusals because the specimens were substituted.

[Example: If one of the 100 random tests was substituted, "1" would be entered in Column 10 of the Random row.]

■ **Section III, Column 11. "Shy Bladder" ~ With No Medical Explanation** ~ This column requires the count of the number of tests reported by the MRO as being a refusal because there was no legitimate medical reason for an insufficient amount of urine.

[Example: If one of the 100 random tests was a refusal because of shy bladder, "1" would be entered in Column 11 of the Random row.]

■ **Section III, Column 12. Other Refusals To Submit To Testing** ~ This column requires the count of refusals other than those already entered in Columns 9 through 11.

[Example: If the company entered "100" as the number of random specimens collected, however it had five employees who refused to be tested without submitting specimens: two did not show up at the collection site as directed; one refused to empty his pockets at the collection site; and two left the collection site rather than submit to a required directly observed collection. Because of these five refusal events, "5" would be entered in Column 11 of the Random row.]

TIP ~ Even though some testing events result in a refusal in which no urine was collected and sent to the laboratory, a "refusal" is still a final test result. Therefore, your overall numbers for test results (in Column 1) will equal the total number of negative tests (Column 2); positives (Column 3); and refusals (Columns 9, 10, 11, and 12). Do not worry that no urine was processed at the laboratory for some refusals; all refusals are counted as a testing event for MIS purposes and for establishing random rates.

■ **Section III, Column 13. Cancelled Tests** ~ This column requires a count of the number of tests in each testing category that the MRO reported as cancelled. You must not count any cancelled tests in Column 1 or in any other column. For instance, you must not count a positive result (in Column 3) if it had ultimately been cancelled for any reason (e.g., specimen was initially reported positive, but the split failed to reconfirm).

[Example: If a pre-employment test was reported cancelled, "1" would be entered in Column 13 on the Pre-Employment row. If three of the company's random test results were reported cancelled, "3" would be entered in Column 13 on the Random row.]

■ **TOTAL Line. Columns 1 through 13** ~ This line requires you to add the numbers in each column and provide the totals.

Section IV. Alcohol Testing Data

This section summarizes the alcohol testing conducted for all covered employees (to include applicants). The table in this section requires alcohol test data by test type and by result. The categories of test types are: Pre-Employment; Random; Post-Accident; Reasonable Suspicion / Reasonable Cause; Return-to-Duty, and Follow-Up.

The categories of results are: Number of Screening Test Results; Screening Tests with Results Below 0.02; Screening Tests with Results 0.02 Or Greater; Number of Confirmation Test Results; Confirmation Tests with Results 0.02 through 0.039; Confirmation Tests with Results 0.04 Or Greater; Refusals due to "Shy Lung" with No Medical Explanation, and Other Refusals to Submit to Testing; and Cancelled Results.

TIP ~ Be sure to enter all pre-employment testing data regardless of whether an applicant was hired or not. Of course, for most employers pre-employment alcohol testing is optional, so you may not have conducted this type of testing. You do not need to separate "reasonable suspicion" and "reasonable cause" alcohol testing data on the MIS form. [Therefore, if you conducted only reasonable suspicion alcohol testing (i.e., FMCSA, FAA, FTA, and PHMSA), enter that data; if you conducted both reasonable suspicion and reasonable cause alcohol testing (i.e., FRA), simply enter the data with no differentiation.] PHMSA does not authorize "random" testing for alcohol. Finally, you may leave blank any row or column in which there were no results, or you may enter "0" (zero) instead. Please note that USCG-regulated employers do not report alcohol test results on the MIS form: Do not fill-out Section IV if you are a USCG-regulated employer.

■ **Section IV, Column 1. Total Number of Screening Test Results** ~ This column requires a count of the total number of screening test results in each testing category during the entire reporting year. Count the number of screening tests as the number of

screening test events with final screening results of below 0.02, of 0.02 through 0.039, of 0.04 or greater, and all refusals. Do not count cancelled tests in this total.

[Example: A company that conducted twenty pre-employment tests would enter "20" on the Pre-Employment row. If it conducted fifty random tests, "50" would be entered. If that company did no post-accident, reasonable suspicion, reasonable cause, return-to-duty, or follow-up tests, those categories will be left blank or zeros entered.]

■ **Section IV, Column 2. Screening Tests With Results Below 0.02** ~ This column requires a count of the number of tests in each testing category that the BAT or STT reported as being below 0.02 on the screening test.

[Example: If seventeen of the company's twenty pre-employment screening tests were reported as being below 0.02, "17" would be entered in Column 2 on the Pre-Employment row. If forty-four of the company's fifty random screening test results were reported as being below 0.02, "44" would be entered in Column 2 on the Random row. Because the company did no other testing, those other categories would be left blank or zeros entered.]

■ **Section IV, Column 3. Screening Tests With Results 0.02 Or Greater** ~ This column requires a count of the number of screening tests in each testing category that BAT or STT reported as being 0.02 or greater on the screening test.

[Example: If one of the twenty pre-employment tests was reported as being 0.02 or greater, "1" would be entered in Column 3 on the Pre-Employment row. If four of the company's fifty random test results were reported as being 0.02 or greater, "4" would be entered in Column 3 on the Random row.]

■ **Section IV, Column 4. Number of Confirmation Test Results** ~ This column requires entry of the number of confirmation tests that were conducted by a BAT as a result of the screening tests that were found to be 0.02 or greater. In effect, all screening tests of 0.02 or greater should have resulted in confirmation tests. Ideally the number of tests in Column 3 and Column 4 should be the same. However, we know that this required confirmation test sometimes does not occur. In any case, the number of confirmation tests that were actually performed should be entered in Column 4.

[Example: If the one pre-employment screening test reported as 0.02 or greater had a subsequent confirmation test performed by a BAT, "1" would be entered in Column 4 on the Pre-Employment row. If three of the four random screening tests that were found to be 0.02 or greater had a subsequent confirmation test performed by a BAT, "3" would be entered in Column 4 on the Random row.]

■ **Section IV, Column 5. Confirmation Tests With Results 0.02 Through 0.039** ~ This column requires entry of the number of confirmation tests that were conducted by a BAT that led to results that were 0.02 through 0.039.

[Example: If the one pre-employment confirmation test yielded a result of 0.042, Column 5 of the Pre-Employment row would be left blank or zeros entered. If two of the random confirmation tests yielded results of 0.03 and 0.032, "2" would be entered in Column 5 of the Random row.]

■ **Section IV, Column 6. Confirmation Tests With Results 0.04 Or Greater** ~ This column requires entry of the number of confirmation tests that were conducted by a BAT that led to results that were 0.04 or greater.

[Example: Because the one pre-employment confirmation test yielded a result of 0.042, "1" would be entered in Column 6 of the Pre-Employment row. If one of the random confirmation tests yielded a result of 0.04, "1" would be entered in Column 6 of the Random row.]

TIP ~ Column 1 should equal the sum of Columns 2, 3, 7, and 8. The number of screening tests results should reflect the number of screening tests you have no matter the result (below 0.02 or at or above 0.02, plus refusals to test), unless of course, the tests were ultimately cancelled. So, Column 1 = Column 2 + Column 3 + Column 7 + Column 8. Certainly, double check your records to determine if your actual screening results count is reflective of all these counts.

There is no need to record MIS confirmation tests results below 0.02: That is why we have no column for it on the form. [If the random test that screened 0.02 went to a confirmation test, and that confirmation test yielded a result below 0.02, there is no place for that confirmed result to be entered.] We assume that if a confirmation test was completed but not listed in either Column 5 or Column 6, the result was below 0.02. In addition, if the confirmation test ended up being cancelled, it should not have been included in Columns 1, 3, or 4 in the first place.

■ **Section IV, Columns 7 and 8. Refusal Results** ~ The refusal section is divided into two refusal groups—they are: Shy Lung ~ With No Medical Explanation; and Other Refusals To Submit to Testing. When an individual does not provide enough breath at the test site, the company requires the employee to have a medical evaluation to determine if there exists a medical reason for the person's inability to provide the appropriate amount of breath. If there is no medical reason to support the inability as reported by the examining physician, the employer calls the result a refusal to test: Refusals of this type are reported in the "Shy Lung ~ With No Medical Explanation" category.

Finally, additional reasons exist for a test to be considered a refusal. Some examples are: the employee fails to report to the test site as directed by the employer; the employee leaves the test site without permission; the employee fails to sign the certification at Step 2 of the ATF; the employee refuses to have a required shy lung evaluation. Again, these are only four examples; there are more.

■ **Section IV, Column 7. "Shy Lung" ~ With No Medical Explanation** ~ This column requires the count of the number of tests in which there is no medical reason to support the employee's inability to provide an adequate breath as reported by the examining physician; subsequently, the employer called the result a refusal to test.

[Example: If one of the 50 random tests was a refusal because of shy lung, "1" would be entered in Column 7 of the Random row.]

■ **Section IV, Column 8. Other Refusals To Submit To Testing** ~ This column requires the count of refusals other than those already entered in Columns 7.

[Example: The company entered "50" as the number of random specimens collected, however it had one employee who did not show up at the testing site as directed. Because of this one refusal event, "1" would be entered in Column 8 of the Random row.]

TIP ~ Even though some testing events result in a refusal in which no breath (or saliva) was tested, there is an expectation that your overall numbers for screening tests (in Column 1) will equal the total number of screening tests with results below 0.02 (Column 2); screening tests with results 0.02 or greater (Column 3); and refusals (Columns 7 and 8). Do not worry that no breath (or saliva) was tested for some refusals; all refusals are counted as a screening test event for MIS purposes and for establishing random rates.

■ **Section IV, Column 9. Cancelled Tests** ~ This column requires a count of the number of tests in each testing category that the BAT or STT reported as cancelled. Do not count any cancelled tests in Column 1 or in any other column other than Column 9. For instance, you must not count a 0.04 screening result or confirmation result in any column, other than Column 9, if the test was ultimately cancelled for some reason (e.g., a required air blank was not performed).

[Example: If a pre-employment test was reported cancelled, "1" would be entered in Column 9 on the Pre-Employment row. If three of the company's random test results were reported cancelled, "3" would be entered in Column 13 on the Random row.]

■ **TOTAL Line. Columns 1 through 9** ~ This line requires you to add the numbers in each column and provide the totals.

DOT Agency Rules ■

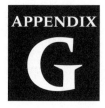
The following pages contain a short summary of some of the operating adminis-trations' requirements. These summaries are reproduced from DOT's *Urine Speci-men Collection Guidelines.*

Federal Motor Carrier Safety Administration (FMCSA) ■

Covered employee: A person who *operates (i.e., drives)* a Commercial Motor Vehicle (CMV) with a gross vehicle weight rating (gvwr) of 26,001 or more pounds; or is designed to transport 16 or more occupants (to include the driver); or is of any size and is used in the transport of hazardous materials that require the vehicle to be placarded.

Types of tests for drugs: Pre-employment, random, reasonable suspicion, post-accident, return-to-duty, and follow-up.

Types of tests for alcohol: Pre-employment (optional), random, reasonable suspicion, post-accident, return-to-duty, and follow-up.

Definition of accident requiring testing: Any accident involving a fatality re-quires testing. Testing is also required in accidents in which one or more motor vehicles are towed from the scene or in which someone is treated medically away from the scene *and* a citation is issued to the CMV driver.

Reasonable-suspicion determination: One trained supervisor or company of-ficial can make the decision based upon specific, contemporaneous, articulable observations concerning the appearance, behavior, speech, or body odors of the employee.

Pre-duty alcohol use prohibitions: Four (4) hours prior to performance of duty.

Actions for BACs 0.02–0.039: The employee cannot be returned to duty until the next day or the start of the employee's next regularly scheduled duty period, but not less than 24 hours following the test.

Employee training: Employer must provide educational materials explaining drug and alcohol regulatory requirements and employer's policies and procedures for meeting regulation requirements. Distribution to each employee of these educational materials and the employer's policy regarding the use of drugs and alcohol is mandatory.

Supervisor training: One hour of training is required on the specific, contemporaneous physical, behavioral, and performance indicators of probable drug use. One hour of training is also required on the specific, contemporaneous physical, behavioral, and performance indicators of probable alcohol use.

Reportable employee drug and alcohol violations: No requirements to report violations to FMCSA.

Other: Drivers are prohibited from using alcohol for 8 hours following an accident (as just described) or until they have undergone a post-accident alcohol test, whichever occurs first.

Federal Railroad Administration (FRA) ■

Covered employee: A person who performs *hours of service* functions at a rate sufficient to be placed into the railroad's random testing program. Categories of personnel who normally perform these functions are *locomotive engineers, trainmen, conductors, switchmen, locomotive hostlers/helpers, utility employees, signalmen, operators,* and *train dispatchers.*

Types of tests for drugs: Pre-employment, random, reasonable suspicion, reasonable cause, post-accident, return-to-duty, and follow-up.

Types of tests for alcohol: Pre-employment (optional), random, reasonable suspicion, reasonable cause, post-accident, return-to-duty, and follow-up.

Definition of accident requiring testing: FRA's post-accident testing rule requires urine and blood specimen collection from surviving employees and also tissue from deceased employees (these collection procedures go well beyond the normal Part 40 procedures). For surviving employees, these specimens are collected at an independent medical facility. FRA regulation, 49 CFR Part 219 Subpart C, stipulates the level of events requiring testing and who has to be tested. The collected specimens are analyzed only at FRA's contract laboratory. Post-accident testing provides FRA with accident investigation and usage data.

Reasonable-suspicion determination: One trained supervisor can make the decision for alcohol testing based upon specific, contemporaneous, articulable observations concerning the appearance, behavior, speech, or body odors of the employee. A decision to conduct a drug test requires two supervisors (only the on-site supervisor must be trained).

Reasonable-cause determination: Employers are authorized to use federal authority to test covered employees after specific operating rule violations or accidents/incidents that meet the criteria in 49 CFR Part 219 Subpart D.

Pre-duty alcohol use prohibitions: Four (4) hours prior to performance of duty or after receiving notice to report for covered service, whichever is the shorter period.

Actions for BACs 0.02–0.039: The employee cannot be returned to duty until the start of the employee's next regularly scheduled duty period, but not less than 8 hours following the test. Railroads are prohibited from taking further disciplinary action under their own authority.

Employee training: Employer must provide education materials that explain the requirements of the FRA rules as well as railroad policies and procedures with respect to meeting these requirements.

Supervisor training: A total of 3 hours of training is required: 1 hour on the specific, contemporaneous physical, behavioral, and performance indicators of probable drug use; 1 hour of similar training on probable indicators of alcohol use; and 1 hour of training on how to determine if an accident qualifies for post-accident testing.

Reportable employee drug and alcohol violations: No requirements to report violations to FRA. Engineers, who are the only certificate holders in the rail industry, will have their certificates reviewed for suspension or revocation by the employer when a FRA violation occurs. Note that a FRA alcohol violation occurs at 0.04% or greater. When a locomotive engineer is in a voluntary referral program, the counseling professional must report the engineer's refusal to cooperate in the recommended course of counseling or treatment.

Other: Anyone with direct or immediate supervisory authority over an employee may not collect that person's urine, saliva, or breath.

Refusal to test results in a mandatory minimum 9 month removal from covered service. During this 9 month period, there is no prohibition against the employee working a non-covered service position if agreeable to the employer.

Locomotive engineers (or other employees certified as a locomotive engineer at the time of the alcohol or drug violation) required both alcohol and drug return-to-duty tests and both alcohol and drug follow-up tests.

Locomotive engineers who have a DUI are required by Part 240 to be evaluated to determine whether they have an active substance abuse disorder. A DUI is not considered to be a violation of FRA regulations if it occurred during the employee's off-duty time; therefore, any testing would be conducted under employer authority.

Employers must provide a *voluntary referral program* that allows an employee to self-refer for treatment, and a *co-worker report program* that allows one employee to refer another for treatment before the employer identifies a problem. Both of these *employee assistance programs* guarantee that employees will retain their jobs if they cooperate and complete the required rehabilitation program. For an engineer who is in a voluntary referral program, the counseling professional must report the engineer's refusal to cooperate in the recommended course of counseling or treatment to the employer.

Federal Aviation Administration (FAA) ■

Covered employee: A person who performs *flight crewmember duties, flight attendant duties, flight instruction duties, aircraft dispatch duties, aircraft maintenance* or *preventive maintenance duties; ground security coordinator duties; aviation screening duties;* and *air traffic control duties.* Note: Anyone who performs these duties directly or by contract for part 121 or 135 certificate holders, *sightseeing operations* as defined in 135.1(c), and *air traffic control* facilities not operated by the government are considered covered employees.

Types of tests for drugs: Pre-employment, random, reasonable cause, post-accident, return to duty, and follow-up.

Types of tests for alcohol: Pre-employment (optional), random, reasonable suspicion, post-accident, return to duty, and follow-up.

Definition of accident requiring testing: Accident means an occurrence associated with the operation of an aircraft which takes place between the time any person boards the aircraft with the intention of flight and all such persons have disembarked, and in which any person suffers death or serious injury, or in which the aircraft receives substantial damage. Testing must occur if employee's performance either contributed to the accident or cannot be completely discounted as a contributing factor of the accident. The decision not to test an employee must be based on a determination, using the best information available at the time of the determination, that the employee's performance could not have contributed to the accident.

Reasonable cause determination (drugs): Two of the employee's supervisors, one of whom is trained, shall substantiate and concur in the decision to test the employee. If the employer is not an air carrier operating under 14 CFR Part 121 and has 50 or fewer employees, a single trained supervisor can make the determination. A trained supervisor makes the determination based upon specific contemporaneous physical, behavioral, or performance indicators of probable drug use.

Reasonable suspicion determination (alcohol): One trained supervisor makes the determination based upon specific, contemporaneous, articulable observations concerning the employee's appearance, behavior, speech, or body orders.

Pre-duty alcohol use prohibitions: Eight (8) hours prior to performance of flight crewmember duties, flight attendant duties, and air traffic controller duties. Four (4) hours prior to performance of other duties.

Actions for BACs 0.02–0.039: If the employer chooses to return the employee to covered services within 8 hours, the BAC retest must be below 0.02.

Employee training (drugs): An employer must train all employees who perform safety-sensitive duties on the effects and consequences of prohibited drug use on personal health, safety, and work environment, and on the manifestations and behavioral cues that may indicate drug use and abuse. Employers must also implement an education program for safety-sensitive employees by displaying and distributing informational materials, a community service hot-line telephone number for employee assistance, and the employer's policy regarding drug use in the workplace that must include information regarding the consequences under the rule of using drugs while performing safety-sensitive functions, receiving a verified positive drug test result, or refusing to submit to a drug test required under the rule.

Employee training (alcohol): Employers must provide covered employees with educational materials that explain the alcohol misuse requirements and the employer's policies and procedures with respect to meeting those requirements. The information must be distributed to each covered employees and must include such information as the effects of alcohol misuse on an individual's health work, personal life, and the signs and symptoms of an alcohol problem and the consequences for covered employees found to have violated the regulatory prohibitions.

Supervisor training (drugs): One hour of training is required on the specific, contemporaneous physical, behavioral, and performance indicators of probable drug use. In addition, supervisors must receive employee training as defined. Reasonable recurrent training is also required.

Supervisor training (alcohol): One hour of training is required on the physical, behavioral, speech, and performance indicators of probable alcohol misuse.

Reportable employee drug and alcohol violations: Each employer must notify the FAA about any covered employee who holds a certificate issued under 14 CFR Parts 61 (pilots and flight and ground instructors), 63 (flight engineers and navigators), or 65 (air traffic control tower operators, aircraft dispatchers, airframe or power plant mechanics, and repairmen) who has refused to take a drug or alcohol test. The MRO may report a positive or refusal (i.e., adulterated, substituted results or no medical explanation for providing an insufficient specimen) on behalf of the employer.

Each employer must notify the FAA about any safety-sensitive employee who is required to hold an airman medical certificate issued under 14 CFR Part 67 who has a positive drug test result, an alcohol test result of 0.04 or greater, or who has refused to submit to testing. The MRO may report a positive or refusal (i.e., adulterated, substituted results or no medical explanation for providing an insufficient specimen) on behalf of the employer.

Each employer must not permit an employee who is required to hold a medical certificate under Part 67 to perform a safety-sensitive function to resume that duty until the employee has received a new medical certificate issued by the FAA federal air surgeon *and* the employer has ensured that the employee meets the return to duty requirements of Part 40. (Medical certificates are not operating certificates but employees cannot continue to perform airman duties without a medical certificate.)

According to FAA's regulation 14 CFR Part 121 Appendix I, Section VII. C.1 and 2, when a MRO verifies a drug test result or a SAP performs the initial evaluation, they must ask the employee whether he or she holds or would be required to hold an airman medical certificate issued under 14 CFR Part 67 of this chapter to perform a safety-sensitive function for the employer. [This requirement only applies to MROs and SAPs who provide services for FAA regulated employers.] If the employee answers in the affirmative, the employee must obtain an airman medical certificate issued by the federal air surgeon dated after the drug and/or alcohol violation date.

The SAP must wait until the employee obtains his or her airman medical certificate before reporting to an employer that the employee demonstrated successful compliance with the SAP's treatment and/or education recommendations.

Federal Transit Administration (FTA) ■

Covered employee: A person who performs a *revenue vehicle operation; revenue vehicle and equipment maintenance; revenue vehicle control or dispatch (optional); Commercial Drivers License non-revenue vehicle operation;* or *armed security duties.*

Types of tests for drugs: Pre-employment, random, reasonable suspicion, post-accident, return-to-duty, and follow-up.

Types of tests for alcohol: Pre-employment (optional), random, reasonable suspicion, post-accident, return-to-duty, and follow-up.

Definition of accident requiring testing: Any accident involving a fatality requires testing. Testing following a non-fatal accident is discretionary: If the employer can show the employee's performance could not have contributed to the accident, no test is needed. Non-fatal accidents that may require testing must have disabling damage to any vehicle or immediate medical attention away from the scene to meet the testing threshold.

Reasonable-suspicion determination: One trained supervisor or company official can make the decision based upon specific, contemporaneous, articulable observations concerning the appearance, behavior, speech, or body odors of the employee.

Pre-duty alcohol use prohibitions: Four (4) hours prior to performance of duty.

Actions for BACs 0.02–0.039: If the employer chooses to return the employee to covered service within 8 hours, the BAC re-test must be below 0.02.

Employee training: Employer must provide education with display and distribution of informational materials and a community service hot-line telephone number, if available.

One hour of training on the effects and consequence of prohibited drug use on personal health, safety, and the work environment, and on the signs and symptoms that may indicate prohibited drug use. Distribution to each employee of the employer's policy regarding the use of drugs and alcohol with signed receipt is mandatory.

Supervisor training: One hour of training is required on the specific, contemporaneous physical, behavioral, and performance indicators of probable drug use. One hour of training is also required on the specific, contemporaneous physical, behavioral, and performance indicators of probable alcohol use.

Reportable employee drug and alcohol violations: No requirements to report violations to FTA.

Other: Anyone with direct or immediate supervisory authority over an employee may not collect that person's urine, saliva, or breath.

Pipeline and Hazardous Materials Safety Administration (PHMSA) ■

Covered employee: A person who performs on a pipeline or liquefied natural gas (LNG) facility an *operation, maintenance, or emergency-response* function.

Types of tests for drugs: Pre-employment, random, reasonable cause, post-accident, return-to-duty, and follow-up.

Types of tests for alcohol: Post-accident, reasonable suspicion, return-to-duty, and follow-up.

Definition of *accident* requiring testing: An accident is one involving gas pipeline facilities or LNG facilities or involving hazardous liquid or carbon dioxide pipeline facilities.

Reasonable-suspicion determination: One trained supervisor can make the decision based upon signs and symptoms.

Reasonable-cause determination: One trained supervisor can make the decision based upon reasonable and articulable belief that the employee is using prohibited drugs on the basis of specific, contemporaneous physical, behavioral, or performance indicators of probable drug use.

Pre-duty alcohol use prohibitions: Four (4) hours prior to performance of duty.

Actions for BACs 0.02–0.039: If the employer chooses to return the employee to covered service within 8 hours, the BAC retest must be below 0.02.

Employee training (drugs): Employer must provide EAP education with display and distribution of informational materials; display and distribution of a community service hot-line telephone number; and display and distribution of the employer's policy regarding the use of prohibited drugs.

Employee training (alcohol): Employer must develop materials that explain policies and procedures (as well as names of those who can answer questions about the program) and distribute them to each covered employee.

Supervisor training: One hour of training is required on the specific, contemporaneous physical, behavioral, and performance indicators of probable drug use. One hour of training is also required on the specific, contemporaneous physical, behavioral, and performance indicators of probable alcohol use.

Reportable employee drug and alcohol violations: No requirements to report violations to PHMSA.

U.S. Coast Guard (USCG) ■

Covered employee: A person who is *on board a vessel* acting under the authority of a *license, certificate of registry,* or *merchant mariner's document.* Also, a person *engaged* or *employed on board a U.S. owned vessel* and such vessel is required to engage, employ, or be operated by a person holding a license, certificate of registry, or merchant mariner's document.

Types of tests for drugs: Pre-employment, periodic, random, reasonable cause, and post-serious marine incident (SMI), return-to-duty, and follow-up.

Types of tests for alcohol: 49 CFR Part 40 alcohol-testing requirements do not apply to the maritime industry. 46 CFR Part 4.06 requires post-SMI chemical testing for alcohol use. 33 CFR Part 95.035 allows for a marine employer or a law enforcement officer to direct an individual to undergo a chemical test for intoxicants when reasonable cause exists or a marine casualty has occurred.

Definition of incident requiring testing: An SMI is defined in 46 CFR 4.03-2. In general, an SMI is: a discharge of 10,000 gallons or more of oil into the navigable waters of the United States, whether or not resulting from a marine casualty; a discharge of a reportable quantity of a hazardous substance into the navigable waters or into the environment of the United States, whether or not resulting from a marine casualty; or a marine casualty or accident required to be reported to the Coast Guard, involving a vessel in commercial service, and resulting in any of the following: one or more deaths; an injury to any person (including passengers) that requires professional medical treatment beyond first aid, and, in the case of a person employed on board a commercial vessel, which renders the person unable to perform routine vessel duties; damage to property in excess of $100,000; actual or constructive total loss of any inspected vessel; or actual or constructive total loss of any uninspected, self-propelled vessel of 100 gross tons or more.

Reasonable-cause determination (drugs): The marine employer must have a reasonable and articulable belief that the individual has used a dangerous drug. This belief should be based on the direct observation of specific, contemporaneous physical, behavioral, or performance indicators of probable use and where practicable based on the observation of two persons in supervisory positions.

Reasonable-cause determination (alcohol): The employee was directly involved in the occurrence of a marine casualty or the individual operated a vessel and the effect of the intoxicant(s) consumed by the individual on the person's manner, disposition, speech, muscular movement, general appearance, or behavior is apparent by observation.

Pre-duty alcohol use prohibitions: Four (4) hours prior to performance of scheduled duty.

Employee training: Employer must provide education with display and distribution of informational materials and a community service hot-line telephone number. Distribution to each employee of the employer's policy regarding the use of drugs and alcohol is mandatory. Training must include the effects of drugs and alcohol on personal heath, safety, and work environment and manifestations and behavioral cues that may indicate drug and alcohol use and abuse.

Supervisor training: One hour of training is required on the effects of drugs and alcohol on personal heath, safety, and work environment; and manifestations and behavioral cues that may indicate drug and alcohol use and abuse.

Reportable employee drug and alcohol violations: Results of all post-SMI tests and positive drug test results for all mariners who hold a license, certificate of registry or merchant mariner's document must be reported to the nearest Coast Guard officer in charge, marine inspection.

Index ■

Substance Abuse Program Administrators Association (SAPAA), 2, 48, 300, 301
Substance Abuse Program Administrators' Certification Commission (SAPACC), 48
Substituted specimen, 98
 HHS criteria for substituted urine, 122–123, 128–129
 MRO review, 162–165
Subutex, 145, 250
Supervisors
 training of, 34
 use of as specimen collectors, 58
Supplies. *See* Collection supplies
Surfactant, as adulterant, 97, 126
Sweat analysis, 14, 201

T
TAC, 145
Temazepam, 145, 231
Temperature, urine specimen, 72–73
Temporary leave, testing following, 27–28
Test subversion, criminalization of, 19
THC. *See* Marijuana
Third parties, access to MRO records, 186
Third-party administrators (TPAs), 47, 53
Tissionex Pennkinetic, 146
Tolectin, 124
Tolmetin, 162
Traizolam, 231
Tramadol, 265
Tranxene, 145, 231, 232
Treatment arrangements, 284
Triazolam, 232
Tussigon, 146
Tylenol, 146
Tylox, 147, 260

U
Unemployment benefits, 19
Unfit drivers, mandatory reporting of, 166–167
Unionized workplaces, 20
Unsafe practice testing, 28–29
Urinary tract infections, 96
Urine, incorporation of drugs into, 206
Urine analysis
 advantages/disadvantages of, 203–205
 alcohol, 220–221
 for amphetamine/methamphetamines, 227
 for cocaine, 235
 collection supplies for, 62–63
 in conjunction with hair analysis, 205
 detection times, 202–203
 dilute specimen, 126–127, 128
 fatal and correctable flaws, 104–105
 fees, 50
 for marijuana, 240–241
 point-of-collection tests, 89, 90
 regulations, 201
 substituted specimen, 128–129
 types of invalid specimens, 124–125
 validity testing, 108–109
Urine collection procedure

after-hours testing and, 86
for alcohol testing, 86–87
concerns regarding, 206–207
directly observed, 76–79
donor cannot urinate into container, 71
donor identification, 68–69
donor with catheter, 71–72
for drugs, 67–86, 206–207
specimen security before shipment, 75
timing of, 207
transmittance of CCF copies 2 and 4, 75–76
Urine Specimen Collection Guidelines, DOT, 295
Urine Specimen Collection Handbook, HHS, 295
Urine specimens
 abnormal physical characteristics, 73, 125, 160–161
 adulterants found in, 95–98
 different or abnormal, 73, 125, 160–161
 packaging of before shipment, 75
 security of prior to shipment, 75
 temperature of, 72
U.S. Coast Guard, 15, 407–408
 authorization of blood tests, 215
 contact information for, 296
 periodic drug tests, 32
 reporting of test results to, 174
 requirements for employer policies, 33
 return-to-duty process, 286–287
 supervisor training requirements, 34

V
Validity testing, 107–111
 hair validity testing, 109
 oral fluid validity testing, 109
 point-of-collection tests, 90–91
 urine validity testing, 108–109
Valium, 145, 231, 232
Varenicline, 169
Venlafaxine, 265
Versed, 231, 232
Vicks VapoInhaler, 144, 226, 229
Vicodin, 146
Vinegar, as adulterant, 99
Vitamin B, as adulterant, 99
Vitamin C, as adulterant, 99
Voice reporting, automated, 182
Volume, urine specimen, 73
Vyvanse, 144

W
Warfarin, 169
Water loading, 98
Web-based reporting, 183
Weight loss, marijuana, 239
Workers' compensation benefits, 19
Written testing policies, 33–34

X
Xanax, 145, 231, 232

Z
Zebutal, 144
Zydone, 146